SEXUAL BEHAVIOUR, DISCLOSURE AND BEHAVIOUR CHANGE AMIDST HIV INFECTED MEN

THE AUTHOR

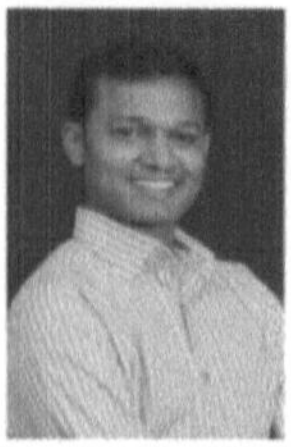

Dr. Sony Thomas, completed his MSW from College of Social Work, Nirmala Niketan, (CSWNN) Mumbai (2005) and completed a Certificate course in Advanced Social Research Methodology' and was awarded the PhD Degree from the Mumbai University in 2011.

He started his work in the field of HIV/AIDS with his MSW dissertation (unpublished) on "Awareness amongst Tamil migrants in Dharavi, Mumbai". In 2005, he worked as a Project Coordinator with CSWNN in its pilot project CHIRAG towards providing community based care and support for people living with HIV/AIDS. He then worked as a Zonal Program Manager for project Saksham supported by GFATM Round 7, towards organizing trainings and supervision of counselors and Master trainers working in the field of HIV/AIDS, deputed by NACO. He currently works with FPA Inida, on sexual reproductive health issues, as the Training Co-ordinator.

SEXUAL BEHAVIOUR, DISCLOSURE AND BEHAVIOUR CHANGE AMIDST HIV INFECTED MEN

–Author–

Dr. SONY THOMAS

2014

Scholars World

A Division of

Astral International Pvt. Ltd.

New Delhi-110 002

ISBN 9789351308430

Published by : **Scholars World**
A Division of
Astral International Pvt. Ltd.
– ISO 9001:2008 Certified Company –
4760-61/23, Ansari Road, Darya Ganj
New Delhi-110 002
Ph. 011-43549197, 23278134
E-mail: info@astralint.com
Website: www.astralint.com

Laser Typesetting : **SSMG Computer Graphics**
Delhi - 110 084

Printed at : **Replika Press Pvt. Ltd.**

PRINTED IN INDIA

ACKNOWLEDGEMENT

It gives me an enormous sense of accomplishment as I lay my finger tips to rest after over 40 months of tireless perseverance in methodical exploration and disciplined documentation. I dedicate this thesis as a tribute to the dreams of my family and to their incessant motivation throughout this voyage.

The genesis of this research sprouts with the wisdom and keen interest of Dr. Mary Alphonse, whose dedicated service in the upholding the rights of PLHIV, envisaged the quality of this dissertation. Every tireless discussion on the thesis encouraged critical learning, insightful interpretation and also helped building a holistic perspective on the issue.

The exodus of this study was fuelled by the "Award of NACO Research Fellowship on HIV/AIDS for the year 2008-09" through its letter vide T11020/20/2008-NACO (R&D), as attached in the Appendix. This recognition has certainly been very instrumental in the conduct of this study.

My sincere thanks to the CHIRAG team, who have been instrumental, not just in contributing their observations into the construction of this study but also for their sincere assistance in the conduct of interviews. Out goes my admiration to Mr. Anil, Mr. Sanjay K. Pawar and Ms. Meghna Jethva, who captured various facets of the study very sensitively and skilfully in their interviews.

In exploring the respondent's sexual lives and disclosure patterns, every interviewee by their free diffusion of thoughts, has opened up a new world to me. A world that was startling, audacious and precarious, yet practically empathetic. This research is memoir of quite a few lives battling with their own conscience, in trying to follow what is socially desirable... one of whom although critical and facing death each day, ceaselessly enquires on the completion of this study. If these chronicles can somehow be instrumental in stimulating its readers in exploring remedies for intervention and in transforming the quality of services offered to PLHIV, this toil shall be considered more than rewarded!

Hats off to you all once again!!

SONY THOMAS

ABSTRACT

Background

Sexuality and Livelihood are the root issues that snowball into contemporary social problems. Under the paradigm of sexuality, humans around the globe are particularly threatened by the tentacles of Sexually Transmitted Infections, of which HIV/AIDS has been labelled the most threatening pandemic of this century. Information and Services on Sexuality and Reproductive Health for PLHIV are important emerging issues has constantly attracted social scientists in exploring the extent and intensity of the problem, in order to sort out appropriate social work intervention and coping strategies. The predominant route of HIV transmission has been reported to be the sexual route and men are claimed to be the perpetrators of the virus. Therefore to control this epidemic, intervening organizations focus on reforming the sexual indulgences of PLHIV. An understanding on the sexual behaviours and behaviour change of PLHIV, is amplified in this research and it also aims to break the culture of secrecy that surrounds their sexuality related issues. The objective of this study is to understand the socio-economic, health profile and sexual practices of the HIV infected respondents and study their sexual practices, disclosure and behaviour change attempts.

This explorative study was conducted in 3 Phases using non random purposive sampling method. In Phase 1, the counsellor's perception of the MLHIV's sexual practices were explored and assessed. Herein, 85 counsellors working in ART and ICTC of MDACS and MSACS were interviewed for this. Based on the variables identified here, the interviews with MLHIV were structured for Phase 2. The sample selected for this phase includes 152 MLHIV in Mumbai, who were on ART, since at least 6 months selected purposively in a non random manner. The findings from both these Phases were triangulated in the focus group discussion conducted with the spouses of MLHIV in Phase3. Two such FGDs were conducted with the spouses of the MLHIV respondent's, interviewed in Phase 2. The sample size, in all the 3 phases were ceased, when the researcher observed saturation in data gathered. The goal of the study is therefore not to generalise the findings, but pave way to understand the nuances in experiences and practices of MLHIV.

Results

The findings of the study show high significance between the respondent's age and their duration of stay in Mumbai, also their educational achievement and income. The consolidated health status of only 16.4 percent respondents was found to be 'good' after the onset of ART. The better health of the respondent was found to hold significance with variables like younger age, higher income, reduced frequency of extramarital sexual relations and sexual partners.

The respondent's sexual history chronologically sequenced, depict the inception of sexual fantasies around the age of 17, which proceeded towards penetrative sexual debut around the age of 20. The respondents got married by the age of 26 and got tested positive for HIV at the age of 33. They had to soon initiate ART around the age of 34, due to low CD_4 count. The respondents got their spouses tested only after all this around the age of 35 years, pointing out the paradox in the HIV test amongst women.

Most of the MLHIV respondents (93.1 percent) had at least one or more sexual partners before marriage with about a fifth of them having more than 10 sexual partners. The major factors that influence pre marital sexual relationship include peer influence (94.8 percent), relaxation and enjoyment (94.8 percent), experimentation (94 percent), alcohol influence (88.9 percent), easy access and availability of sexual partners (85.9 percent), happened in an intense relationship (79.3 percent). Most respondents had sexual relationship with brothel based partners (64.4 percent) in comparison to non brothel based partners (31.1 percent). Only 7 percent of these respondents practiced the use of condoms consistently, and all of these were with 'regular partners' from 'brothels'.

More than half of the respondents (56.6 percent) had extra marital sexual relations and majority of them had less than 10 sexual partners. The major factors that influence the decision for extra-marital sexual relations include relaxation and enjoyment (100 percent), peer influence (90.7 percent), variety / wanted a change (90.7 percent), alcohol influence (87.2 percent), porn film influence (84.9 percent), dissatisfaction with spouse (84.7 percent), embarrassment to perform varied types of sexual acts with spouse (81.5 percent), restrictions in having sex at home (81.4 percent), experimentation (79.1 percent), spousal disinterest in sex (79.1 percent), menstruation periods of spouse (79.1 percent), child bearing phase of spouse (70.9 percent), menopause of spouse (65.2 percent) and to maintain HIV negative status of spouse (65.1 percent). More respondents had their sexual partners often from brothels (55.8 percent) than non-brothel based partners (40.7 percent).

The level of sexual satisfaction as rated by the respondents was found to be highly satisfactory within marriage (67.6 percent) than their indulgences outside marriage (48.2 percent). Half of the respondents (52 percent) were the initiators of sexual activity every time with their sexual partners. Oral sex was performed by 57.9 percent of the respondents and anal sex by 47.3 percent of them.

The incidences of the respondent's desire to have sex was found to reduce by half after the HIV test and consequently further, after the onset of ART. The respondent's frequent indulgences in penetrative sex also reduced one-fourth times after the onset of ART. The respondent's incidence of consistent condom use increased 6 times after HIV detection and 12 times after ART onset. Only one tenth of the MLHIV 'often' disclose their HIV positive status to their sexual partners outside marriage, after their HIV test. While after ART onset, about one fourth of the respondents reported disclosure.

Before undertaking the HIV test, most respondents (92.1 percent) admitted having one or more sexual partners outside marriage, which reduced to 59.2 percent after their HIV test and further reduced to 36.9 percent after the onset of ART. It was found that 92.8 percent of the respondents had more than one sexual indulgence outside their marriage, before undertaking the HIV test, which reduced to 58.5 percent after HIV test and further reduced to 36.2 percent after the onset of ART. Although the average frequency of sexual relations with spouses did not change after ART, about one fourth of the respondents (26.9 percent) claimed to have abstained from sexual relations. None of the respondents claimed to be a gay but homosexual sexual relations was observed in the case of 14.4 percent of the respondents before the HIV test, which reduced to 3.4 percent after the onset of ART.

The attitudes of the male respondents towards sexuality was measured on a 14 point Likert scale and the findings denote 74.3 percent of the respondents to hold moderate level of sexist attitude and 25 percent of the respondents demonstrated high level of sexist attitude.

Thus in the MLHIV interviews, the following hypotheses were proven true:

1. Earlier the sexual initiation, greater the number of sexual partners
2. Men have had more multiple sexual partners before the knowledge of their HIV status
3. HIV test counselling is the first exposure to respondent's education on HIV
4. Men have rarely ascertained the STI/HIV status of their sexual partners outside marriage
5. Men indulging in high risk behaviour have more sexist views about women
6. Onset of ART helps behaviour change

The counsellor's interviews reveal that their explorations about MLHIV's penetrative sexual behaviours are very limited. There were more MLHIV, who practiced alternate sexualities than that perceived by the counsellors. Even with regard to spousal disclosure, more MLHIV have disclosed their status to their spouses than that perceived by the counsellors. The counsellors held correct perceptions about minimal disclosure of MLHIV to their non-spousal partners as well as on the kind of prevention strategies (A-B-C) practiced by their MLHIV.

The interviews with spouses triangulate the findings from the MLHIV interviews about limited voluntary spousal disclosure and behaviour change strategies used. According to the spouses, they discovered the HIV status of their husband either through self during pregnancy or through the HCP when the husband is admitted. Their reaction to the knowledge of HIV infection has either been negative or naive. Most spouses declared the precautionary measures they take, like abstinence, reduced frequency of sexual intercourse, non penetrative sex and condom use, in order to prevent HIV super-infection.

In conclusion, the findings emphasized the need for health care providers, especially counsellors, to understand the sexual behaviour patterns among HIV positive individuals, which is influenced by gender disparities. The areas that need counsellors due attention and behaviour assessment skills have been suggested in the Counsellor-Counselee road map.

CONTENTS

LIST OF TABLES

LIST OF FIGURES

Chapter 1

INTRODUCTION

The breadth and scope of the Human Immunodeficiency Virus (HIV) infection is incredibly vast; from medical implications to biological research, from sociological effects to sexual and reproductive behaviour, from individual psychology to interpersonal communication, HIV has ramifications affecting each of these realms. With the development of a cure that may be years away, and out of the purview of contemporary virology, social scientists must continue to endeavour to define new branches of study regarding the disease while simultaneously refining what is currently understood.

The onset of HIV and its congeniality with sexual behaviour has constantly fascinated social scientists to explore the extent and intensity of the problem, in order to sort out appropriate social work intervention and coping strategies. Increasing efforts have been undertaken by the socio-medical professionals to understand the constructs, dimensions and manifestations of sexuality in order to curb the recurrent HIV related psycho-social problems. The increasing availability of treatment options for people living with HIV (PLHIV), has given growing recognition of their sexual and reproductive needs and aspirations, as essential factors in promoting their human rights. The rapid progression of HIV epidemic in the last decade, is largely attributed to the 'unprotected and unsafe sexual practises' of HIV infected men (Klitzman, 2004). Understanding the Male Sexuality and exploring its association with the 'acquisition and spread' of HIV, is therefore ascribed to be the major paradigm of this research intervention.

In exploring the male sexuality, this study seeks to explore and understand the sexual behaviour patterns amongst HIV infected men, which in turn will contribute to an insight on the contemporary sexual practices within the community of PLHIV. The 'HIV status disclosure' of infected men unfolds an arena to negotiate safer sexual practices and thus retard the spread of HIV. Hence this study aims to also investigate the 'HIV status disclosure' attempts and process, initiated in the context of a sexual relationship and to then comprehend the impact of such a revelation. According to some epidemiologists, a change in risk indulgences of PLHIV is the only available vaccine to arrest the growth and spread of HIV infection (Gunter R., et al, 2008). Further, 'Behaviour change' is determined as the goal in all the national and international efforts to stop the spread of AIDS. Hence this research in conclusion, aspires to determine the perception and practice of 'behavioural change' amidst HIV infected men and also to identify the factors influencing such a change in behaviour.

This study conducted amidst HIV infected men residing in Mumbai, who are on Anti Retroviral Treatment (ART) regimen, follows both a qualitative and a quantitative methodology. The onset of Free ART roll out was intended to reduce the multiplication of the virus amidst PLHIV so that they can lead a healthy life (free from Opportunistic Infections) for a prolonged duration of time. Further adherence to this treatment regimen is also aimed to encourage non risky behaviour practices amongst PLHIV so that the drug resistant virus is not transmitted to the uninfected community. Experts felt that the same purpose of keeping low the viral load within the PLHIV and curbing the spread of HIV infection in the community will also be a guiding force of 'HIV status Disclosure', which is essential to overcome stigma and discrimination. An evidential exploration to assess if the free ART rollout has influenced behaviour change and disclosure amongst PLHIV is intended in this study. Whether men feel socially bound to their sexually responsible behaviour with the onset of free ART and free counselling needs to be ascertained. The factors either internal or external, which may influence such a change needs to be studied.

The findings made herein will be helpful to have better understanding on the contemporary sexual practices of men on ART, which in turn will help develop appropriate intervention tools in counselling for behaviour change. This will impact the positive prevention of the spread of HIV amidst the general community and help minimise cases of re-infection amongst PLHIV.

1.1. Scheme of Study Chapters

This study comprises of 12 chapters wherein the first 6 chapters take an account of the available secondary data and the next 5 chapters focuses on analysing primary data. The last 2 chapters search for possible strategies related to findings of the study.

This first chapter is an 'Introduction' to the study paradigm and establishes a link between the theoretical concepts of Sexual behaviour, Disclosure and Behaviour Change. The second chapter on 'sexuality' exposes the central theme of the discussion of this study and makes an attempt to understand male sexual behaviour in the context of HIV. The third chapter speaks of 'Self Disclosure' and its impact on sexual behaviour. The fourth chapter focuses on the role of sexual behaviour change in an attempt to revert the spread of HIV/AIDS. The various researches conducted across the globe on the issue of sexual behaviour, disclosure and behaviour change and its inter linkages is noted in Chapter 5, 'Literature Review, Rationale and Objectives.'

The relevance of the study in the contemporary situation of HIV/AIDS, the reason of choosing the issue along with the objectives, is also discussed here. In Chapter 6, the methodology of identifying the sample for the study and data collection techniques is explained.

Chapters 7 to 11 are the analysis of the primary data gathered on Sexual behaviour, Disclosure and Behaviour change respectively, wherein Chapter 7 reflects the findings from the counsellors interviews, Chapters 8 to 10 explain the findings from the MLHIV interviews and chapter 11 marks the MLHIV's spousal perception and reactions. The major findings of this study is thematically summarised in Chapters 11 along with the researchers recommendations. This study ends with a 'Road Map' for the counselling training in Chapter 12 for appropriate intervention.

1.2. Selecting the theme for the study

Sexuality and Livelihood are the root issues that snowball into varied grave social problems. Sexuality has become a largely discussed theme within globalization, largely because of the AIDS outbreak. Economic changes under globalization have increasingly commoditised sexuality through sex trade and prostitution. Modernisation has resulted in dispersed understanding of sexual behaviour and sexual identity, making way for irrational understanding of oneself which often conflict bitterly with traditional mores (Robles, 1998). Human sexuality refers to a whole range of behaviour associated with psycho-biological phenomena of sex. Under the paradigm of sexuality, humans around the globe are largely endangered by the tentacles of Sexually Transmitted Infections, of which, HIV has been labelled the most threatening pandemic of this century. Furthermore, the rapid and trajectory spread of HIV has been largely associated with 'illicit' sexual practices (Panda, 2002).

The NACO press release on World AIDS Day 2010 claim that the national adult prevalence of HIV has gone down to 0.31 percent. In the year 2010, total number of PLHIV in India was estimated at 24 lakhs; almost 50 percent of the previous estimate of 52 lakhs in the year 2004 (NACO, 2010). This estimation is however is debated by many organizations, since a large magnitude of the epidemic is believed to be spreading outside the projected pool of knowledge. Findings for the last few years affirm a paradigm shift of the epidemic from 'high-risk' and 'urban population' to 'young males', 'household women' and 'rural areas'. Thereby the earlier stress exclusively the on "Risk groups" has changed attention to identifying and preventing "Risk Behaviours", in wider populations. Such 'generalisation' and 'feminisation' of the HIV epidemic has raised concerns on the sexual and reproductive wellbeing of the population (NACO, 2007).

Young men are the hardest hit by HIV and the spread of infection amongst them is rising exponentially. Majority (90 percent) of the infection occurs in the sexually active and economically productive age group of 15 to 44 years. Globally, most young men have begun sexual intercourse by the age of 18 years. With sexual activity often initiated in adolescence – within and outside marriage – the sexual and reproductive needs of this group are often underestimated (UNAIDS, 2004). The varied access available for urban youth to accomplish their sexual needs, have been well documented. As the young body reaches maturity, sexual drives are strong but social sanctions of our cultural patterns are imposed against its expression. Furthermore, being denied frank and scientific information on sex from either parents or teachers, lead them to seek incorrect information from unreliable and undesirable sources. Exploration and Experimentation with one's own sexuality is on the rise amongst the young. This is also a formative stage of relationships with the opposite sex and in carrying out health damaging activities. In the absence of proper channels of guidance, all the above factors lead to the practise of under-cover/ high risk sexual behaviour (Nair, 2004).

1.3. HIV and Sexual Behaviour

HIV is commonly spread through four major routes namely transfusion of HIV infected blood and blood products, sharing HIV infected injecting equipments, vertical transmission from HIV infected mothers to children and through unsafe/ unprotected sex. However the Government and Intervening agencies have played a vital role in curbing the spread of HIV through the first 3 modes of transmission. i.e.

1. Transmission of HIV through blood and blood products/organs have been minimised by blood safety mechanisms being implemented in blood banks.
2. The use of sterilised equipments, needle exchange programs, universal safety precautions and post exposure prophylaxis has reduced the risk of transmission in occupational exposures or through needles, syringes other medical equipments.
3. Vertical transmission of HIV has been negated to a great extent by introducing Nevirapine and safe feeding counselling under the PPTCT programme (UNAIDS, 2004).

However no reliable mechanism could be introduced to curtail the reduction of unsafe sexual practices. The Intervening agencies only tool to prevent HIV transmission through unprotected sex, dwells in counselling and educating PLHIV on the A-B-C Model of **A**bstinence – **B**eing Faithful – **C**onsistent and Correct use of Condom.

Yet predominantly, more than 84 percent of HIV transmission is spread through heterosexual route leading to the spread of infection from the High risk groups to the General population. Studies show that 80 to 90 percent of married women infected acquire HIV from their polygamous husbands (UNAIDS, 2004).

The increasing number of new infections clearly indicates that PLHIV are continuing to indulge in unsafe sexual practices. Thus implying that Abstinence messages or by Condom promotion techniques have not proved effective to contain their sexual behaviours. Therefore the lesson learnt is that sexual practices can't be governed by 'Radical Approaches' of restrictive policies on abstinence or by embedding moral values. Currently operating HIV interventions, in the framework of *'disease'* and *'death'* may not ensure participation of PLHIV in reproductive and sexual health programmes and is less likely to improve the quality of sexual life of men and women (Heise, 1995). All these factors exhibit the need for encouraging dissemination of information on alternative forms of safer sexual practices to PLHIV. According to Peter Piot, the former director of UNAIDS, "The impact of HIV on the sexuality of infected youth and their coping skills needs to be theoretically addressed in order that the progress of sexual transmission of HIV could be contained or reversed. Only then can we achieve the Millennium Development Goal 6: Combat HIV/AIDS by 2015" (UNAIDS, 2001).

1.4. Male PLHIV and Sexual Behaviour

Although an HIV positive test result typically prompts people to avoid transmitting HIV to others, there are often impediments to implementing or sustaining safer sexual behaviour (Nyblade, 2000). The HIV epidemic in the developing countries is increasingly being understood to be a consequence of the sexual and social subordination of women in those countries. This is evidenced by a pattern of infection in which men are the vectors of infection and women the principal subjects of infection. Married men who have multiple sexual partners are infecting their wives, who are prevented by economic and social restraints from protecting themselves from infection. Men are claimed to be the perpetrators of the virus. Therefore, in response to control this epidemic, intervening organizations have started to solely focus on reforming safer sexual indulgences of "men in risk behaviour" and invoke preventive messages to 'HIV infected men' (Foreman, 1998).

Male PLHIV confront problems because of their inability to adequately manage their sexual behaviour as soon as they are tested HIV infected. The tendency to spread the infection to their sexual partners or spouses, distances themselves from their earlier engaged high risk behaviours with them. This leads to apprehensions and anxiety within them since their immediate abstinence or safe sex practices may be questioned by the sexual partner. Thus emerging the dilemma between the need to disclose self HIV status and practise safe sex or remain undisclosed and enjoy the liberty to practise unsafe sex (Nyblade, 2000). This feature shall be discussed elaborately in Chapter 3 on Disclosure.

In the absence of any well informed adult intervention on handling one's sexuality without the risk of transmitting the infection and also with regards to the healthy disclosure of one's status to enhance safer practices in the relationship, male PLHIV may continue unsafe practices or resort to illicit sexual practices or even resort to alcohol and drugs. Under the influence of which, either the skills to negotiate safer sex practices is compromised and thus they tend to transmit the virus or men become fatalistic in the spread of the infection (Jackson, 2002).

1.5 ART and Sexual Behaviour

Highly active antiretroviral therapy (HAART) became available freely in Mumbai since 2001. Although HAART regimens may not be effective for all infected persons due to drug-resistant strains of HIV and unmanageable adverse effects, many PLHIV have substantially lowered their HIV RNA levels (i.e., viral load) through strict adherence to treatment regimens. Consequently, the incidences of AIDS and deaths due to AIDS have decreased considerably in countries in which HAART has been widely available (Nicole, 2004). Further discussions on these research findings are explained in Chapter 5.

Apart from beneficial clinical effects, treatment advances may have unintended effects on sexual behaviour. Some evidence suggests that since HAART became available, the prevalence of unprotected sex and the incidence of sexually transmitted infections (STIs), including HIV, have increased, mostly among men who have sex with men (MSM). Some with a low viral load may feel protected from transmitting HIV, sexually. Recent evidence does suggest that a low viral load may reduce the level of infectiousness of HIV-positive persons receiving HAART. As these information moves into the public domain, it may influence people's 'beliefs about HIV transmission' and lessen concern about engaging in safe sex. Researches mentioned in Chapter 5 explain, how people who hold these beliefs may be more likely than their counterparts to engage in unprotected sex. Given that taking HAART and having an undetectable viral load do not eliminate the possibility of transmitting HIV, it is important to examine whether use of HAART and beliefs about HAART and viral load are associated with sexual risk taking (Nicole, 2004).

The onset of ART has increased PLHIV's quality of life and appears to have rekindled their interest in sexuality and elevated their views to reconsider their decision on having children. Some couples wish to 'replace' their children who have died of HIV/AIDS through procreation. The role of antiretroviral therapy (ART) in continuing and reversing the practice of sexually 'high risk' behaviours among PLHIV in India is unknown. This study makes an attempt to explore the sexual practices that male HIV infected male youth pursue to satisfy their thirst for sexual orgasms. The inter-linkages between sexual behaviour and disclosure and behaviour change will be explored. The researcher is anxious to know if risks taken under sexual behaviour are related to any specific factors in oneself or outside oneself. What are the trends in disclosure amidst various sexual partners? Does disclosure mean an admission of high risk behaviour? How is disclosure and behaviour change interrelated? Thus this search is done with the hope to understand the sexuality and sexual practices amongst the infected men who are also on ART, which will enable intervening organizations to draw specific programs for the men in different age groups, who suffer from the HIV infection.

Conclusion

As the HIV epidemic continues to amplify in India, there is a growing need for HIV prevention interventions particularly amongst PLHIV. Information and Services on sexuality and reproductive health for PLHIV are important emerging issues in the advent of increasing occurrences of STI and HIV infection. Sexuality issues of PLHIV are usually avoided due to pervasive sensitivities and the surrounding stigma on their sexual behaviour. An understanding on the sexual needs and rights of PLHIV, amplified in this research, aims to break the culture of secrecy that surrounds sexuality related issues of HIV infected persons. It's a utopia that this research will be beneficial in improvising the existing interventions in dealing with the epidemic.

Chapter 2
SEXUALITY

This chapter seeks to explore the concept of sexuality as the central theme of this research and provides an in-depth understanding on male sexuality. It depicts how male sexuality was looked upon in history both in ancient cultures across the globe and its evolution in India. It further provides a glimpse of the well recognized Freudian concept of sexuality and the feminist's perspective on male sexuality. The theoretical frame of male sexuality, its definitions and congeniality with HIV are also cited. In conclusion, the attitudes, myths and misconceptions about male sexuality, the high risk behaviours of men and the factors influencing these high risk behaviours are listed.

2.1. Understanding sex

Sex is a chromosomal categorisation of any species based on their reproductive functions into groups of female (who can reproduce) and male (who cannot reproduce). It is also understood as the manifestation of instincts or desires. Sex is colloquially attributed to the act of sexual intercourse. The word 'Sex' can evoke a kaleidoscope of emotions, from love, lust, excitement, and orgasm to tenderness, longing, anxiety and disappointment. On another level, sex is seen as a hormone-driven bodily function designed to perpetuate the species (Alfred, 1981).

Vaginal intercourse is often given the lofty position in literature as the ultimate sexual event. However, pleasurable activities ranging from casual intimacies such as kissing and caressing to more intense types of physical contact designed to produce orgasm, can complement intercourse or stand alone as a means for gratification. The penis and vagina are not the only tools for sexual enjoyment; people can have intense pleasure without any direct genital contact. The mouth, breasts, anal area, hands and other sensitive spots on the skin are significant sources of erotic sensation. Even the friction of bodies rubbing together, can bring sexual pleasure. Sexual activity does not always demand having a partner either. Masturbation, viewing sexually stimulating materials and creating fantasies, may all be avenues for sexual gratification (Alfred, 1981).

The preliminary phase of sexual response is 'sexual desire', also called lust or libido. Desire is the wish for sex sparked by a sight, sound, taste, touch, or smell, or it may also be ignited by a memory or fantasy. Desire occurs before any physical signs of sexual readiness take place in the body, leading to arousal and orgasm, but this isn't always the case. Arousal can also lead to desire, and desire can linger on its own indefinitely. Rosemary Basson found that the sex drive of men tends to be goal-oriented, setting its sights on intercourse and orgasm. This drive is propelled by frequent sexual fantasies and thoughts (Basson, 2006).

2.2. Definitions of sexuality

Human sexuality is how people experience and express themselves as sexual beings; the awareness of themselves as males or females; the capacity for erotic experiences and responses. It can also be the manner in which one is attracted to another i.e. what they feel can be heterosexual *(attracted to the opposite sex)*, homosexual *(attracted to the same sex)* or bisexual *(attracted to both sexes)*. It can also cover cultural, political, legal and philosophical aspects. It also refers to issues of morality, ethics, theology, spirituality or religion and how they relate to all things sexual (Alfred, 1981).

2.3. Psychosocial dimension of sexuality

Sexuality in humans generates profound emotional and psychological responses. Some theorists identify sexuality as the central source of human personality. Psychological studies of sexuality focus on psychological influences that affect sexual behaviour and experiences. Early psychological analyses were carried out by Sigmund Freud, who conjectured the concepts of erogenous zones, psychosexual development, and the Oedipus complex (David, 1975), which has been elaborated further in the section on 'Historical Perspectives'. Human sexuality can also be understood as part of the social life of humans, governed by implied rules of behaviour and the status quo. Sexuality is also influenced by social norms, including the effects of politics and mass media.

2.4. Physical dimension of sexuality

The physical transformations that human body undergoes as one ages, also have a major influence on sexuality.

a. The impact of aging on Sexual Response

Advancing years leave their mark on the body, mind, and emotions. Many of the physical changes that come with age have noticeable effects on the sex organs and the sexual cycle. Declining hormone levels and changes in neurological and circulatory functioning may lead to sexual problems such as erectile dysfunction or vaginal pain. Half of men, ages 50 and older, report at least occasional erection problems with increasing age, while, many women contend with issues of vaginal dryness and a lagging libido after they pass menopause, when the ovaries stop producing oestrogen.

Table 1 Possible age-related sexual changes in women and men

Such physical changes often mean that the intensity of youthful sex gives way to

	Women	Men
Physical changes	Decreased blood flow to the genitals. Lower levels of estrogens and testosterone. Thinning of the vaginal lining. Loss of vaginal elasticity and muscle tone.	Decreased testosterone. Reduced blood flow to the penis. Less sensitivity in the penis.
Desire	Decreased libido. Fewer sexual thoughts and fantasies.	Decreased libido. Fewer sexual thoughts and fantasies.
Arousal	Slower arousal. Reduced vaginal lubrication and less expansion of the vagina during arousal. Less blood congestion in the clitoris and lower vagina. Diminished clitoral sensitivity.	Greater difficulty achieving an erection, maintaining an erection, or both. Erections aren't as rigid.
Orgasm	Delayed or absent orgasm. Less intense orgasms. Fewer and sometimes painful uterine contractions.	Longer time required to reach orgasm. Smaller volume of semen and less forceful ejaculation. Less intense orgasms.
Resolution	Body returns more rapidly to an un-aroused state.	Body returns more rapidly to an un-aroused state. More time is needed between erections.

(Berer, 2003)

more subdued responses during middle and later life. But the emotional by-products of maturity like increased confidence, better communication skills, and lessened inhibitions, can help create a richer, more nuanced, and ultimately satisfying sexual experience. These physical changes should provide an impetus for developing a new and satisfying style of lovemaking, i.e., based more on extended foreplay and less on intercourse and orgasm.

b. Impact of menopause on Sexual Response

While midlife brings many changes for women, menopause is clearly a physical milestone. Menopause and the preceding months or years (known as pre-menopause) are marked by hormonal fluctuations, which can provoke a host of symptoms from insomnia and irritability to dry skin and a thicker midriff. Many of these effects — vaginal changes and loss of libido, in particular, can wreak havoc on a woman's sex life.

In the strictest sense, men don't normally experience the precipitous drop in reproductive hormones, that marks a woman's midlife. Although testosterone (the hormone responsible for a man's libido and fertility as well as his deep voice and facial hair), does taper off with age, the process is gradual. Men may notice changes in their sex lives after they reach their 50's. Erections may require more direct stimulation, the need to ejaculate is less urgent, and the rest period between ejaculations grows longer. However, none of these effects need interfere with a satisfying sex life, provided the man and his partner understand these changes and integrate them into their lovemaking.

An exception to the typical pattern of declining testosterone levels is a disorder called 'hypogonadism', which can strike at any age. In this condition, the testes don't produce enough testosterone to maintain normal male functions and characteristics.

c. Impact of sexual dysfunction on Sexual Response

Sexual dysfunction can be defined as any aspect of the sexual response that causes the partner dissatisfaction or distress. The focus here is not on the problem of dysfunction, but on the fact that this condition troubling to the people involved. It occurs in both sexes and includes:

a) Sexual desire disorder: The absence of sexual fantasies, thoughts, behaviour or low libido and avoidance of certain types of sexual activity because of anxiety.

b) Sexual arousal disorder: The lack of sexual excitement, including absence of vaginal lubrication and other physical indications of arousal.

c) Orgasmic disorder. Difficulty or delay in reaching orgasm, or absence of orgasm after sufficient stimulation.

d) Sexual pain disorders: Genital pain during sexual intercourse (dyspareunia). This category includes nonspecific pain in the vulva (vulvodynia) and involuntary spasm of the vagina (vaginismus) that prevents penetration.

d. Sexual dysfunction in Men

a) Erectile dysfunction: The inability to produce an erection that's sufficient for intercourse since penile tissue becomes less elastic, blood flow diminishes, and nerve communication slows. Although this is a relatively uncommon problem for young men, about half of men ages 40–70 have partial or complete erectile dysfunction. Often, erectile problems stem from illnesses that become more prevalent with age or the medications used to treat these illnesses.

b) Ejaculatory disorders: Rapid or premature ejaculation occurs when the man ejaculates before or immediately after penetration, or before the couple has achieved a mutually satisfying sexual experience. Delayed ejaculation, is when a man isn't able to reach orgasm. Certain antidepressant medications, particularly selective serotonin reuptake inhibitors, can cause delayed ejaculation.

2.5 Types of Sexual Identities

1. **Asexual** in its broadest sense, is the lack of sexual attraction or the lack of interest in and desire for sex. Asexuality is distinct from abstention of sexual activity and from celibacy, which are behavioural;

2. **Homosexuality** is romantic and/or sexual attraction or behaviour among members of the same sex or gender. The consensus of the behavioural and social sciences and the health and mental health professions is that homosexuality is a normal and positive variation in human sexual

orientation. The most common adjectives in use are *lesbian* for women and *gay* for men.

3. **Heterosexuality** consists of sexual behaviour, practices, and identity predicated on exclusive preference or desire for the opposite sex.

4. **Bisexuality** is sexual behaviour or an orientation involving physical and/or romantic attraction to both males and females. It is one of the three main classifications of sexual orientation, along with a heterosexual and a homosexual orientation. People who have a distinct but not exclusive preference for one sex over the other may also identify themselves as bisexual.

5. **Pansexuality** (also referred to as omnisexuality) is a sexual orientation, characterized by the potential for aesthetic attraction, romantic love, or sexual desire towards people without regard for their gender identity or biological sex. Some pansexuals suggest that they are gender-blind; that gender and sex are insignificant or irrelevant in determining whether they will be sexually attracted to others. It encompasses all kinds of sexuality; not limited or inhibited in sexual choice with gender or practice.

6. **Polysexuality** refers to people who are attracted to more than one gender or sex but do not wish to identify as bisexual because it implies that there are only two binary genders or sexes. Polysexuality should not be confused with pan sexuality; *pan* meaning *all*, and *poly* meaning *many*, though not necessarily all.

7. **Transsexualism** is an individual's identification with a gender inconsistent, or not culturally associated with their biological sex. A medical diagnosis is made if a person experiences discomfort as a result of a desire to be a member of the opposite sex, or if a person experiences impaired functioning or distress as a result of their gender identity; concurrently prominent with sex reassignment surgery.

2.6 Philosophy of sexuality

Among the many topics explored by the philosophy of sexuality are procreation, contraception, celibacy, marriage, adultery, casual sex, flirting, prostitution, rape, homosexuality, masturbation, seduction, sexual harassment, sadomasochism, pornography, bestiality, and paedophilia. All of these on the one hand, are related, to the human desires and activities that involve the search for and attainment of sexual pleasure or satisfaction and, on the other hand, the creation of new human beings. For it is a natural feature of human beings that certain sorts of behaviours and certain bodily organs are employed either for pleasure or for reproduction, or for both. Given the fact that sexual activity is carried out voluntarily by all persons involved, assuming that no harm to third parties exists, then that the sexual activity is morally permissible (Parker, 1995).

The pessimists in the philosophy of sexuality, such as St. Augustine , Immanuel Kant, and Sigmund Freud, perceive the sexual impulse and acting on it to be unbefitting the dignity of the human person; they see the essence and the results of the drive to be incompatible with more significant and lofty goals and aspirations of human existence.

They fear that the power and demands of the sexual impulse make it a danger to harmonious civilized life; and they find in sexuality a severe threat to relations with, and our moral treatment of, other persons, and to our own humanity. (Brett, 1999)

On the other side of the divide are the metaphysical sexual optimists like Plato, Bertrand Russell, and many contemporary philosophers perceive nothing especially objectionable in the sexual impulse. They view human sexuality as just another dimension of our existence as embodied or animal-like creatures; they judge that sexuality, which in some measure has been given to us by evolution, will be conducive to our well-being if we diminish it from our intellectual propensities. These philosophers praise rather than fear the power of an impulse that can lift us to various high forms of happiness. (Brett, 1999)

2.7 Historical perspectives of sexuality

According to Brett Kahr (1999), virtually every action, position, or disposition can be found in the literature or on the pottery or cave paintings of our ancient ancestors who lived five thousand years ago. A brief glance at the historical writings reveal an intimate acquaintance with such diverse aspects of sexual behaviour as marriage, divorce, adultery, incest, child sexual abuse, onanism , mutual masturbation, fellatio, cunnilingus, sodomy, vaginal, anal or inter-femoral intercourse, rape, prostitution, contraception, menstrual purification, celibacy, pornography, heterosexuality, homosexuality, bisexuality, circumcision, impotency, pregnancy testing, sexual therapy, aphrodisiacs, mechanical aids, infectious diseases, paraphilia in its many forms, kissing, cuddling, fondling, and caressing. Historians from Suetonius to William Gibbon to Michel Foucault have always relished a healthy appetite for details about sex through the ages, within recent years, sexuality has become an increasingly professionalized field of enquiry.

2.8 Sex in Ancient cultures

The way sex is perceived not only differs from region to region but also differs in small areas within every region. From the most prudish to the most risqué sexual behavioural patterns has been a subject of intense scrutiny for years.

Sex in Ancient Egyptian Cultures

In ancient Egypt, girls could be deflowered in arranged marriages at six years of age. But the ancient women had to endure further indignities: in particular, the socially sanctioned sharing of their men with both male and female lovers. If a Babylonian wife could not bear a child, she would be forced to supply her own husband with a substitute spouse. The Egyptians could divorce their wives if they could not prove their fertility.

"The **Great Rite**" was known to be performed in **Egyptian** times and in **pre-Roman Europe**. In this ritual sex, the male becomes the fertilizing force and the woman the land. By ritual intercourse in the fields or in a temple, the fields of a country were fertile for the next year. It was also a way of showing a King's sovereignty in a rather explicit way. The Queen was considered the human embodiment of the Earth or the country. If a King could get the Queen pregnant, this sympathetic magic would ensure that the land would become fertile and the nation would be prosperous. The history of sex in ancient cultures had **material purposes** rather than gratifying physical desires

The history of sex in ancient cultures also included the roles sex could play in the life of the **lower classes**. In the Middle East, sacred **prostitutes** worked as priestesses in temples to **Goddesses of Love and War**. One of their sacred duties was to take soldiers fresh from battle and get them through the culture shock of coming back home to live a normal life. Sacred prostitution lasted through the **Greek civilization** and through **Rome**. Sex was considered a release of your personal and magical store of energy. This was why having virgins attend some other sacred duties like tending a sacred flame was essential.

Sex in Ancient Roman Cultures

Homosexuality was practiced in **ancient Rome and** was even more open, than it is now. Homosexuality was such a norm that there was not even a name for it. **Public bath houses** were hot beds for homosexual behaviour. Unlike today where the man would be considered a pervert or abnormal for such behaviour, it was not out of the norm to find sexual partners in the bath house and have sexual relations there. Homosexuality was a huge part of life for most men in Rome, especially those **in power**, to be the active sexual partner and show **manliness**, which was a prized Roman virtue (Dover, 1988).

It was acceptable for a man to have sex with women and male prostitutes as well as slaves, as long as he was the active partner. However, it must be noted that while slaves were seen as simply things and the master could penetrate them whenever he wanted, it was looked down upon to have sex with your slave for pleasure. Rather, the act of penetration was seen as a punishment akin to a beating.

Emperor **Nero** was the first to actually marry a male. Of the first twelve emperors of Rome, only one, Claudius, did not have a male lover. All of the other emperors had man or boy lovers (Pitt, 1992). While males experienced sexual openness and the ability to have both male and female lovers, **female homosexual relations were not an accepted sexuality**. Female lovers were considered disgusting and vile. Even a woman who took an active role in sex was considered disgusting. There are even reports of husbands killing their wives for homosexual affairs. Thus open sexuality in ancient Rome did not extend towards females (Manniche, 1987). Sexuality in ancient Rome was very erotic and more open than what we have today, but **it was still private**.

Sex in Ancient Japanese Cultures

Japanese are known for their seemingly humble nature and their great technological achievements. The 2005 movie 'Memoirs of a Geisha' has sparked some interest in sex in Japanese culture. This film has given the world a glimpse of ancient views and Japanese ways of sex at the different hierarchical levels. These **animations** show the sexually liberated Japan highlighting some sexual and erotic fantasy. It is this that might deceive the world into thinking that sex in Japanese culture is rife and explorative, in a way that one can buy magazines showing nude women in vending machines without embarrassment. It was here that prostitution was also legalised.

There are many ways that the Japanese dress that has sexual connotations to their past and gives a glimpse of sex in Japanese culture. Geisha (high class prostitutes) has sparked great interest due to their exotic appearance and interesting way of life. There are many **'love hotels'** in Japan; these are built due to the lack of space in the many Japanese homes. They are a practical solution especially if you are young couple who wished to just go out and have sex in a private setting (Rossiaud,1984).

Sex in Ancient Chinese Cultures

Sex was not a taboo subject in ancient China. The **Taoists'** religious literature documents the importance of sex to **good** health vitality and **immortality**. In order for men and women to give each other their yin (female gender) and yang (male gender) essences, sex was very important and the different sexual positions had different purposes. The Taoists' believed that men should ejaculate as little as possible to maintain a high level of 'jing' (sexual energy), as **semen was believed to be rich in 'jing'** (Stone, 1987). **Homosexuality** was considered unhealthy but it was not forbidden. Lesbianism was more common (Stone, 1987).

Women also played an important role in sexual relations and sex was not seen as beneficial unless the woman also received pleasure. Ancient texts like the **Book of Changes**, or **I Ching**, are full of sexual imagery. The I Ching contains detailed descriptions of sexual organs and behaviours and its message is that sexual union is harmonious and life-giving (Stone, 1987).

In the early history of sex in China, when Taoism was the common doctrine, **women were on equal footing with men**. That began to change when **Confucianism** took over and women became inferior to men. Confucianism is inherently sexist and men were seen as the gender in control. Sex was seen only as a means of procreating and frowned upon if engaged in for the sake of pleasure. Husbands and wives only had physical contact behind closed doors. The Taoist philosophy later made a comeback but eventually intertwined with Confucianism and Buddhism (Tannahill, 1980).

Sex in ancient American Culture

One of the surviving American tribes – Caddo consists of matrilineal clans. In winter, both men and women would wear deerskins. During the summer, they stayed virtually naked. Men had elaborate hair decorations and women painted themselves and had tattoos. There was no formal wedding ceremony. If a man desired a woman, he would try to find the best gift he could manage and give it to a woman. If she accepted, they'd have sex and considered the act of sex 'marriage'. Sometimes these marriages would only last a few days and women were allowed to accept gifts from several different men, and also engage in sexual relations with those different men with no repercussions.

Another American tribe – Calusa was characterized by marriages within in the family. The chief had many wives and was polygamous. He also married his sibling sisters. The Cerokee tribe too had had matrilineal clans. Children were not considered blood relatives of their fathers, but only a blood relative to their mother. Both men and women had a high degree of sexual freedom. After marriage, the couple goes to live with her mother and in divorce the man had to return home to live with his own mother.

The Chickasaw tribe too had matrilineal clans and had practices as above. If a man's brother died, he could marry his brother's widow. If he did not, the widow would go without a husband for four years. At puberty, girls were sent to menstrual huts and each month after that during menstruation (Tannahill, 1980).

Sex in ancient Africa

According to Ibo tribe of Nigeria, all women must be marital virgins and the groom's relatives would physically examine the bride on the wedding day. In the Potok tribe young women undergo a public cliterodectomy. The Turu of Tanzania is infamous for the number of extra marital affairs, a high divorce and assault rate. Men treat marriage as a business enterprise. The Yoruba of Nigeria follows the painful practice of female circumcision. Having a number of wives is a sign of wealth for men, not infidelity, and polygamy is encouraged (Maman, 2000).

Sex in ancient Asia

The Tre-ba of Tibet was a polyandrous society where only one marriage is allowed for all brothers in a family. The Muria tribe of the Bastar region in India had a system called Ghotul where children above the age of 6 are encouraged to have sex with each other. They are punished if they have sex with one person for more than 3 consecutive days. Boys are known to carve out penises and genitals in wood and gift it to the girls. Women are however not allowed to return to the Ghotul after marriage and couples have to maintain strict monogamy after marriage. The Dahari tribe of India has a system where wives are bought by a family and all the brothers are allowed to have sex with her. If the family has more money then they can purchase more wives (Tannahill, 1980).

Sex in Ancient Indian Culture

India played a significant role in the history of sex, from writing the first literature that treated sexual intercourse as a science. It may be argued that India pioneered the use of sexual education through art and literature. As in all societies, there was a difference in sexual practices in India between common people and powerful rulers, with regards to indulging in hedonistic lifestyles that were not representative of common moral attitudes.

Sexuality in the Indus Valley civilization is the practice of fertility rituals. The epics of ancient India, the Ramayana and Mahabharata, support the view that in ancient India, sex was considered a mutual duty between a married couple, where husband and wife pleasured each other equally, but where sex was considered a private affair. Polygamy was practiced during ancient times by rulers as a way of preserving dynastic succession, while common people maintaining a monogamous marriage (Tannahill, 1980).

Historical evidence shows that men and women in many parts of ancient India, mostly dressed only the lower half of their bodies, as a matter of tropical climatic necessity. The philosophical work on Kama Shastra, or 'love science', was intended as both an exploration of human desire, including seduction and infidelity, and a technical guide to pleasing a sexual partner within marriage. The Tantric school of Indic/Hindu philosophy formed at some point in this period, and part of the philosophical system was the idea that sex, as a basic and powerful desire experienced by all humans, could be utilised as a way of achieving enlightenment. It is also during this period that some of India's most famous ancient works of art were produced, often freely depicting nudity, romantic themes or sexual situations. Examples of this include the depictions at Khajuraho temples and Ajanta, which were used to remind people of the romantic duty that married couples should perform as part of dharma.

2.9. Sexual Practices in Medieval times

What exactly differentiated men from women and why the species evolved into the two sexes, unsurprisingly confounded Victorian theorists such as Herbert Spencer and Patrick Geddes, who constructed a stereotypical dyadic model. Other than the different sex organs and physical differences, men were considered the active agents, who expended energy while women were sedentary, storing and conserving energy. Such beliefs laid the groundwork for the separation of spheres for men and women. According to the model, since men only concerned themselves with fertilization, they could also spend energies in other arenas. On the other hand, woman's heavy role in pregnancy, menstruation (considered a time of illness, debilitation, and temporary insanity), and child-rearing left very little energy left for other pursuits. As a result, women's position in society came from biological evolution - she had to stay at home in order to conserve her energy, while the man could and needed to go out and hunt or forage.

During the Middle Ages, any acts of the flesh would be tarnished by depressing affects of shame and disgust by the Church fathers. St. Augustine condemned sexuality, as did many other clerics. Origen of Alexandria worried so much about the sinfulness of sex that he castrated himself in order to become more fully abstinent. Interestingly, one can trace the etymology of the word "pudenda" (which means to be ashamed), or female genital region, to this medieval period of history (Keuls, 1985). The Stoics and the Neo-Platonists exerted a terrific influence, urging asceticism and self-control at every turn, accentuating Plato's ideas on the supremacy of the soul over the body. If a man experienced a nocturnal emission, he would be required to intone thirty-seven psalms upon awakening, ever mindful of Seneca's injunction that *"pleasure is a vulgar thing, petty and unworthy of respect, common to dumb animals"* (Keuls, 1985).

By this time, the wild abandon of the Tiberian and Caligulan orgies disappeared and the ability to control libidinal impulses became more pronounced. But sexual activity could only be practiced according to a harsh set of rules and restrictions. Thus, during the Middle Ages, the notion of abstinence days took root, and for many years Christians could not make love on Wednesdays, Fridays, Saturdays, or Sundays, as well as during the forty-day periods of fasting before Easter and Christmas, and after Whitsuntide. Some adhered to religious dictates so forcefully that they refrained from lovemaking during the wife's breast-feeding period, which could last for a year or more (deMause, 1974).

During the Renaissance, the segregated single-sex monasteries and nunneries began to collapse, and men would routinely live with one another on a full-time basis, without fleeing to homosexual lovers. As scientific discovery began to take root, and magical thinking started to vanish, men could no longer blame their bad feelings on the stars or on the gods in quite the same compulsive way, and the so-called "weaker vessels" became the obvious targets. Renaissance men regarded women as objects of obscurity, who must be probed and prodded by a "rapier and dagger man" (Keuls, 1985).

2.10 Sex in Medieval India

Islamic and Hindu doctrine believed in sexual freedom within the context of marriage and the right to polygamy. The liberality of pre-colonial India had allowed individuals scope of sexual freedom within the home, while imposing strict seclusion from public life. With the influence of colonial morality, women were comparatively free to mix with men (not related to them) and also the freedom to explore their sexual identities. These new ideas of 'temperance' and good conduct overlay and reinforced ideas of asceticism and yogic self-containment, the *'brahmacharya'* of ancient tradition.

In ancient India, homosexuality was known and 'The Laws of Manu' (1st century BC) prescribe certain punishments for homosexual intercourse, with the degree of severity depending on gender, social and marital status. On the other hand, the Kama Sutra describes, without apparent reprobation, sex between a man and a person of a 'third gender', (eunuch/hijras). In any case, the modern status of homosexuality as a taboo is probably also connected with Victorian morality and the influence of Islam, which consider homosexuality a fundamental sin. Sexual dualism has been well recognized by "Kama Sutra' in its concepts of 'Ardhanarishwara', a form in which Siva is represented as half-male and half-female, typifying the male and female energies. Tantric rituals describe elaborate rites that include anal penetration as a method to brutally awaken the coiled up energy (kundalini) leading to enlightenment and perception of realities of a transcendental order. The Shushruta, a treatise on medicine describes the *'wounding of the lingam with the teeth as one of the causes of a disease treated upon in that work'* (Tannahill, 1980). Like many things, sexuality has gone from acceptable to unacceptable times throughout history. In some ways, **acceptance of alternate sexuality is like fashion**, since in some centuries it is in, and in some centuries it is out.

2.11. Sexuality in 18th and 19th Century

The greatest advances in researches on sexuality were in the eighteenth century. In 1760, AndrŽ Tissot, a Swiss physician from Lausanne, published his infamous anti-masturbation tract, urging generations of children to refrain from touching themselves. This subscribed to the misguided belief that masturbation causes blindness and insanity. Tissot also advised the boys and girls to forbid the adults from molesting them as well. Until this time, mothers and nurses routinely resorted to masturbation in order to put their children to sleep. (Tannahill, 1980)

One can now begin to see a cycle emerging through the centuries whereby one generation will indulge in manifold passions, and the next crop will rebel, re-enacting that age old battle of the Freudian Titans, namely, the id and the super-ego. But though on the surface it seems that sex will always be a minefield of progression and regression, there was glimmers of hope in the Victorian era during the nineteenth century. Throughout the nineteenth century, people struggled to situate themselves between conservative and liberal poles. On the outrageously awful side, women underwent surgery to remove some of their rib bones so that they could fit more snugly into their restrictive and hazardous corsets; and young boys had to survive the application of leeches to their genital region, a practice which doctors recommended in order to reduce the likelihood of penile erections. Women suffering from hysteria would be subjected to the odious practice of clitoridectomy, or in some cases, cauterization of the clitoris; and young Victorian men would be wrapped in sheets, or chained to walls, or fitted with metal-toothed penis rings to prevent masturbation. And untold numbers of men eliminated tea, coffee, alcohol, chocolate, oysters, eggs, cheese, asparagus, and flesh meats from their diets, on medical advice, in the hope that these ostensibly tempting foods would reduce the awful urge to touch one's penis. Women adopted not only their husbands' surnames, but they stripped themselves of any personal identity by assuming their husbands' Christian names as well. After the **People's Republic of China** was formed, homosexuals had to go underground because they were persecuted. In modern-day China, homosexuality is slowly becoming accepted and recently, sodomy was decriminalized. Furthermore, the government **no longer classifies homosexuality as a mental illness** (Dover, 1988). The Indian Judicial system overturned the old British law stating that 'homosexual intercourse is illegal' (Roazen, 1969).

2.12 SEXUALITY IN CONTEMPORARY WORLD

In the twentieth century, the chastity belts, bridles, branks, corsets, beheadings, burnings, penis rings, and anti-masturbation tracts of yesteryear have disappeared; and a semblance of equality between men and women, as well as a deep appreciation of children and of children's rights and welfare emerged (Miles, 1994).

Globally, women can now seemingly assume control of their own bodies and of their own reproductive capacity, as evidenced by the legalization of abortion, as well as the recognition of rape within the context of marriage. Prior to this time, a husband could fornicate with his wife with full impunity, irrespective of the wife's wishes. Women can now work at high level posts, and they can even delegate their childcare to fathers, who can act as primary caretakers. In spite of widely existing taboo on sexual matters, this century emerges with increasing de-stigmatization of masturbation, homosexuality, pre-marital sexuality, children born out of wedlock, childlessness and the emergence of the 'New Man' who now has the capacity to wash dishes, change nappies, and cry in public with relative ease. For those individuals who experience difficulty with sexual roles and gender stereotypes, one can now offer sexual education, sex therapy, and psychoanalysis or psychotherapy, as treatments for psychosexual or relational difficulties.

Of most importance, the sexual futures of the children are protected by recognizing the cruelty of child abuse. After thousands of years of polymorphous sexual activity throughout human history, men and women of this century have a greater likelihood of enjoying modern genital love. The sexual partner is not treated as part-objects for the gratification of self desires. With the growth of psychotherapeutic and psychoanalytical treatment facilities, and with the continuous improvement in the quality of child care, couples can derive greater fulfilment and satisfaction.

With increased exposure to world culture due to globalisation, and the proliferation of progressive ideas due to greater education and wealth, India is beginning to ironically go through a western-style sexual revolution of its own, especially in cosmopolitan cities. The entertainment industry of modern India plays an expressive role of Indian society in general. Historically, Indian television and film has lacked the frank depiction of sex; until recently, even kissing scenes were considered taboo. Currently, some Indian states show soft-core sexual scenes and nudity in films. Indian cinema, mainly the Hindi speaking Bollywood industry, fascinated by the process of glamorisation of Hollywood films, is also beginning to add sexual overtones to films.

Some anthropological research has suggested that in Afghanistan (especially Kandahar), India, Pakistan, Bangladesh, Sri Lanka, Morocco and elsewhere, men's sexual desires for other men is understood as universal, and not the characteristic of one or more sexual minorities (deMause, 1974). According to this research, a man's display of sexual interest in another man in social environments in which this understanding is shared may not be seen as a sign of difference from the societal mainstream. Belief in the ordinariness and ubiquity of male same-sex desire may be freely acknowledged. In other cultural settings, same-sex desire may be openly acknowledged in spaces socially defined as male but denied in formal or mixed gender spaces (e.g., in India) (deMause, 1974). The current debate on Sexuality as such and Homosexuality is vibrant in India, with homosexual identity is fast coming out of the closet and asserting itself. Under the construct of homosexual males, studies point out that an individual may have sexual variations over a period of time and not have a steady sexual identity or belong to a distinct group of people with a common circumscribed behaviour pattern.

2.13 Psychological Perspective Sexuality: Freudian

According to Freud, sexuality covers much wider than genital intercourse and whatever shape or form of one's sexuality eventually takes, it inevitably has its roots in the infantile sexuality, which is described in terms of psycho-sexual development in the first few years of a life. This theory of sexual drive posits that from birth, humans have instinctual sexual appetites (libido) which unfold in a series of stages. Each stage is characterized by the erogenous zone ie. the source of the libidinal drive during that stage. These stages in order are: oral, anal, phallic, latency, and genital. Freud believed that if, during any stage, the child experienced anxiety in relation to that drive, that themes related to this stage would persist into adulthood as neurosis. (Deutsch, 1973).

Freud observed that, at somewhat predictable points during early development, children's behaviour often orients around certain body parts (the mouth during breast-

Table 2 Freud's model of psychosexual development

Stage	Age Range	Erogenous zone(s)	Consequences of Fixation
Oral	0-18 months	Mouth	Orally aggressive: Signs include chewing gum or ends of pens. Orally Passive: Signs include smoking/eating/kissing/fellatio/cunnilingus Fixation at this stage may result in passivity, gullibility, immaturity and manipulative personality
Anal	18-36 months	Bowel and bladder elimination	Anal retentive: Obsession with organization or excessive neatness Anal expulsive: Reckless, careless, defiant, disorganized, Coprophiliac
Phallic	3-5 years	Genitals	Oedipus complex (in boys only according to Freud) Electra complex (in girls only, later developed by Carl Jung)
Latency	6 years-puberty	Dormant sexual feelings	(People do not tend to fixate at this stage, but if they do, they tend to be extremely sexually unfulfilled.)
Genital	Puberty and beyond	Sexual interests mature	Frigidity, impotence, unsatisfactory relationships

(deMause, 1974)

feeding, the anus during potty-training, and later the genitals). Freud suggested that humans are born "polymorphous perverse", meaning that infants can derive sexual pleasure from any part of the body. It is only through socialization that libidinal drives are focused into adult heterosexuality. According to his theory, each child passes through five psychosexual stages. During each stage, the libido has a different erogenous zone as the source of its drives. However, in the pursuit of satisfying these sexual urges, the child may experience failure or reprimands from its parents or society and may thus come to associate anxiety with this erogenous zone. In order to avoid this anxiety, the child becomes preoccupied with a phenomenon Freud termed 'fixation'. Freud believed the fixation persists into adulthood and underlies the personality structure and psychopathology, including neurosis, hysteria and personality disorders. Freud called this psychosexual infantilism. (Roazen, 1985)

2.14 Foucault's Sado-Masochistic Paradigm:

Foucault, critiqued Freudian theory arguing that an implicit concept of sado-masochism emerges, because it supplies the mechanism that makes power productive in "libidinal" sense. Power implies the existence of inequality, subordination, humiliation, or pain, and it is primarily the concept of sado-masochism that can account for the conversion of such an experience of displeasure, whether it is inflicted on others or on the self, into a source of pleasure (deMause, 1974). He makes no attempt here to distinguish a masochistic from a sadistic manner of mixing pleasure and power. On the contrary, he stresses the inter-changeability of the dominant and subordinate positions in the "spirals of power and pleasure", with the result that both pleasure and power are exchanged freely between them. It is not just that these spirals place the subject in differing positions, some of which are sadistic and others masochistic. Instead, each position in the spiral is indeterminately sadistic and masochistic, or both at the same time, because attached to each position is a certain pleasure and a certain power.

2.15. Feminist Concepts of sexuality and their perceptions of sexuality

There is quite a debate between feminists amongst their perspectives on male sexuality. Liberal Feminists claim that inequality stems from unequal participation in spheres outside of the family, primarily education and paid labour force. According to Radical feminists, patriarchy, women's oppression and domination by men, is the fundamental oppression and hence seek to replace existing gender roles based on the characteristics of sexes. They focus specifically on the male physical, psychological and social control of female sexuality as the basic cause of female subordination. Cultural feminists believe that male sexuality is selfish, violent and women-hating; linking male sexuality as committing violence against women in pornography or sex work. They advocate lesbianism as a personal and political choice that expresses ultimate rejection of patriarchy and demand separation from men (male values) in every way. (Bordo, 1994)

Numerous feminists have contended that one hundred years of sexological theory and research has remained indifferent to or even tried to contain women especially, young girls', long struggle for control over their lives and their sexuality. Western feminism claims that male sexuality (understood as mostly sexual harassment/ dominance and sexual violence against women) is not biologically determined but socially constructed. Yet in its place, the feminists substituted an equally essentialist idea, of male sexual needs now redefined as 'male power needs' (Bordo, 1994). According to these feminists, the need to dominate and exercise power in sexual activity determines the nature of male sexuality. Within such a 'feminist' world picture, women are portrayed mostly as powerless and helpless, low in sexual drive and most vulnerable in sexual matters; and the biologism of sexology quietly re-enters through the back door.

A group of feminists believe that pornography and the sex industry constitute the most serious forms of degradation for women in our culture. According to them, men are exposed to pornography in their adolescence from where they get an understanding of their sexuality in the social sphere. Feminist philosophers argue that pornography violates the moral imperative to treat women as autonomous, rational subjects. According to Alison Assiter, the Master-Slave dialectic seems to capture the relation between people in pornographic eroticism, where one person becomes a body desired by the other, but this is not reciprocated. Women here are treated as objects for another. To treat someone as merely a body for another's use, without recognizing that she too is a subject with desires, is to treat someone as a slave, as a subhuman creature or object, and therefore violates her dignity as a human being (Assiter, 1988). Susan Bordo writes, *"The woman in porn abdicates her will, her sexual discrimination, her independence, in order to become a mute body for the man"* (Bordo, 1994). This expression and fulfilment of sexual desire under patriarchy involves men taking control of women's bodies in a way that fails to respect women as persons. Assiter also argues that *"the role of the wife in marriage is very like that of the slave"* for the wife's social identity is subsumed by her husband, who holds social power, and thus she is not a social subject in her own right (Assiter, 1988). LeMoncheck states, *"men in sex treat woman as an object and dehumanizing her because she is perceived as a person whose will, seductiveness, and power is subordinate to men"* (LeMoncheck 1997).

With regards to male sexual relationships with sex workers, feminists claim that some of the actions are always morally problematic, but some of them are acceptable when they are part of a larger relationship involving mutual respect. Nussbaum writes, *"Denial of autonomy and denial of subjectivity are objectionable if they persist throughout an adult relationship, but as phases in a relationship characterized by mutual regard they can be all right, or even quite wonderful* (Nussbaum, 1999). In other words, some actions in which we use another's body sexually are consistent with recognizing the person so used as an end and do not involve treating her as a mere object.

Feminists who embark upon "gender equality education" (sex education being a part of it) in response to the increasingly active sexual activities among teenagers, are oriented towards abstinence and monogamous marriage (Nussbaum, 1999). By now, the two grand polarities—that between man and woman, and between normal and abnormal—have come to constitute the field of sexological research and feminism, as the most basic essential facts of human sexuality and both are believed to find their most socially desirable state in the institution of marriage.

Feminist sex radicals, on the other hand, lay open the often troubling, irrational, or perverse nature of sexual desire and fantasy. In other words, what arouses sexual desire rarely obeys the walk-in-the-sunset type of marital sexual bliss, nor does it follow the dictate of conscious feminist pursuit of sexual equity, but often includes inappropriately submissive, aggressive, hostile, or deviant impulses. Feminists feel that it is the need to dominate and exercise power in sexual activity that determines the nature of male sexuality. Feminism provides the 'discourse of victimology' for women and an 'image of righteousness' for the State to institute more rigid rules to govern all forms of sexual expression. Their approaches claim that new sex education be oriented toward abstinence and monogamous marriage. In fact, when sex therapy and sexology, discuss sexual harmony, sexual expression, or sexual satisfaction, the 'sexual' should always be framed within monogamous marital relationships (LeMoncheck 1997).

As evident from feminist perspective, this research will explore if the sexual drives and initiation in a marital relationship is 'Male' based and understand the level of female satisfaction. The inclination of MLHIV to alternative sexuality shall also be studied.

2.15.1 Social Constructs of Human sexuality

Human sexuality is how people experience and express themselves as sexual beings. It comprises of a broad range of behaviours, processes, and societal topics. Biologically, sexuality encompasses sexual intercourse and sexual contact in all its forms, as well as medical concerns about the physiological or even psychological aspects of sexual behaviour. Sociologically, it covers the cultural, political, and legal aspects; and philosophically, it spans the moral, ethical, theological, spiritual or religious aspects. The sexual meanings (meanings of the erotic dimension of human sexual experience), are social and cultural constructs, they are made subjective only after cultural and social mediation. Being the main force conditioning human relationship, sex is essentially political for the construction of a "sexual universe" is fundamentally linked to the structures of power. The construction of sexual meanings by social institutions (like religion, marketing, educational system, psychiatry, etc.), control and shape relationships.

The components of sexuality is summed up in the P's of sexuality—**Practices, Partners, Pleasure/Pain, and Procreation**. The first two refer to aspects of behaviour—how one has sex and with whom; while the others refer to the underlying motives. However, there is an additional 'P' of sexuality that is the most important—**Power**. The power underlying any sexual interaction, heterosexual or homosexual, determines how all the other P's of sexuality are expressed and experienced. Power determines whose pleasure is given priority and when, how, and with whom sex takes place. Each component of sexuality is closely related to the other but the balance of power in a sexual interaction determines its outcome (Weiss, Gupta, 1998). The unequal power balance in gender relations that favours men, translates into an unequal power balance in heterosexual interactions, in which male pleasure supersedes female pleasure and men have greater control than women over when, where, and how sex takes place. An understanding of individual sexual behaviour, thus necessitates an understanding of gender and sexuality as constructed by a complex interplay of social, cultural, and economic forces that determine the distribution of power.

Internal Influencers of Sexuality

An individual constructs their sexuality based on the knowledge ascertained on different types of sexuality, social and family beliefs and practices, personal attitudes and values. Thus all these concepts build into the individual's sexual behaviour and practice. The experience from this behaviour builds new knowledge and thus the cycle of Human Sexuality is a constant exploration.

2.16 External Influencers of Sexuality

The expression of sexuality is externally influenced by ethical, spiritual, cultural, and moral concerns.

Figure 1 Internal Influencers of Human Sexuality

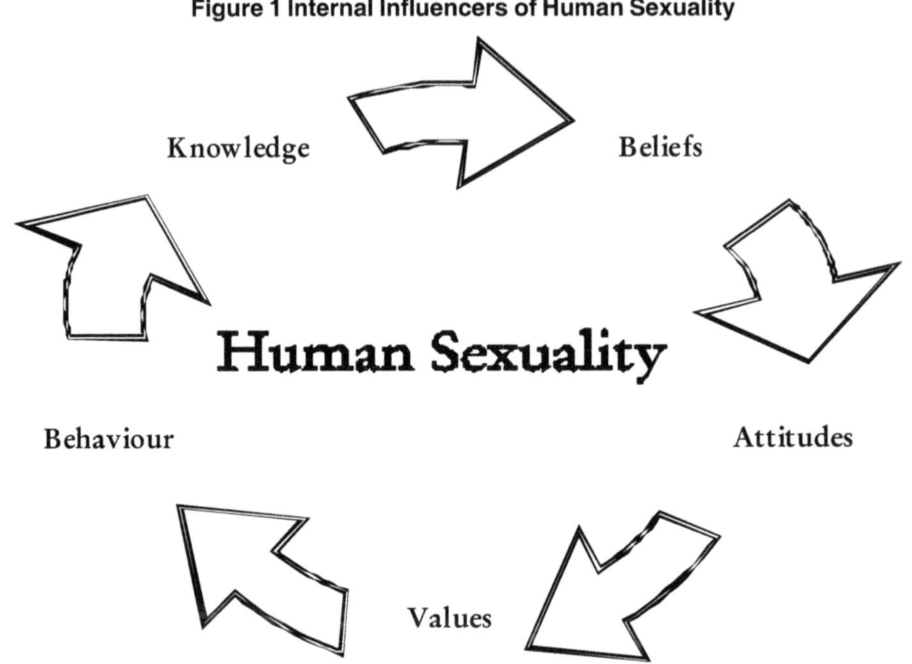

Cultural aspects

Human intelligence and complex societies have produced among the most complicated sexual behaviours of any animal. Most people experiment with a range of sexual activities during their lives, though they tend to engage in only a few of these regularly. Some enjoy many different sexual activities, while others avoid sexual activities altogether for religious or other reasons. Some societies and religions view sex as appropriate only within marriage. However, most societies have defined some sexual activities as inappropriate (wrong person, wrong position, wrong place, etc.).

Moral Aspects

Human sexual behaviour is also governed by social rules that are culturally specific and vary widely. These social rules are referred to as sexual morality (what can and cannot be done by society's rules) and sexual norms (what is and is not expected). Sexual ethics, morals, and norms relate to issues including deception/ honesty, legality, fidelity and consent. Some activities, known as sex crimes in some locations, are illegal in some jurisdictions (sodomy law and adult-adult incest), including those conducted between (or among) consenting and competent adults. Hiding one's homosexual or heterosexual status from their partner, soliciting sex outside marriage, engaging in various sexual activities as a business transaction, other aspects of the adult industry include, telephone/ internet sex operators, strip clubs, pornography are all considered immoral (Altman, 2000). Nearly all developed societies consider it a serious crime to force someone to engage in sexual behaviour or to engage in sexual behaviour with someone who does not consent (called as sexual assault, and if sexual penetration occurs, it is called rape). Laws regulating the minimum age at which a person can consent to have sex are frequently the subject of political and moral debate. Some cultures consider engaging in sexual activity without a partner, through masturbation or sexual fantasy, as immoral.

Religious norms

Religion shapes sexual values with 'sacred' law that articulates a range of acceptable sexual behaviours and practices like whom an individual should marry, the types of sexual expression allowed, non-use of contraception, etc.). In many countries, "sacred" laws continue to have a powerful impact on current secular law (Altman, 2000).

Figure 2 External Influencers of Sexuality

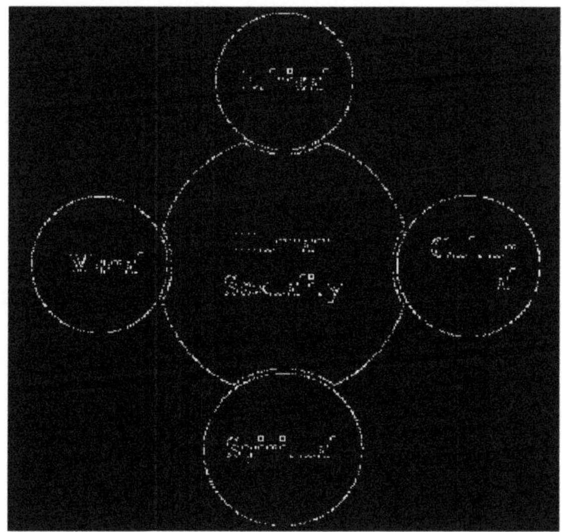

The other external aspects influencing one's sexuality include:

Impact of Alcohol on risky sex

Men in all cultures use alcohol and recreational drugs of various kinds as social dis-inhibitors before the sexual activity. Alcohol, lowers self-control, heightens self-delusion and makes previous decisions about safe sex harder to stick to. It is not that alcohol deprives men of the ability to control their sexual behaviour; but that it gives them an excuse to behave in ways which they know would be otherwise unacceptable. Thus the use of Alcohol supersedes the internal and external influencing factors, to indulge in sexual practices that would not be performed in a normal state of mind.

Impact of Westernization

Heterosexual division of a society or of social spaces refers to a process whereby the gender-based spaces in traditional non-Westernised societies (which are divided into men's spaces, women's spaces and third gender spaces) are abolished as part of Westernization and is replaced with heterosexual, mixed-sex spaces. This is also accompanied by introducing hetero-normative values in the society, thus changing the character of a society from 'gender segregation' to 'sexual orientation segregation'.

Economics, laws, and politics

Economics shape sexual values and become part of a culture's tradition. Although some laws are designed to protect people against sexual abuse (e.g., rape, paedophilia, incest), some laws also regulate sexual conduct between consenting adults and may favour one gender or sexual orientation over another. In some countries (e.g., Belarus, Cyprus, Romania), a homosexual or bisexual orientation is outlawed and discrimination is permitted. But laws can protect sexual practices as well. In some countries (e.g., Denmark, Holland, Sweden, and Ukraine), the legal rights of people with these sexual orientations are protected

In this context, the various factors influencing male sexual behaviour in our study setting shall be explored and its attributes in practice would be identified.

2.17 THEORIES ON SEXUALITY

Considering the external and internal factors influencing sexuality, a few theories have been proposed, on how ones sexuality is evolved. These theories have been classified principally on whether the perspectives of sexuality being psychological or social. Sexuality has been understood in the context of these two major theories namely:

A. Social Psychology Theories which consists of **Self-perception theory, 'Over-justification' hypothesis and Cognitive dissonance theory**

B. Social Exchange Theory

A. Social Psychology Theories of Sexuality

Male sexuality has to be understood considering the psychosocial factors like the sexual context and interpersonal interactions, which influence sexual functioning, as explained by the following theories:

a) Self-perception theory. Self-perception theory is based on the premise that people make attributions about their own attitudes, feelings and behaviours by relying on their observations of external behaviours and circumstances in which those behaviours occur.

For example: A 50-year-old woman married since 25 years, had the drive to be sexual about once per week throughout her marriage, her husband has had the drive to be sexual three times per week. This has resulted in the husband always being the initiator. This woman now observes her own behaviour and sees that she has only engaged in sex when asked. Even though she was often receptive to the initiation and enjoyed the encounters, her self-perception is that she has little desire and is not a sexual person because she hardly ever thinks of it on her own and never initiates. Her husband has a similar perception about her. **(Bem, 1965)**

In line with this self perception theory, the study shall explore if the perception of the male PLHIV on 'sexual fantasies' interferes with their 'sexual performance' within marriage. And to ascertain if it is this perceived dissatisfaction that lead men to seek sexual satisfaction outside marriage.

b) "Over-justification" hypothesis. This theory predicts that when an external reward is given to a person for performing an intrinsically rewarding activity, the person's intrinsic interest will decrease (Lepper, Greene, & Nisbett, 1973).

For example: In this case, if the 50-year-old woman responds to her husband's sexual initiation and the result is that she experiences a reward, such as relief from guilt (a form of negative reinforcement), relief from criticism from her husband, or gratitude and more housework done by him, the actual enjoyment of the sexual encounter may decline for her. This woman is now likely to interpret her enjoyment as being primarily from the reward instead of the actual activity. **(Bem, 1965)**

It will be interesting to explore if it is the external rewards of the MLHIV to their sexual partners, (in cash or kind), influence exchange of sexual favours outside marriage.

c) Cognitive Dissonance Theory, states that an inconsistency between two 'cognitions' or between 'cognition' and a 'behaviour' will create such discomfort in a person that they will alter one of the cognitions or behaviours in order to restore consistency and reduce this distress (Festinger, 1957).

For example: If this same woman responds to her husband's advances but does not perceive any external reward for this, that is, no relief of guilt, no reduction in whining, no gratitude etc., the need for cognitive balance or consistency between her observed behaviours and thoughts would lead her to attribute her behaviour to intrinsic enjoyment of sex. **(Bem, 1965)**

Many women, falling under self-perception or over-justification theory, would perceive sex as a chore or an obligation rather than an enjoyable experience and consider themselves sexually inadequate. In addition, many couples in long-term relationships would misinterpret the natural decrease in excitement and passion as being a symptom of a bad marriage.

B. Social Exchange Theory (SET)

SET is one of the social science theories that have been applied to the study of human sexuality. This theoretical perspective is useful for understanding sexuality within a relationship context, including why two people choose each other as sexual partners, which partner has more influence on what sexual activities they do together, sexual satisfaction, and the likelihood that one or both partners seek sexual activity outside the relationship. The exchange approach is applicable to all types of sexual dyads, ranging from the prostitute-client relationship (where exchange is very explicit and salient) to a couple married for many years (where the exchange is more implicit).

A social exchange framework, very broadly, refers to any conceptual model or theoretical approach that focuses on the exchange of resources (material or symbolic) between or among people and/or refers to one of the major exchange concepts, which are rewards, costs, and reciprocity. Some exchange theorists also consider the fairness or equity of the exchange, which refers to the relative rewards and costs for both partners.

Rewards and costs are two key concepts included in the social exchange framework. Rewards are defined as exchanged resources that are pleasurable and gratifying. Costs are defined as exchanged resources that result in a loss or punishment (Thibaut & Kelley, 1959). Costs also include foregone opportunities because of being in the particular relationship or interpersonal transaction. Reciprocity is another key concept of social exchange and refers to the notion that we give something back (and do not hurt) to those who have given to us (Gouldner, 1960). In many intimate relationships, sexual rewards and costs are sometimes exchanged for other resources in the relationship, such as intimacy, love, favours, and money. This research will also explore the cost and rewards involved in sexual behaviour.

2.18 Male Sexual Orientation

Views of Essentialists vs. Social Constructionists

The above theories help define the male sexual orientation and its nuances. There arises a debate on the male sexual orientation as to whether it follows an essential biological paradigm or if it is socially constructed. In Western cultures, a male who displays sexual attraction to other men may be classified as *bisexual* or *homosexual.* In a number of other cultures, a male is defined by his (putatively internal) gender; in such a culture, a masculine gendered male (of any sexual orientation) might simply be labelled a *man*, and males putatively gendered as feminine (transvestites of any sexual preference, flamboyantly effeminate males who are believed to indulge in receptive anal sex, and transsexuals) would not be considered 'men' but would be classified as members of the 'third sex', *i.e. partly male and partly female* (Connell, 1995).

Essentialists maintain that people across time and cultures, can be neatly divided into sexual identities determined on the basis of the sex of the partner desired as heterosexual, homosexual, or bisexual, claiming these identities represent natural divisions. They claim that there have always been equivalents of 'homosexual' identity in all times and all cultures. Social constructionists argue that sexual identities, especially those based on the sex of the partner, have been socially constructed, and are thus culturally specific. They claim that in all times and cultures, only passive sex by effeminate/ transgendered males (third sex) was identified as a separate category, and rather than a sexual identity, these were considered gender identities.

Historian David Greenberg, in the nineteenth century, argues that the concept of homosexuality did not exist prior to the mid-nineteenth century. He argues that *"the production and dissemination of a medical discourse in the recent past gave birth not just to the concept of a homosexual person, but also to homosexuals themselves, and at the same time, to their anti-twins, heterosexual persons"* (Connell, 1995).

Ideas of gender and sexual orientation are closely linked. The putatively *homosexual* identity exhibits some continuity with third sex identities and is more closely associated by some modern Western stereotypes with putative femininity in males. The contemporary *heterosexual* identity is arguably more closely associated with putative masculinity and may reflect earlier delineations of mainstream men's spaces.

While there is no division on the basis of the Western pattern of sexual orientation, there is a strong division of the male population between masculine-gendered males and feminine-gendered males. While the former are referred to as "men", the latter are known as members of the third gender, regardless of their sexual orientation (Masenja, 1993). The third sex is considered a separate gender category, and its members are not considered men or women but rather members of a neutral or intermediate gender. Thus, sexual relations between a man and another man are not treated as equivalent to sexual relations between a man and a member of the third gender.

In this regard the Kinsey's grading of male sexuality is widely accepted as it gives a holistic understanding towards the classification in male sexual orientation.

2.19 The Kinsey's Scale of grading sexuality in Males

According to Dr. Kinsey, males do not represent two discrete populations, 'heterosexuals' and 'homosexuals'. The world is not to be divided into sheep and goats ie. not all things are black nor all things are white. It is a fundamental law of taxonomy that nature rarely deals with discrete categories. The living world is a continuum in each and every of its aspects and cannot be categorised into separated pigeon holes. Thus persons should not characterized as heterosexual or homosexual, but as individuals who have a certain amount of heterosexual experience and certain amounts of homosexual experience (Pukar, 2004). The following figure explains that sexuality is rarely very exclusive as homosexual or heterosexual behaviour but of its nuances and shades.

Figure 3 Kinsley's scale of human sexuality

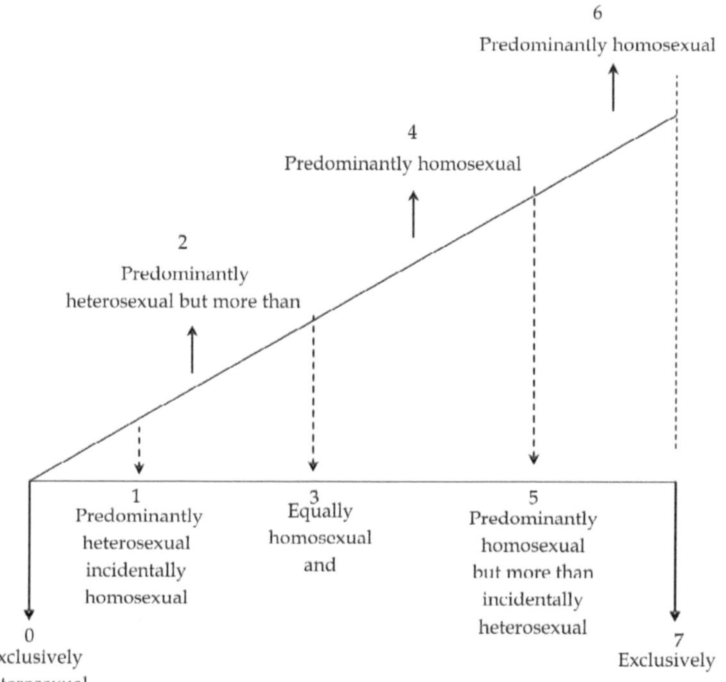

However, the male sexual orientation, which is a social construct, is debated to be different from the male sexual identity, which is a genetic composite. Thus, while the orientation defines the behaviour, the sexual identity defines ones personality.

2.20 Male Sexuality Identity

Male sexuality is associated with masculinity, which is a character that specifically describes men and can have degrees of comparison 'more masculine', 'most masculine'. The opposite can be expressed by terms such as 'unmanly', 'epicene or effeminate'. Masculinity has its roots in genetics; therefore while masculinity looks different in different cultures, there are common aspects to its definition across cultures. Machismo, a form of westernized masculine culture, includes assertiveness or standing up for one's rights, responsibility, selflessness, general code of ethics, sincerity, and respect.

While men do have a relative freedom compared to women, particularly in sexual and reproductive behaviours, lack of access to income earning opportunities has made men's role as heads of household and breadwinners a precarious one. With a majority of men reduced to figurehead authority, male identity and sense of self-esteem are threatened. Patriarchy does not mean that men only have privileges but also many responsibilities. Patriarchy used to be closely linked to male entitlement to control all essential resources, to 'own' and decide over the means of production. In contrast, male responsibility is normatively constituted, making men's roles and identities confusing and contradictory (Ortner and Whitehead 1989).

According to Connell (1995) the male gender is constructed round at least two conflicting characterisations of the essence of manhood: first, being a man is natural, healthy and innate; second, a man must stay masculine; he should never let his masculinity falter. Thus, a man is not born masculine, but acquires and enacts masculinity, and so becomes a man. Masculinity is composed of a number of elements, identities and behaviours that are not always coherent. They may be competing, contradictory and mutually undermining, they may vary across cultures, and they may have multiple and ambiguous meanings which alter according to context and over time (Connell, 1995). There are strong and weak masculinities, violent and non-violent ones, etc. Masculinity (and femininity), just like gender and sexuality does not simply reflect a biological 'given' but is largely a product of cultural and social processes (Connell 1995; Gagnon and Parker 1995; Bourdieu 1998). Thus neither masculinity nor sexuality are constant factors but change along with different historical and social structures. Linked to this, masculinity has to be constantly reasserted in the continuous denial of 'femininity' or 'feminine qualities' (Seidler, 1991). In order to exercise domination and reject feminine qualities, men are obliged to play their prescribed roles (Bourdieu 1998).

Drawing on Kopytoff 's distinction between existential and role-based identities sheds light on the link between different types of male identities. According to Kopytoff, some identities are based on what a person ***is*** (= existential identity), others are based on what a person ***does*** (farmer/craftsman = role-based identity). Some of these identities are negotiable; others are not (Kopytoff, 1990).

The existentially based identity is composed of features that are intrinsic, or 'immanent' in a cultural definition of what it is to be male or female – and not negotiable. The existential identity indicates a state of being rather than of doing. It is difficult to renegotiate, relatively immutable, and surrounded by strong sanctions that punish deviant behaviour. In contrast, features of role-based identity may be negotiated and the identities themselves relinquished with no sanctions. Following these distinctions, a man's sexual identity is closely linked to his (culturally defined) sexuality:

Thus in order to understand the role of male sexual behaviour in the AIDS epidemic the focus should fall on the social and cultural context, in which the sexual activity is shaped and constituted. The male sexual orientation and identity are thus concepts, which although distinct, are yet interconnected. In the light of this understanding of theories and concepts of male sexuality, the study now proceeds to look into its coherence with the HIV infection. For the HIV/AIDS prevention campaigns that lead to behaviour change can only be successful if proper attention is given to the wider socio-economic context, and to issues of sexuality (Parker, 2001).

2.21 CONGENIALITY OF MALE SEXUALITY AND HIV

According to Peter Piot, "Men are a key to reducing HIV transmission and have the power to change the course of the AIDS epidemic". Heterosexual men are often seen as the driving force behind the epidemic. The view is that gender inequalities permit men to dictate the terms of sexual intercourse, which results in victimizing women with unprotected sex (UNAIDS, 2001). Such a discussion on Male sexuality, on one hand, is helpful in moving gender based intervention approaches away from focusing exclusively on women as has been the case in the past (sex workers and pregnant mothers). On the other, it runs the danger of essentialising the category 'men' and deflects attention away from the complexities of multiple masculinities. It was only with the September 1994 Cairo International Conference on Population and Development (ICPD) that a focus on men, their role as responsible partners and also their own sexual and reproductive health needs became clear. It recognised the need to address and involve men in order to improve women's reproductive health (UNAIDS, 2001). However, there is no generally accepted clarity or agreement about how men should be approached or integrated into existing HIV-prevention or reproductive health programmes.

Dar es Salaam from UNAIDS speaks of the need to focus the HIV intervention program on men stating that the challenge in the field of HIV prevention and reproductive health remains of involving men and overcoming their resistance to such involvement. Efforts here are charged with considerable difficulties because they may threaten established male privileges as well as men's existential sexual identities. One opportunity lies in focusing on men's own vulnerability to infection. Most men have not considered their own vulnerability, since historically women have been encouraged to pay attention to their health because of their childbearing capacities (UNAIDS, 2003). With the A-B-C approaches still being considered 'best practice' in HIV/AIDS prevention activities by many organisations it seems that the gendered effects of socio-economic change and in particular the implications for male identities, masculinities and sexualities have been totally overlooked. And so have male vulnerability and male self-interest in avoiding HIV/ AIDS (Cornwall, 1994).

2.22 ATTITUDE TOWARDS MALE SEXUALITY

With a majority of men not having been able to develop new role-based identities and with male sexual activity generating categories of masculinity, the need for men to pursue their existential identities seems to have become essential to their self-esteem. It also clarifies why male sexual activity is so important, and why greater emphasis is placed on sexual relations and even risky behaviour (Kopytoff, 1990). Men seem to use measures like establishing their authority, thus developing masculinist discourses, being sexually aggressive and violent. This attempt to regain control and authority over women seems to run counter to the promotion of gender equality and women's empowerment (Willott and Griffin 1996).

On the other hand, there are also men who actually abandon their immediate realm of authority (the household) and seek new forms of affirmation (in the arms of other lovers) (Morrell 2001). Domination is not inscribed in men's nature nor does masculinity remain static. They change along with different historical and social structures, the complexity of contemporary life, etc. (Connell, 2002). This approach provides space for optimism, precisely because it acknowledges the possibility of intervening in the politics of masculinity to promote new types of masculinities that may embrace gender equality. These sexist attitudes of men will be explored in this research.

Myths and Misconceptions

The myths regarding male sexuality have been particularly tenacious because men have traditionally not talked about their sexual feelings and experiences honestly and openly, with their sexual partners. There have been positive signs recently that this is changing with men's movement beginning to redefine what it means to be a man, and qualities of gentleness, caring, and vulnerability are valued (Caldwell, 2000). More men are beginning to discuss their sexuality more openly, and this will benefit both them and their partners.

In some cultures it is acceptable for men to have multiple sexual partners or sex with a person, who is not their spouse, whereas a woman in the same culture who has sexual relations outside of marriage may be stigmatized, punished, or socially ostracized even if she has been raped. Many other types of sexual taboos exist some of which are nearly universal, while others rare. For example, many cultures have laws or taboos regarding sex or marriage with close family members (such as fathers with daughters or mothers with sons), but cultures vary in what they consider to be "too close" a relation (for example, some cultures allow first cousins to marry, while others do not). Many cultures also have taboos regarding sex during menstruation, pregnancy, or lactation.

Middle-aged and older adults no longer accept such myths as "Sex is only for young people" and "Sex isn't important to older adults." The once widespread myths that "people in their 60s and beyond wouldn't want to have sex" are fading away.

Here are a few commonly observed myths about to Male Sexuality (Ortner, 1989; Weiss, 1998):

- All sexual contact must lead to intercourse
- Foreplay is only for teenagers
- Sex is the way to demonstrate love.
- A girl cannot get pregnant the first time she has sexual intercourse.
- Having a male withdraw his penis from a female's vagina before he ejaculates or "comes" (*coitus interruptus*) is a good way to prevent pregnancy.
- Having sexual intercourse while standing up, urinating after intercourse or jumping up and down after intercourse will prevent pregnancy.
- All teenagers are having sexual intercourse these days.
- Very few men are virgins.
- Men must always initiate sexual activity.
- Males have stronger sex drives and are more interested in sex than females.
- The man must be in charge of the sexual activity
- A male always wants and is always ready to have sex.
- There's something wrong with a *guy* who hasn't had sex by the time he is 18.
- Oral-genital sex between a man and a woman is a sign of homosexuality.
- One is a homosexual if he has had sex with, or even had a "sexy" dream about, someone of the same sex.
- Homosexuality is abnormal
- You can tell if a person is a homosexual by looking at him or her.
- AIDS is a "gay" or homosexual disease.
- Condoms don't work.
- A large penis is important for sexual enjoyment.
- Top of Form
- Bottom of Form
- Bottom of Form
- Sex requires an erection.
- Bottom of Form
- Sex is over when the man ejaculates.
- Bottom of Form
- Bottom of Form
- Men in relationships don't masturbate.
- Having an orgasm while asleep, a "nocturnal" orgasm, is a sign of sexual problems.

- Nocturnal emissions/ Loss of semen weakens the body
- Masturbation is restricted almost exclusively to males, Masturbation can cause a number of physical and mental problems like warts, pimples, acne and insanity.
- "If the passion is gone, something is seriously wrong."
- Circumcision increases the sexual power of men

This study shall also aim to understand the attitudes of men in these contexts.

2.23 FACTORS INFLUENCING HIGH RISK BEHAVIOURS IN MEN

HIV is commonly spread through unprotected sexual contact with an infected person, by direct blood contact through contaminated needles (primarily for illicit drug injection or in healthcare settings without proper sterilization procedures), during birth or breastfeeding (for infants born to HIV-infected mothers), or through transfusions of infected blood. Any behaviour which exposes the risk of acquisition of blood, breast milk, seminal or vaginal fluid of an HIV infected person is termed as a 'High Risk Behaviour'. While everyone is biologically susceptible to infection with HIV if exposed to the virus, this does not mean that everyone is equally at risk from the virus. ie. a gay having unsafe sex is at much greater risk of becoming infected with HIV than a heterosexual having unsafe sex.

Some commonly observed High Risk Behaviours include, sexual relationships with more than one sex partner (casual or steady), sex without protection (anal, vaginal and oral) or inconsistent condom use, Sharing needles or having sex with someone who does have history of STI, Use of drugs or alcohol while having sex, Blood transfusion, organ transplant, tattoo, body piercing. In the health care setting, health care workers can be infected with HIV after being stuck with needles containing HIV-infected blood or, less frequently, after infected blood gets into a worker's open cut or a mucous membrane (for example, the eyes or inside of the nose).

Heterosexual men are often seen as the driving force behind the epidemic. The view is that gender inequalities permit men to dictate the terms of sexual intercourse and this result in unprotected sex with women being the major victims. Majority of men feel that it is quite legitimate to have 'outside' partners. Most men argue that 'zero grazing' and sticking to one partner aren't possible, simply because 'it is against a man's nature'. Even if the sale of condoms has increased, condoms are hated, and men have myriads of excuses for not using them. The sexual performance, the control over women – not to mention the pleasure derived from it, seems fundamental to male identity. Thus, neither sticking to one partner nor using condoms, which are standard lines of argument in HIV/AIDS prevention activities and campaigns, are acceptable solutions to most men.

The groups commonly involved in male sex work like masseurs, transgender, young migrant men and gays, practicing male sex work for survival, or men with other occupations practicing male sex work are at a high risk for acquiring STIs including HIV (Coleman, 1992). Dandona reports that the probability estimates for acquiring HIV by men who sell sex were 6.7 times higher compared with women who sell sex.

MSM in India can be divided into various subgroups: self-identified MSM (gay identified, kothis, panthis), behaviourally MSM with no identity, bisexual men, and male-to-female transgender (hijras) are vulnerable because of their occupations/ profession, and often engage into 'survival sex'; work is often intermittent and irregular for these men and they may actually have to offer sex in exchange for money.

The variables noted by various studies, which seem to influence high risk behaviours in men have been briefed below:

Psychological Factors: Research in the North reveals specifically male depression caused by economic marginalisation and lack of self-esteem. These depressions are characterised by increased aggressive behaviour, lack of self-control, overconsumption of alcohol and often suicide (Sabo and Gordon 1995). A study from Tanzania argues that frustrations and inner disturbances may even result in men raping children and women. Possessing no means to change their economic status, many seem to be responding by developing macho attitudes and resorting to physical violence against women. Other variables that hold strong clinical implications such as the experience of childhood sexual abuse or problematic substance abuse profiles are found to be associated with a high-risk sexual profile (Masenja, 1993).

Adolescence: Mounting research suggests that men with a history of sexual activity during childhood are more likely than those without such a history, to have engaged in high risk sexual practices, in contracting HIV. High-risk sexual behaviour in adolescents appears to be influenced by the sexual attitudes of peers, and young people select friends whose attitudes about sex are consistent with their own attitudes (Shajahan and Cavanagh 1998).

Early sexual exposure: Research conducted on high-risk behaviours among heterosexual African American men reported having had anal sex with men, inconsistent condom use during anal sex, and unprotected oral sex. An increasing 'risk for HIV' was found to be associated with decreasing 'age at first sexual experience'. The age group of young adults is also a strong marker for HIV risk. Epidemiological surveillance among MSM as young as 15-20 years yields high rates of new HIV infections (Rutz et al 1997).

Education: Less well studied in literature is the effect of socioeconomic status on sexual HIV risk, although a few populations based studies found a strong association between HIV infection and low educational attainment among MSM (Catania, et al., 2001).

Homosexuality: A series of individual-level demographic variables have been found to be associated with high-risk sexual behaviour and/or HIV infection among MSM. The HIV status itself is conceptualized as a demographic variable, among men. Many studies have detected a strong association between HIV seropositivity and greater sexual risk among MSM. A significant number of PLHIV across the globe report that they continue to engage in unprotected behaviour with their sexual partners putting them at the risk of HIV (Valleroy et al., 2000). The notions of masculinity that emphasize sexual domination over women as a defining characteristic of manhood contribute to homophobia and the stigmatization of men who have sex with men. The stigma and fear that result force men who have sex with men to keep their sexual behaviour secret and deny their sexual risk, thereby increasing their own risk as well as the risk of their partners (UNAIDS, 1999).

Machismo: Not all sexual acts between men convey an equal risk for HIV infection; it therefore stands to reason that men who have eroticized the most risky sexual practices (for example, unprotected receptive anal intercourse) are at the greatest risk for HIV transmission. Similarly, many different epidemiological studies have found that men with greater numbers of sexual partners (especially high-risk sexual partners), are more likely to be HIV seropositive. Men who can demonstrate greater skills at using condoms, who have ready access to condoms and lubricants, and who report a greater sense of self-efficacy at being able to use condoms consistently also typically report lower rates of sexual risk taking. Men are challenging the notion of "use a condom every time" as an unworkable long-term strategy and are gambling with very high stakes indeed to define a set of effective "harm reduction" strategies (Stillion, 1995).

Alcohol : Of the contextual levels variables, perhaps the best studied is that of sex under the influence of alcohol and drugs. Although the behavioural data concerning the associations between alcohol or drugs during sexual activity are still far from uniform, both sero-prevalence and sero-incidence data strongly support the argument that men who also use drugs are a vulnerable population for HIV infection (Stall, 2000).

Experimentation: Sex also occurs in a physical, emotional, and socio-cultural context, and these variables are also understood to influence whether high risk sex occurs. Other mood states transitory depression, use of sex as a coping strategy, emotional attraction between partners, the desire to engage in 'time out behaviour', and the trait of 'sensation seeking' have also been identified as important components to high risk sexual events.

Culture : Culture is widely assumed to have an effect on sexual practice, although relatively little research has been done to describe the specific ways in which culture functions to shape sexual practice in diverse subcultures of 'males' (Bandura, 1997). It is widely assumed that among men who do not identify as gay and among who fear of disclosure and/or violence is high, the safe sex practices are attenuated.

ART : The emergence of HAART combination drugs to fight HIV infection are said to have profoundly changed the calculations that PLHIV use to gauge sexual risks and has contributed to increased indulgence in high-risk sexual behaviours (Bouhnik, 2002).

Fatalism : Elford coined the term "AIDS burnout", by virtue of which PLHIV may not adopt safe sex regimens as a lifelong strategy, but as an adaptation to a temporary health crisis. In fact, some have argued that no group of men can be expected to adopt condoms as a permanent and universal sexual strategy. HIV concordant couples, indulge in a sexual expression that assumes that no further harm could result from HIV transmission between individuals already infected with HIV. HIV negative insertive partners are unlikely to be infected by positive receptive partners (Ekstrand, et al., 1999).

Stage of HIV Infection : Studies show that patterns of risk behaviour vary according to HIV disease stage, which are marked by changes in physical functioning and quality of life. A number of studies find that the period immediately preceding the acquisition of HIV is characterized by high rates of risk behaviours. Such behaviour increases the likelihood of rapid spread of HIV during the time when transmission risk is greatest and the individual is least likely to be aware that he or she is infected with HIV. For many affected individuals, risk behaviours decrease following a diagnosis of HIV. (Stillion, 1995).

Health: The risk behaviours for HIV transmission is often related to the individual's state of health. When individuals with HIV experience long periods of asymptomatic HIV infection, they often revert to risk behaviours. CD4 counts below 200 µL, resulting in a formal diagnosis of AIDS, are associated with decreased sexual and drug-related risk behaviours, but resurgence is possible during later-stage disease. Reductions in transmission risk behaviours seem to relate to both passage of time and decline in health (Stillion, 1995).

Migratory status: More episodes of unprotected sex were reported by established immigrant men compared with recent immigrants in western studies. Recent immigrants were, less likely to be HIV-tested, encounters institutional barriers of linguistic isolation, lacks health insurance, and avails medical care irregularly. These populations have greater access to sex workers, which increases their risk to infections (Rutz et al 1997).

Religion : Previous studies have shown a positive relationship between religiosity and the practice or adoption of protective health behaviours, including reduction of illicit drug use among hard-core injecting drug users. Most studies hypothesize high religiosity to be associated with a lower likelihood engaging in risky behaviours for HIV transmission (Weiss and Gupta, 1998).

Masculinity norms: First, prevailing norms of masculinity that expect men to be more knowledgeable and experienced about sex, put men, particularly young men, at risk of infection because such norms prevent them from seeking information or admitting their lack of knowledge about sex or protection, and coerce them into experimenting with sex in unsafe ways, and at a young age, to prove their manhood (UNAIDS, 1999).

Need for a change: It is believed that variety in sexual partners is essential to men's nature and that men will seek multiple partners for sexual release. a hydraulic model of male sexuality that seriously challenges the effectiveness of prevention messages that call for fidelity in partnerships or a reduction in the number of sexual partners (Mane, Rao Gupta, and Weiss 1994; Heise and Elias 1995).

Sexual dissatisfaction with spouse: Accumulated anger, hurt, disappointment, distance and resentment can fester and extinguish the flames of desire with spouse. Overwhelming, concern about sexual performance by spouse obscures pleasure and leads to sexual dysfunction, performance anxiety is a particularly insidious issue affecting aging couples. Performance anxiety is common, in women, who have experienced pain during sex (dyspareunia) in the past. They may be worried that sex will be uncomfortable again, and this anxiety can decrease lubrication. In turn, this makes sex painful, which heightens their anxiety and further interferes with lubrication. Ultimately, some women decide to avoid sex. The worry about having sagging breasts or potbelly can discourage the spouse from having sex, needless to say, these conditions don't leave much room for inspired lovemaking. For men, episodes of impotence can undercut confidence in their manhood.

Lack of a partner: It may seem obvious that not having a partner *(either being a widower or divorced /separated)* is an impediment to an active sex life.

Women's Vulnerability: Research supported by ICRW and conducted by researchers worldwide has identified the different ways in which the imbalance in power between women and men in gender relations curtails women's sexual autonomy and expands male sexual freedom, thereby increasing women's and men's risk and vulnerability to HIV (Bruyn et al. 1995).

Culture of silence that surrounds sex dictates the fact that "good" women are expected to be ignorant about sex and passive in sexual interactions. This makes it difficult for women to be informed about risk reduction or, even when informed, makes it difficult for them to be proactive in negotiating safer sex (Carovano, 1992). Second, the traditional norm of virginity for unmarried girls that exists in many societies, paradoxically, increases young women's risk of infection because it restricts their ability to ask for information about sex out of fear that they will be thought to be sexually active. Virginity also puts young girls at risk of rape and sexual coercion in because of the erroneous belief that sex with a virgin can cleanse a man of infection and because of the erotic imagery that surrounds the innocence and passivity associated with virginity. In addition, in cultures where virginity is highly valued, research has shown that some young women practice anal sex, in order to preserve their virginity placing them at increased risk of HIV (Weiss and Gupta, 2000). Third, the role of power in sexual decision-making surrounds sex, accessing treatment services for sexually transmitted diseases can be highly stigmatizing for adolescent and adult women (Weiss, 2000; Bruyn et al. 1995). Also since motherhood is considered to be a feminine ideal, using barrier methods or non-penetrative sex as safer sex options presents a significant dilemma for women (Elias 1995; UNAIDS 1999). Women's economic dependency also increases their vulnerability to HIV. Research has shown that the economic vulnerability of women makes it more likely that they will exchange sex for money or favours, less likely that they will succeed in negotiating protection, and less likely that they will leave a relationship that they perceive to be risky (Gupta 1994).

Further to the above factors, men in many societies are socialized to be self-reliant, not to show their emotions and not to seek assistance in times of need or stress. Their pleasurable past experiences with non-spousal relationships may also influence their illicit indulgences. Health ailments of the spouse inclusive of heart disease, diabetes, cancer, and arthritis can have a serious, lasting impact on your sexuality. Treatments for OI or ART can also alter sexual functioning (WHO, 1999).

These are the factors influencing high risk sexual behaviours in men, which need to be ascertained further.

Conclusion

If men are to be key actors in reducing HIV transmission, they need to develop a concern about their own sexual health before they can be concerned about the health of their partner. As long as men have not recognised their own vulnerability and are not aware that their sexual behaviour, they can be lethal to themselves, and cannot be expected to adopt a more responsible behaviour. Also, men will not be inclined to 'involvement' unless they see for themselves what the benefits of behaviour change are. From this point of view, the notion of 'self-efficacy' may constitute an important determinant in male sexual behaviour. With the urgent need to make a halt to the HIV/AIDS epidemic, a focus on men, their vulnerability and the promotion of male self-efficacy should constitute a first step.

This chapter spoke about behaviours associated with ones sexuality, while one's disclosure of their risk behaviours or their HIV/STI status have been untouched here. The next chapter opens the window to understanding the process and benefits of status disclosure with sexual partners.

Chapter 3

DISCLOSURE

INTRODUCTION

The prevention and control of HIV infection depends on the success of strategies to prevent new infections and treat currently infected individuals. HIV testing and counselling serves as both a critical prevention and treatment tool in the control of the HIV epidemic. Within HIV testing and counselling programmes, focus is placed on the importance of HIV status disclosure among HIV-infected clients, particularly to their sexual partners. This focus on disclosure is with the intent to equip PLHIV and their sexual partners to practice preventive measures. For any HIV infected person, the first and most obvious being fear is of the medical implications of the disease itself and the next biggest fear is that of disclosure.

The process of self-disclosure is not an easy activity to take part in. This process is a complex communication phenomenon and researchers for the past 30 years, continue to analyze it (Klitzman et al, 2004). The focus of this chapter is to inform the reader of self-disclosure within interpersonal communication and discuss an array of different areas concerning self-disclosure. These areas of discussion include: a definition of self-disclosure, functions of self-disclosure, goals, influencing factors, benefits, risks, and process of self-disclosure in the context of HIV.

3.1. Definition of SELF - DISCLOSURE

Self-disclosure in psychology is a process of providing personal information to another individual. The information that is disclosed about oneself may include one's thoughts, feelings, past experiences, and future plans. According to Derlega (1986), self-disclosure plays a major factor in intimate relationships and has been described as a component that can establish and stabilize a relationship. The process of self-disclosure involves an appropriate time and place, various levels of intimacy, and a person whom one feels comfortable to disclose to (Borchers, 1999).

Jourard (1975) defines self-disclosure as making ourselves "transparent" to others through our communication. According to Culpert (1968) Self-Description involves communication that levels 'public layers' whereas Self-Disclosure involves communication that reveals more private, sensitive, and confidential information. Pearce & Sharp (1973) make an interesting distinction among three related terms: self-disclosure, confession, and revelation. Wherein 'Self-disclosure' is voluntary communication of information about one's self to another, 'Confession' is forced or coerced communication of information about one's self to another and 'Revelation' is unintentional or inadvertent communication of information about one's self to another. According to Fisher & Adams (2003), all possible knowledge about oneself can be classified into two categories: public knowledge (what other people know) and private knowledge (what only we know). Hence, when one self-discloses information to another, he/she makes public the private information of him/herself.

3.2. SELF DISCLOSURE – THEORETICAL FRAMEWORK

Behavioural researchers have initiated developing theories on disclosure only in the last century. The following five major theories attempt to explain the process of Self Disclosure as a concept and process. These theories have been classified based on their focus on Individual, Society and Structural systems

A. Focus on Individual : Johari Window Model

B. Focus on Society : Social Penetration Theory, Theory of Reciprocity

C. Structural Systems : Disease Progression Theory, Consequence Theory

A. Focus on Individual

1. The Johari Window Model

One way to view the process and functioning of self-disclosure at the 'Level of Individual' is the Johari Window, named after Joseph Luft and Harry Ingham. The four panes of the window is a way of showing how much information we know about ourselves and how much others know about us (Borchers, 1999). The four panes include the open pane, blind pane, hidden pane, and unknown pane:

Known to Self	Unknown to Self
Known to Others	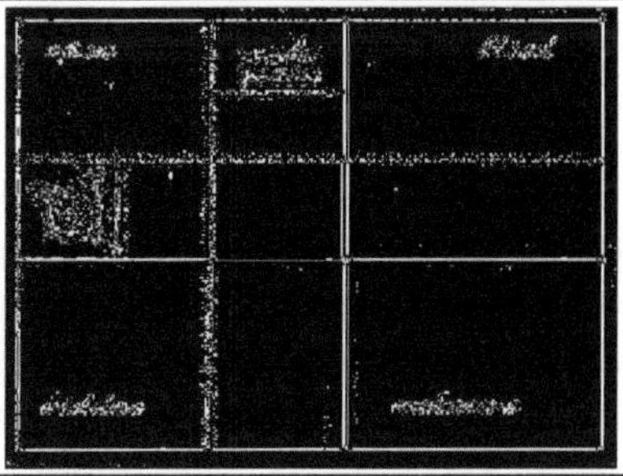
Unknown to Others	

Open: The open pane includes basic information about one's conscious self - our attitudes, behaviour, motivation, values and way of life - of which we are aware and which is known to others. We move within this area with freedom, for example, one's physical appearance, the occupation and hair colour are included in the open pane.

Hidden: The hidden pane keeps information such as one's dreams and ambitions private. Our hidden area cannot be known to others, unless we disclose. This we freely keep within ourselves, and that which we retain out of fear. The degree to which we share ourselves with others (disclosure) is the degree to which we can be known.

Blind : The blind pane is information that one cannot see of oneself or which one may not know but the other individuals can see. When others say what they see (feedback) and we are able to hear it; in that way we are able to test the reality of who we are and are able to grow.

Unknown: We are more rich and complex than that which we and others know, but from time to time something happens - is felt, read, heard, dreamed - something from our unconscious is revealed. Then we "know" what we have never "known" before. Finally, the unknown pane is the window in which information about the self is unknown by the individual and others. A hidden talent one may encompass is an example of the unknown pane.

It is through disclosure and feedback that our open pane is expanded and that we gain access to the potential within us represented by the unknown pane. Borcher (1999) states, "It is through self-disclosure, we open and close panes so that we may become more intimate with others." This is an important model that is being attempted to be operationalized amongst couples living with HIV or even those PLHIV who plan to get married. This model is pictorially represented as below:

A. Focus on Society

1. Social Penetration Theory (SPT)

Psychologists Altman and Taylor (1973) proposed that closeness occurs through a gradual process of self-disclosure, and closeness develops if the participants proceed in a gradual and orderly fashion from superficial to intimate levels of exchange. Self-disclosure is the act of revealing more about oneself, on both a conscious and an unconscious level. Only through opening one's self to the main route to social penetration – in self-disclosure – and thus becoming vulnerable to another person, can an intimate relationship develop.

Social penetration is perhaps best known for its onion analogy, which describes the multilayered nature of personality. Self-disclosure is referred to in terms of breadth and depth, the latter of which is described in units of layers. When one peels the outer skin from an onion, another skin is uncovered. The outer layer of personality contains the public self, which is accessible to anyone who wants to look. The public self layer has a myriad of details which help to describe who one is, such as height, weight, gender, and other public information which takes little questioning to discover. Below the surface layer, however, the personality holds more private information like beliefs, faith, prejudices, and general relationship information. Within the inner core are values, self-concept, and deep emotions. The inner core is the unique private domain of individuals, which, although invisible to the rest of the world, has a profound impact on the areas of life which lie closer to the surface. The key components of this theory are:

- Peripheral items are exchanged more frequently and sooner than private information.
- Self-disclosure is reciprocal, especially in the early stages of relationship development.
- Penetration is rapid at the start but slows down quickly as the tightly wrapped inner layers are reached.
- De-penetration is a gradual process of layer-by-layer withdrawal

Critique: According to Taylor (1973), the SPT made no mention of gender differences, for there is a great deal of evidence that females disclose personal information more often and sooner than males. Male relationships can often be characterized by breadth without a high degree of depth, often resulting in more casual relationships. Females on the other hand seek the need for a human connection, which results in more frequent self-disclosure to establish the needed connection.

2. Theory of Reciprocity :

If one's goal is to get the other to disclose information, that one must start the conversation by disclosing, thereby making the other person feel a sense of obligation to reciprocate and disclose. When one person engages in self-disclosure it is through the norm of reciprocity that the other person listening also self-discloses information about what he/she is thinking, feeling. This enables a sense of trust, deepens in the relationship and allows each person to understand one another accurately (Cunnhingam, 1981).

B. Focus on Structural aspects

The theories formulated herein account the systemic aspects responsible for disclosure and holds the belief that the control on disclosure does not purely rest with oneself but are bound to disclose due to structural needs (Kalichman, 1998).

3. Disease Progression Theory:

According to the disease progression theory, individuals disclose their HIV status only when they become symptomatic. It is theorized then that as HIV progresses to AIDS, individuals can no longer keep their HIV status a secret. Disease progression often results in hospitalizations and physical deterioration, which, in some cases, mandates individuals to explain their illness (Kalichman, 1998). Not only would hospitalization require explanation, but if death is imminent, or if individuals fear that they will need additional assistance to manage their illness, they may disclose as a means of accessing additional needed resources (Holt et al., 1998). Conversely, delaying disclosure may be a way to normalize one's life and to protect others from pain (Babcock, 1998).

4. Consequence Theory

The consequence theory of HIV disclosure suggests that disease progression influences disclosure through individuals' perception of the consequences anticipated as a result of disclosure (Serovich, 2001). As the disease progresses the need to evaluate the consequences of disclosure becomes more pronounced. PLHIV are likely to disclose their status to significant others and sexual partners only when they feel that the rewards for disclosing outweigh the associated costs.

3.3 GOALS OF SELF DISCLOSURE

The above theories point out the goals of self disclosure, which is to gain knowledge or information, about the other person, as well as to get to know oneself. Another goal is achieving a 'sense of support' and confirmation of 'self-worth'. The perceived truthfulness of one's disclosures symbolizes and demonstrates a commitment of pursuing and maintaining a close relationship. Therefore through self-disclosure, when an individual's 'true self' is accepted by another, this acceptance leads to love, trust, commitment, and intimacy, thus leading to a successful relationship. If the goals of self-disclosure are not successful, conflict of the relationship and conflicts within the self may arise (Kalichman, 1998). Duck and Pittman (1994) stated that the primary goal of self-disclosure is the maintenance of one's mental health. Jourard (1961) feels that through self-disclosure people are able to validate one another's thoughts and feelings so as to understand more fully how we conform to the world around us.

3.4. SELF DISCLOSURE IN THE CONTEXT OF HIV

Disclosure in the context of HIV is understood as "the act of informing another person/s of the HIV-positive status of an individual". There is a strong stigma that accompanies the disclosure of an HIV diagnosis. A positive sero-status can suggest to others an adoption of negative behaviours notoriously associated with sero-conversion, i.e., injection drug use, or unprotected sexual intercourse (Kalichman & Nachimson, 1999). It can also imply that death is imminent and proximal (Katz, 1997). Reluctance to physically touch or share space with a PLHIV has also been noticed (Green, 1995; Wight, 2006); and the uninfected general population continues to hold incorrect, specious beliefs about the degree to which HIV is communicable (Crawford, Travers, 1999). Considering these perceptions and behaviours, disclosure is daunting, and for some, impossible. Yet, researches on PLHIV suggest that over a period of time, the need to widen those private communication boundaries and to discuss one's sero-status steadily increases (Derlega, 2003; Kalichman, 2003). Disclosure becomes an eventuality of living with the disease, and the need to include others in the HIV status diagnosis supersedes the need to prevent stigmatization.

One of the foremost concerns for PLHIV is how, when, where and to whom to disclose their HIV status. Disclosure could happen at home, in a healthcare setting or within the community so that support is readily available. 'Whom to tell' about the

HIV status and 'how to tell' can be a very complex and personal decision. Although there is generally no one right time, the disclosure happens whenever the individual feels ready or when s/he is legally required to do so. An act of disclosure may be done by the PLHIV him/herself or by another person, with or without the consent of the PLHIV.

Disclosure can occur in many contexts: ie. disclosure within personal relationships (to lovers, partners, spouses, children, friends and other family); disclosure in the workplace (to an employer, other employees, clients); disclosure to health and other service providers (physicians, emergency services, dentists, social workers, insurers, etc.); disclosure in an institutional setting (prisons, schools, etc.), and disclosure to the general public via the media. Disclosure to sex partners is more likely in longer-term, romantic relationships than in casual relationships (one-night stands, anonymous partners, group scenes, etc.). Disclosure also varies depending on perceived HIV status of partners, level of HIV risk of sex activities, sense of responsibility to protect partners (personal vs. shared responsibility) and alcohol or drug use. Disclosure is therefore a process and not just an event, and it is very much a two-way process rather than being solely reliant on the HIV infected individual.

Most PLHIV disclose their status to some, but not all, of their partners, friends and family. Disclosure generally becomes easier the longer someone has been living with HIV, as he/she becomes more comfortable with an HIV positive status. PLHIV may disclose differently with doctors, family, friends, work colleagues, sexual and injecting partners. The traditional message has been that they should always disclose their HIV status to partners so that it provides them with both emotional and practical support. Some decide to become more public and use their stories to advocate with government or media to curb stigma and discrimination against PLHIV or in the interest of eliciting PLHIV friendly services or policies. Some may disclose for educational purposes to neighbours, community and religious groups, schools, other PLHIV, or healthcare providers. Studies reveal that PLHIV find a sense of purpose and increased self-esteem by telling their story (Kalichman, 1998).

Initiation of Disclosure can thus be classified into three broad categories

1. **Self disclosure wherein** the PLHIV voluntarily chooses to notify his/her partner. The disclosure assistance provider guides and prepares the client before disclosure.
2. **Dual disclosure wherein t**he PLHIV chooses to notify a partner in the presence of a health care provider (counselor/ doctor/ social worker). The health care provider supports the client during disclosure and acts as a resource for the partner.
3. **Health Care Provider (HCP) Initiated** is conducted when an individual approaches the HCP to know the HIV status of a spouse / sexual partner, perceiving a threat to acquisition of the infection, ethically the HCP discloses the status of the client valuing the health of the spouse. Herein the disclosure is initiated directly by the HCP with or without consent of the PLHIV. This initiative is debated by many organizations and undertaken only if the PLHIV is adamant not to disclose his/ her status either by self or in the presence of

a health care provider, even after repeated counselling. This initiative is legally permissible in some areas (Dev, 1999).

Discussing and disclosing HIV status among PLHIV is a two-way street. Most people feel that when a person knows that s/he is HIV positive then s/he has an obligation to tell the other person, and counsellors are expected, as a part of their job, to help people with this process. Also, laws in some areas require disclosure of HIV positive status prior to sex. However, both partners should be responsible for knowing each other's status towards positive prevention.

3.5. BENEFITS IN DISCLOSURE

Self-disclosure as seen in the above discussions seems to be a complex process, which demands patience and compassion from both the discloser and receiver. Although there are risks involved in disclosure, researches points out that the benefits outweigh those risks by achieving an intimate and loving relationship with another (Wight, 2006).

Benefits for the Individual

Human beings rely intensely on love, closeness and intimacy as prerequisites to nurture a healthy and happy life. Without self-disclosure participating in a relationship would prove to be difficult, if not impossible. Many benefits regarding self-disclosure that an individual can experience are, gaining information or knowledge of an individual, becoming aware of one's own thoughts and feelings, achieving partner's acceptance and trust. Disclosure provides psychological benefits like increased intimacy with partners and reaffirmation of their sense of self. Many PLHIV who disclose their status find that it reduces anxiety about transmission, so sex can be much more comfortable and relaxed (Wight, 2006).

Disclosure is also fundamental in managing HIV, especially in terms of adhering to complex treatment regimens (Chesney and Smith, 1999). For example, HIV-positive people report that they sometimes skip ART doses, because they could not take a prescribed medication without being observed doing so.

Research has shown that disclosure of stressful events have positive outcomes such as reduced health problems and increased social support (Derlega et al., 1993). Although disclosing HIV infection to family is a taxing experience, it has been reported that social support decreases depressive symptoms among PLHIV and leads to better psychosocial functioning (Hays et al., 1992). It also improved and increased productivity and well-being of PLWHA in Africa and Asia-Pacific region (Klein, 1999).

Social Benefits

Disclosure is an important public health goal for it motivates the sexual partners to seek testing, transform their behaviour and ultimately decrease transmission of HIV. In addition, the potential benefits of disclosure for the individual include increased opportunities for social support, improved access to necessary medical care including antiretroviral treatment, increased opportunities to discuss and implement HIV risk reduction with partners, and increased opportunities to plan for the future (Klein, 1999).

Disclosure of HIV status has become an entry criterion for many treatment programmes in resource constrained settings (Klein, 1999). And, access to other forms of care such as home based care and specific social grants are also dependent upon the disclosure of HIV status. In some instances, disclosure of personal and secret information is necessary to garner resources needed to survive and overcome the daily and stressful demands of the vent such as HIV/AIDS.

3.6. RISKS IN DISCLOSURE

Self-disclosure sometimes works against the individuals in the relationship. This is what makes the process of self-disclosure confusing and difficult.

Risks for the Individual

There is a high degree of vulnerability when an individual self-discloses private information and there is a chance of getting hurt and his 'true self' may be rejected or exploited. Prior to, and during, self-disclosure people tend to experience ambivalence and hence too much or too little of self-disclosure can damage a relationship, especially early on. The information that was disclosed may not be responded to in a positive manner or the information may be used against the discloser, leaving the other person in the relationship to gain power. Studies have shown that fear of violence can have a strong impact on the decision to disclose. The highest rates of disclosure-related violence were reported among women in ANC. HIV-infected women in sero-discordant couples were the most likely to experience violence as a result of disclosure (Wight, 2006).

The most common barriers to disclosure is the fear of loss of sexual intimacy and fear of accusations on infidelity. Studies from both 'developed' and 'developing' countries found that disclosure rates to sexual partners tend to increase over time. Results from both settings also found discrepancies between intention to disclose and actual disclosure behaviour, with actual disclosure rates lower than intended disclosure rates (Klein, 1999).

Social Risks

Many MLHIV feel being the 'vector of disease' and thinks of being a terminal, degenerating and socially stigmatized entity. This can have massive impact upon their self-esteem and feelings of self worth. Disclosers may be avoided, ridiculed, or gossiped about afterwards and prevent them from receiving desperately needed support (Wight, 2006). In addition, people may withhold disclosing stressful events because they do not want to burden their loved ones and friends.

Public health messages have traditionally urged disclosure to all sexual and drug using partners. In reality, some PLHIV may choose not to disclose due to fears of rejection or harm, feelings of shame, desires to maintain secrecy, feelings that with safer sex there is no need for disclosure, fatalism, perceived community norms against disclosure, and beliefs that individuals are responsible for protecting themselves. HIV status disclosure to sexual partners has a number of potential risks for the individual including loss of economic support, blame, abandonment, physical and emotional abuse, discrimination, and disruption of family relationships. (Kalichman, 2001; Wight, 2006)

Sharing one's sero-positive status is a stressful process as PLHIV tend to be stigmatized and discriminated against compared to people with other chronic illnesses. HIV/AIDS disproportionately affects already marginalized individuals (such as gay men, drug users, immigrants from endemic countries, etc.), some of whom may be even further ostracized if they disclose their status (Serovich et al., 1998). In fact, fears of rejection and exclusion from social systems play substantial roles in determining categories of disclosure.

In the case of parents, studies have indicated that they worry about sharing their HIV positive status with their children because they fear that children will not keep it secret or will be treated unjustly afterward. Because of these fears (of rejection), mothers are found to have a 'relatively low' rate of disclosure of their HIV infection to their children compared to other family members. Another issue parents may have to grapple with is the fact that sexual intercourse is the common mode of HIV infection and since sex and sexuality are not topics that parents discuss with their children, parents may feel great discomfort disclosing their status to the children. They may fear that children may ask questions that would be difficult and shameful for them to answer. (Oshi et al., 2005; Armistead et al. 1999)

3.7. FACTORS INFLUENCING DISCLOSURE

In consideration of both the benefits and risks above, PLHIV have to be trained to optimise the benefits and capitalise on the risks associated with disclosure. This can best happen when the factors influencing disclosure are understood and appropriately controlled. The factors associated with disclosure have been classified into three broad classifications namely, individual, social and structural factors as described below.

Individual Factors

The period of time between sero-conversion and disclosure to family/ friends in which the HIV-positive individual is still in the metaphoric closet has great psychological and psychosomatic impact on the individual (Klitz, 1999).

Regarding familial disclosure, individuals are less likely to disclose to their immediate families if their t-cell counts are above 500. However, as these levels drop and individuals transition to an AIDS diagnosis, they are dramatically more likely to disclose during AIDS-related complex (ARC). This relationship between cell count and disclosure will only transpire if an individual perceives that disclosure will lead to social support. In fact, individuals who perceive that their family is likely to support them after disclosing, positively affect their lives are likely to go through the process of revealing their HIV status (Ullrich et al., 2003; Laryea & Gien, 1993; Paxton, 2002; O'Brien et al. 2003).

Negotiating Disclosure: Studies show that disclosure is not a one-time event, but is experienced as a process. In the space between full, open or public disclosure, and non disclosure, a temporal stage is occupied whereby a PLHIV manages their HIV disclosure. For some this 'Unburdening of HIV' and 'Freedom' entails disclosure to some family members. A period of struggle before disclosure is experienced by PLHIV and they take a period of time (up to a few years) to disclose to those closest to them.

During this time, individuals undergo the guilt of not having disclosed to their loved ones (Klitz, 1999).

Intimacy : Taylor (1973) provides insight into the way self-disclosure is linked with developing intimacy or liking, in order to reach a sense of mutual trustworthiness.

Self image: Any disclosure of oneself engages the vulnerabilities of body, mind and soul. Hence Self image, self perception and self confidence issues will be brought forward and dependent upon comfort and skill, will be managed within the discloser's frames of reference for life meaning (Borchers, 1999).

Timing : A challenging issue for many people is the timing of disclosure. If it's not done relatively early, it can become more difficult and cause significant disruption to an ongoing relationship if the partner feels betrayed due to the lack of an early disclosure. PLHIV who have thought through a disclosure plan and have a consistent strategy for managing disclosure are less likely to engage in risky sexual behaviours. The ability to disclose can be related to the degree to which an individual has accepted his or her HIV diagnosis. (Fisher & Adams 2003; Jourard, 1975)

Social Factors

The most significant benefit to disclosure still remains to be satisfaction with familial relationships and friendships. Positive individuals either tell quite quickly after a diagnosis or at the very end of the disease. Results suggest an incredibly high level of satisfaction, relief, and familial closeness after the event (Kalichman et al., 2003).

Reciprocity: Sprecher (2004) examined "disclosure given" and "disclosure received," exploring the way in which reciprocity in such behaviour correlated with the amounts of love and liking. The results marked that although men prefer not to self-disclose, they experienced more satisfaction, liking, and loving when they received self-disclosure from another. Females however, experienced no difference in feelings when either giving or receiving self-disclosure. Partners may be responding favourably to the "other's disclosure" because in their minds what they are receiving is not disclosure but reciprocity to their disclosures. Thus reciprocity also influences the process of disclosure.

Reduction in Stigma: There is evidence to suggest that disclosure can help reduce the stigma associated with HIV/AIDS, both for the HIV-positive person and for others. The public disclosure of his HIV-positive status by basketball star Magic Johnson in 1991 resulted in dramatic increases in demand for HIV testing and counselling and in public awareness and sensitivity to HIV/AIDS that were sustained after one year of follow-up (Kalichman, 1993). It is likely that the cumulative effect of increased disclosure of HIV-positive status across society will further reduce the stigma associated with HIV/AIDS.

Structural Factors

Mason et al. (1995) suggest that cultural identity can be a sufficient obstacle hindering sero-status disclosure. In cultures that are likely to marginalize homosexuality, disclosure of one's sexuality, let alone one's serostatus, is unlikely

(Carrier, 1989); and cultures that emphasize gender typicality, gender adherence, and traditional values are less likely to tolerate an HIV-positive member (Ichikawa & Natpratan, 2006).

Age is another correlate of nondisclosure or disclosure of HIV status. Research suggests a positive correlation between older age and disclosure (Serovich, 2005). As a function of age, emotional, physical, and financial independence from the family (and to a lesser extent, friends) may be a substantial factor in discussing one's status. Also, sheer maturity and the ability to cope with an outcome of support or alienation may be another reason driving the age-disclosure correlation (Petrak, et al, 200).

Jourard (1975) marked that women disclose more than men, first born's are less apt to self-disclose than later-borns, people involved in a specific religion disclose more or less depending on the religion, and white individuals self-disclose more than black individuals.

Costs and benefits: Implicit in the correlates of status disclosure are the costs and benefits of such communication. Secrecy and concealment are negatively correlated with healthy physiology, most notably immunological responses (Glaser, 1988). Even if disclosure is painful, difficult, or temporarily stressful, Pennebaker et al. (1988) claim that there is greater health benefits in revealing rather than nondisclosure. The paradox surrounding disclosure is that although it may attenuate psychological and/or physiological HIV/AIDS malignancies, it ultimately welcomes stigma, possible alienation from friends, and familial recalibration and will ultimately create a polarized familial atmosphere (Serovich et al., 2005). Though some benefits are enjoyed and costs relieved, pre-disclosure benefits are lost (e.g., being considered an ordinary, healthy, HIV-negative person) and the HIV-positive individual must endure a new series of costs (e.g. stigma) (Paxton, 2002).

Power position: Those who self-disclose significant amounts of information appear to be open, free, and trusting of others. However, according to Insel, "The over-disclosers appear to trust everyone because he or she has not learned to discriminate the qualities of different relationships". Further, if someone does self-disclose 'all' during the first interaction, this person typically sends the message that she/he is "needy, wants an intimate relationship, or would like someone to take control". According to Insel, "The under-discloser reveals too little for s/he needs to remain in control" (Elkhal, 2010).

Gender: In a 1998 study of homosexual and bisexual men, researchers found that initially after an HIV diagnosis, most of the men were reluctant and fearful of disclosing their HIV-positive status to others. They used this period as an opportunity to come to terms with their diagnosis before having to contend with the reactions of others. After this PLHIV, there was evidence that disclosure was increasingly used as a mechanism for coping with the disease (Jourard, 1993).

Environment/Context: In many cases, disclosure to potential sexual partners may be more difficult than to trusted friends or family, due to fears of rejection. Some reports have suggested that disclosure to potential anonymous sexual partners may be more difficult due to the environments in which anonymous sex takes place, which often are not conducive to conversation. In these environments, people may tend to rely on non-verbal disclosure signals, which may not be accurate (e.g. the assumption by an HIV-positive gay that if another man wishes to engage in anonymous unprotected intercourse he is also HIV-positive, or the assumption by an HIV-negative man that if another man wishes to engage in anonymous unprotected intercourse he is also HIV-negative).

Past research findings on HIV status disclosure to sexual partners from both developing and developed country settings (Ichikawa et al, 2006; Petrak, et al, 2001), highlight the following factors which influence disclosure:

- Sense of ethical responsibility, to facilitate HIV-preventive behaviour.
- Concern for partner's health, failing health
- Severity of one's illness, need for social support to cope with HIV
- To alleviate the stress associated with non-disclosure
- Anticipation of positive outcomes including increased social support, acceptance, kindness, decreased anxiety and depression, and strengthening of relationships.

In the above researches, the following hypothesis were established

- Disclosure increases with increased relational intimacy.
- Disclosure increases with the need to reduce uncertainty in a relationship.
- Disclosure tends to be reciprocal, incremental and symmetrical.
- Liking is related to positive disclosure, but not to negative ones.
- Positive disclosure does not necessarily increase with the intimacy of the relationship; but negative disclosure is directly related to the intimacy of the relationship.

3.8. DISCLOURE AS A PROCESS - STEPS INVOVLVED

The process of disclosure involving whom and how to disclose, preparedness of receiver to absorb the disclosed fact, benefits of disclosure to self and others can be a very complex and personal decision. There is no one best way to tell someone, just as there is no sure way to gauge their reaction to the news. Firstly, it is important to consider the place for disclosure that is a non threatening environment. Secondly one has to consider the time for disclosure that is comfortable. Although there is generally no 'right time', one should tell when they feel ready or when they are legally required to do so, ie., when being involved in an activity where HIV could be transmitted.

Many women who have kept a secret for a long time feel a sense of relief after telling. Many women find a sense of purpose and increased self-esteem by choosing to disclose their status to close friends and family. For many, telling those closest to them provides them with both emotional and practical support. Some people decide to become more public and use their stories to advocate for others with government or media. Others may disclose for educational purposes to neighbours, community and religious groups, schools, other HIV+ people, or healthcare providers.

People may react differently to the news of HIV status disclosure. Some may immediately embrace and accept the diagnosis, while others may react negatively or need some time to process the information, to overcome fears or preconceived notions they have about HIV. Disclosure is such a multifaceted issue wherein disclosing to an employer is very different from disclosing to a parent, disclosing to a child is unlike disclosing to a friend, disclosing to a potential sexual partner is nothing like any of the above. It is therefore important to try finding someone who can be of support during this difficult time. Thus an alternative support system needs to be built, which furthers their understanding on the issue towards catering to the needs and human rights of PLHIV. This support system may include IEC materials on HIV, contact details of support organisations. The health care worker, social worker, counsellor or peer educators are significant entities, whose assistance and support can be solicited for disclosure.

Disclosure to Friends : Some studies show that friends are the most likely recipients of HIV disclosure, as high as 85-90 percent, while others suggest that disclosure levels to friends are much lower, between 2 to 40 percent depending on the previously mentioned correlates, e.g., age, CD4 levels, etc. (O'Brien et al., 2003; Kalichman et al., 2003).

Disclosure to Family members: Disclosure of HIV status does not seem to occur to multiple family members at the same time. Research suggests that it happens individually, family member by family member (Carl, 1986). Female members, mothers and sisters respectively, are the most likely to know about a sero-positive family member followed by male members, brothers and fathers respectively. Statistics show that on average, between 45 to 55 percent of mothers and sisters, and only about 30 to 40 percent of fathers and brothers are privy to the positive serostatus (Kalichman et al, 2003).

Once an initial member is told, his or her opinion is used as an indicator of whom else to tell. By telling one person, e.g. a brother or mother, he or she becomes the liaison between the positive person and the rest of the family. Often an HIV-positive disclosure is linked to the revelation that the person is not heterosexual, and this can be what refers to as the "double death" with simultaneous HIV and sexual orientation disclosure (Bowes & Dickinson, 1991; Katz; Ullrich et al., 2003). However, generally over time, the likelihood that an individual will disclose to most members of his or her family increases. The research confirms that mothers and sisters are the most likely to know initially and continually over time, followed by brothers, and then fathers. (Serovich & Greene, 1993)

3.9. POST-DISCLOSURE REACTIONS

Reactions vary from person to person and no matter the initial response, support will ultimately come from the family to the positive individual (Kalichman et al., 2003); and the individual will report higher levels of satisfaction than those who do not disclose (Paxton, 2002; Petrak et al., 2001; Serovich et al., 2000). Friends are perceived to provide significantly more support than any individual family members, even mothers (Kalichman et al., 2003). But support is an ambiguous concept—and so, some other studies have framed this post-disclosure period in terms of involvement.

Psychosocial involvement.

Often friends, families, or family members step in during ARC/ disease escalation and become involved either in heightened socio-emotional, or in physical, caretaking roles. Cleveland et al (1985) suggest that over 70 percent of AIDS patients live alone, and over 60 percent have little or no contact with their families. These statistics may have changed since the 1980's and although isolation may have attenuated; it still is an overwhelming theme for many individuals living with AIDS. As AIDS becomes a reality, concerns about stigma change. Death and dying, dependency, undesirable changes in appearance or disfigurement, and changes in personal relationships are the new, pervasive concerns. These initially perceived stigmas turn into fears, where a person living with end-stage AIDS fears isolation and abandonment, pain and suffering, and dependency and loss of control (Ryan, 1984).

Parents, and friends to a varying degree, respond to end-stage AIDS usually with great involvement and great sadness, praying for treatment and a cure (Bunting, 2001; Shehan et al., 2005). Others diminish the above stigma by treating AIDS as if the PLHIV had some other terminal disease like cancer, helping physically or monetarily. Friends follow similar behaviours and roles depending on the friendship (Crandall, 1992).

3.10. HIV Disclosure to Casual and Main Partners

In the previous section disclosure focused on friends and family, while this section will explore the correlates of HIV disclosure to casual and main sexual partners, and the most prevalent ways it is accomplished. It is ultimately the significance of romance with an HIV- positive partner and inviting the risk of transmission into relations that substantially differentiate disclosing to friends and family, from casual and main partners.

Recent studies suggest that of the MLHIV, less than half have disclosed their HIV status to the sexual partners before engaging in unprotected intercourse. Though it would seem a sense of conscience or in-group protection might encourage a higher percentage to disclosure, in actuality, disclosure rates are slightly lower than chance. (Ciccarone et al., 2003; Marks & Crepaz, 2001)

Disclosure to Casual Partners

A more detailed examination on disclosure suggests that casual partners are the least likely to be given warning of HIV serostatus (O'Brien et al., 2003). The reasons for this include one-night stands, anonymous encounters, etc. As such, a sense of de-individuation tends to occur (rendering disclosure unnecessary), which is only augmented when combined with drug and/or alcohol use, and/or an environment such as a bathhouse or backroom (Elwood et al, 2003; Gorbach et al., 2004).

Gorbach (2004) suggest that if a positive individual believes that sero-positive status is a private matter or if he is in denial, disclosure is unlikely to casual partners.

A better health status, i.e., low viral load, adherence to highly active anti-retroviral therapy (HAART), will diminish disclosure rates. In terms of psychosocial factors on disclosure to casual partners, outcome expectancies of hedonism, sero-status assumptions and depression all negatively correlate to disclosure (Parsons et al., 2005). The strongest indicators of disclosure to casual partners are efficacies, namely self and outcome (Stirratt, 2006). The ability to communicate about a stigmatizing topic varies from person to person, and culture to culture (Ciccarone et al., 2003).

MLHIV reported strong negative reactions when they disclosed their status to HIV-negative or HIV-unknown casual partners (Gorbach et al., 2006; Kalichman & Nachimson, 1999; Parsons et al., 2005). When the ultimate interaction goal with a casual partner is to have sex or engage in sexual behaviours, negative reactions, e.g., using two condoms or being rejected, are unwanted (Bailey & Hart, 2006). Self-efficacy may indeed be high, but previous negative experiences with other casual partners may decrease a sense of outcome-efficacy for many positive men.

Disclosure to Main partners

Where casual partners were the least of all categories to experience an HIV disclosure event, main partners were the most likely (O'Brien et al., 2003). It would seem that even though many of the previously mentioned fears about rejection, alienation, and stigma are still very much present, there are superseding issues that provide an impetus for disclosure. The first of these issues is sense of urgency. O'Brien et al. (2003) suggest that as age increases and as CD_4 levels decrease, the tendency to disclose to main partners increases. With a diagnosis transition on the horizon, from asymptomatic HIV to ARC, or from ARC to AIDS, it becomes important to acknowledge infection and prepare the main partner for the implications of deteriorating health. Also, individuals claim that after time, it becomes physically impossible to hide infection because of doctor visits, medications, and symptoms of opportunistic illness from main partners (Stirratt, 2006).

If HIV is contracted through heterosexual encounters or through IV drug use, disclosure to a main partner is unlikely; similar trends exist for individuals who are not sexually active with their main partners (O'Brien et al, 2003)

The psychological factors namely moral obligations and feelings for the main partner seem to also have incredible sway over the tendency to disclose to a main partner. A certain sense of morality exists within some MLHIV, where it is considered unjust or unfair not to disclose to a main partner. Along the same lines, others claim a sense of responsibility to the greater community to protect HIV-negative individuals and prevent the further dissemination of the disease (Parsons et al., 2005; Stirratt, 2006).

Main partners experience significantly more intimacy, emotional bonding, trust, and accountability than casual partners making disclosure a palpable corollary (Halkitis & Wilton, 2006). Individuals report that positive feelings towards, and caring about a partner increases the tendency to admit a HIV-positive status (Gorbach et al., 2004). Some men even include it as a relational turning point that has the potential to cement the relationship or dissolve it. Most positive men believe that the relationship will not survive unless HIV status is revealed in a timely manner (Sadovsky, 1991).

Legal aspects in disclosure

In many states, the law requires HIV status disclosure before knowingly exposing or transmitting HIV to someone else. In the state of Georgia, the law states that an individual who knows s/he is HIV infected with and knowingly engages in intercourse without disclosing their status is guilty of a felony. Penalties vary from state to state. Disclosure to doctors and other healthcare providers will help ensure appropriate care and prescribe symptomatic treatment whenever necessary. However, the employer need not know of the employees HIV status for as long the PLHIV is performing his job, the employer cannot legally discriminate against him (Margolese, 2002)

Conclusion

As Holt et al. (1998) claim in their research, disclosure is antithetically dichotomous; it serves as both stressor and coping mechanism. Ultimately, it is the negotiation of these negative and positive costs and benefits that will predict both the health of important friendships, and one's psychological and interpersonal familial health.

Disclosure can be an extremely stressful process, because it makes one vulnerable to perceived stigma of the both the sexual partners as well as the society. However the strategies individuals use to negotiate and counter the fear of rejection and isolation has been relatively under-reported. The way each person experiences and copes with the illness is reflected in the choice and process of disclosure. This decision is embedded within individual perceptions and the local context of HIV/AIDS.

Disclosure as seen in this chapter is a vast arena and this study shall only focus on disclosure in the context of sexual relationships. In this study the aim of the researcher is to understand the disclosure patterns of MLHIV amongst both their main and causal partners. The factors which influenced discloser as well as the perceived barriers for non disclosure, as collated in this chapter will be ascertained with the study sample to understand the commonalities and differences. The reactions of sexual partners to the MLHIV and how they coped with it will be studied too. Describing and analyzing the internal dialogue of the disclosure event is an essential step in designing effective interventions that will facilitate disclosure. The role of disclosure in behaviour change of MLHIV will be the guiding light for this study. The next chapter in continuation categorically emphasises the understanding and the implementation of behaviour change among MLHIV.

Chapter 4

BEHAVIOUR CHANGE

INTRODUCTION

The HIV infection is invariably understood as the result of human behaviours, and a 'change in behaviour' has long been acknowledged as essential to curbing the spread of infection. In all cases where national epidemics have been reversed, behaviour change based interventions were central to success. There is an urgent need to break the silence about sex since it is observed that 'talking openly' is the first step to reducing denial and bringing about behaviour change. The progress in the public health discourse on sexuality is also not matched by progress in action. This substantial gap is partly because it is easier now to explain the why and what with regard to sexuality, and HIV/AIDS, but it is little known about how to address these issues in a way that has an impact on the epidemic. Sexuality as seen through the public health prism is still a potential determinant of ill health. As a result, safer sex is the mainstream theme within this discourse, while sexual health, pleasure, and rights become peripheral in the context of behaviour change. This chapter helps understand sexual behaviour change in the context of the spread of HIV infection. The various theories of behaviour change in individuals, the factors influencing behaviour change are explained and it ends with the process of behaviour change.

4.1. Behaviour Change in HIV Prevention

Increase in casual and illicit sexual behaviour among men is argued to be the cornerstone in the sexual transmission of HIV in India. Hence, bringing about a change in sexual behaviour is deemed an essential tool in the prevention of the epidemic. Behavioural HIV prevention programs in our country has an objective of promoting accurate individual knowledge, perception of HIV risk and increase the individual's motivation to avoid risky behaviour (NACO, 2006).

HIV Prevention programs with PLHIV or high risk groups build the individual's skill to use prevention commodities properly and to avoid or effectively negotiate risky situations. Within households, HIV prevention programs aim to decrease the stigma associated with both HIV and sexuality, to promote open discussion about sexuality and drug use, and to influence gender roles and norms. At a community level, effective prevention programs seek to increase the value associated with safer behaviours, to support community members to reduce their risk, to build social solidarity and reciprocity, and to reinforce new norms.

Behavioural HIV prevention programs may also seek to achieve results at a broader social or structural level. Such approaches might include direct interventions that introduce prevention tools into particular environments (for example, mandating condom use in brothels), influence the physical environment (improving street lighting to reduce the likelihood of rape), expand clinical services (ensuring access to drug substitution therapy for chemical dependence), or create more supportive legal and policy norms (legalizing same-sex relations). Social or structural interventions might also be indirect, by supporting broader efforts to improve the overall protection and promotion of human rights, to reduce income inequality, and to address gender inequities.

Individuals and groups might change behaviours in any number of ways—including some that may be detrimental to the cause of HIV prevention. When this report refers to behaviour change, it intends to encompass only the range of behaviour changes that reduce the risk of HIV transmission or otherwise promote the development of social, physical, and legal environments that are conducive to risk reduction.

HIV risk reduction interventions now extend beyond basic information giving and sensitising people on risk behaviours, to also include communication with regards to sex among partners, increasing individual's skills in condom use, the perception of lower risk practices as an accepted social norm, and to help people receive support and reinforcement for their efforts at changing (Kelly, 1995).

An important point stressed by this broad overview of approaches to behavioural change communication (BCC) is the need to see different levels HIV prevention initiatives as complementary. Individual BCC approaches have shown an impact, but to stem transmission on a larger scale for longer term maintenance of changed behaviour, community and structural level programmes are also required. In an epidemic where changes are occurring rapidly at the level of the virus, treatment context and within populations at risk, multi-dimensional interventions based on theories and models which address individual as well as contextual and socio-cultural variables are required.

4.2. THEORIES IN BEHAVIOUR CHANGE

The most frequently used theories and models of behavioural change begins with theories that focus on the individual's psychological process, such as attitudes and beliefs, then goes into theories emphasizing social relationships, and ends with structural factors in explaining human behaviour. This separation is artificial as there is inevitable overlap in categories, moving from the strictly 'individual centred' to the macro-level of structural and environmentally focused. These theories help understand the factors influencing behaviour change in PLHIV, the process of change and its sustenance.

The following are few theories based on which behaviour change strategies are best derived from:

A. Theories that Focus on Individuals

B. Social Theories and Models

C. Structural and environmental theories

4.2.1 Theories that Focus on Individuals

As HIV transmission is propelled by individual behaviour, theories on 'how individuals change their behaviour' have provided the foundation for most HIV prevention efforts worldwide. Psychosocial models of behavioural risk can be categorized into 3 major groups: those predicting risk behaviour, those predicting behavioural change and those predicting maintenance of safe behaviour.

Models of individual behavioural change generally focus on stages that individuals pass through while trying to change behaviour.

A1. Health belief model

This model holds the belief that health behaviour is a function of individual's socio-demographic characteristics, knowledge and attitudes. Individual health behaviour is governed by (1) perception of personal susceptibility to disease, (2) severity of disease, (3) perceived efficacy of behaviour in dealing with disease, and (4) perceived barriers to adopting behaviours. According to this model, a person must hold the following beliefs in order to be able to change behaviour:

1. Perceived susceptibility to a particular health problem ("am I at risk for HIV?")
2. Perceived severity of the condition ("how serious is AIDS; how hard would my life be if I am infected?")
3. Belief in effectiveness of the new behaviour ("condoms are effective against HIV")
4. Cues to action ("witnessing the death / illness of a close relative due to AIDS")
5. Perceived benefits of preventive action ("if I start using condoms, I can avoid HIV")
6. Barriers to taking action ("I don't like using condoms").

In this model, promoting action to change behaviour includes changing individual personal beliefs. Individuals weigh the benefits against the perceived costs and barriers to change. For change to occur, 'benefits' must outweigh 'costs'. The 'benefits' seen by PLHIV in changing their behaviour include, perception of risk, beliefs in severity of AIDS ("there is no cure"), beliefs in effectiveness of condom use or benefits in reducing multiple sexual relations (Becker 1974, Harrison et al 1992, Strecher et al 1997).

A2. Social Learning Theory (SLT)

The premise of SLT states that new behaviours are learned either by modelling the behaviour of others or by a direct experience. It focuses on the important roles played by vicarious, symbolic, and self-regulatory processes in psychological functioning and looks at human behaviour as a continuous interaction between cognitive, behavioural and environmental determinants (Bandura, 1977). Central tenets of the social cognitive theory include: "Self-efficacy", the belief in the ability to implement the necessary behaviour ("I know I can insist on condom use with my partner") and "Outcome expectancies" - beliefs about outcomes such as "the belief that using condoms correctly will prevent HIV infection". Specifically, activities focus on the experience people have in talking to their partners about sex and condom use, the positive and negative beliefs about adopting condom use, and the types of environmental barriers to risk reduction.

a) ***Social Cognitive Theory***, a term often used interchangeably with SLT, emphasizes the learner having knowledge, motivation, outcome expectancy and self-efficacy. Self-perception of ability to adopt health behaviours is based on thoughts and beliefs rooted in observational learning experiences. Eg: The curricula '*Be Proud! Be Responsible!*' and '*Focus on Kids*' (O'Leary, 2001)

b) ***Cognitive Behavioural Theory*** emphasizes the learner personalizing knowledge, gaining skills, and having self-efficacy. Individuals are motivated to behave in a way that maintains the consistency of their thoughts and beliefs, and will make behaviour changes to reduce tension caused by conflict among beliefs. Cognitive behavioural theory is one of the foundation theories of '*Reducing the Risk Practices*' (Saffren, 1999).

c) ***Social Inoculation Theory*** emphasizes behavioural rehearsal, where learners become "immunized" by resisting peer pressure to engage in risky behaviour. The curriculum *Postponing Sexual Involvement* by Marion Howard and Marie Mitchell is based on social inoculation theory (Devillly, 2005).

d) ***Social Influence Theory*** emphasizes changing social norms as a way to change the individual. Here public bases its health behaviour decisions on information received from "opinion leaders," who are seen as both having expertise in a topic and being an accessible, trustworthy source. Eg: Modules on *Safer Choices* and *Reducing the Risk.* (Latkin, 1999; O'Leary, 2001)

A3. Theory of Reasoned Action

This theory is based on the assumptions that human beings are usually quite rational and make systematic use of the information available to them. Individual attitudes and motivation determine the likelihood that the individual will engage in a specific health behaviour. People consider the implications of their actions in a given context at a given time before they decide to engage in a given behaviour (Ajzen, 1980). The theory of reasoned action is conceptually similar to the health belief model but adds the construct of behavioural intention as a determinant of health behaviour. Both theories focus on perceived susceptibility, perceived benefits and constraints to changing behaviour. The theory of reasoned action specifically focuses on the role of personal intention in determining whether a 'behaviour' will occur. A person's intention is a function of 2 basic determinants:

- Attitude (toward the behaviour), and
- 'Subjective norms', i.e. social influence.

'Normative' beliefs play a central role in the theory, and generally focus on what an individual believes other people, especially influential people, would expect him/her to do. Eg. If a male has to start using condoms, his attitude might be "having sex with condoms is just as good as having sex without condoms" and the normative belief could be "most of my peers are using condoms; they would expect me to do so as well". Interventions using this theory to guide activities focus on attitudes about risk-reduction, response to social norms, and intentions to change risky behaviours. The significance of 'safe sexual practices by male PLHIV' is a normative belief. It will be interesting to ascertain if this 'behaviour' is influenced by 'attitude' of the MLHIV (Martin et al, 2007).

A4. Stages of change model

This model posits 6 stages that individuals or groups pass through when changing behaviour: pre-contemplation, contemplation, preparation, action, maintenance and relapse. With respect to condom use, the stages could be described as:

(1) Pre-contemplation	: Has not considered using condoms
(2) Contemplation	: Recognizes the need to use condoms
(3) Preparation	: Thinking about using condoms in the next months
(4) Action	: Using condoms consistently for less than 6 months
(5) Maintenance	: Using condoms consistently for 6 months or more
(6) Relapse	: slipping-up with respect to condom use

In order for an intervention to be successful it must target the appropriate stage of the individual or group for eg. raising awareness about condoms at stages 1 and 2. Groups and individuals may pass through all stages, but do not necessarily move in a linear fashion. As with the previous theories, the stages of change model emphasizes the importance of cognitive processes and uses. (Porche,2004; Prochaska, 1992)

A5. AIDS Risk Reduction model

The model identifies 3 stages involved in reducing risk for HIV transmission, including:

1. Acknowledging high risk behaviours
2. **Commitment to change:** Committing to reduce high risk behaviours and increase protective behaviours. This stage is shaped by four factors: perceptions of enjoyment, self-efficacy, social norms and aversive emotions.

3. **Taking action to make the change:** includes aversive emotions, sexual communication, help-seeking behaviour and social factors affect people's decision-making process (Znoj, 2010)

Programmes that use this model focus on: Clients' risk assessment, Influencing the decision to reduce risk through perceptions of enjoyment or self-efficacy and Clients' support to enact the change (access to condoms, social support) (Catania,1990).

These psychosocial theories and constructs were very useful early in the epidemic to identify individual behaviours associated with higher rates of HIV transmission. Overemphasis on individual behavioural change with a focus on the cognitive level has undermined the overall research capacity to understand the complexity of HIV transmission and control. Focus only on the individual psychological process ignores the interactive relationship of behaviour in its social, cultural, and economic dimension thereby missing the possibility to fully understand crucial determinants of behaviour. Aggleton (1996) points out that, in many cases, motivations for sex are complicated, unclear and may not be thought through in advance (Porche,2004). Societal norms, religious criteria, and gender-power relations infuse meaning into behaviour, enabling positive or negative changes as evident from the theories and models listed below.

4.2.2 Social Theories and Models

A main difference between individual and social models is that the latter aim at changes at the community level. According to this perspective, effective prevention efforts, especially in vulnerable communities that do not have the larger societal support, will depend on the development of strategies that can enlist community mobilization to modify the norms of this peer network to support positive changes in behaviour (Kelly, 1995). A greater interest in the context surrounding individual behaviour led to increased numbers of interventions guided by the following theories and models.

B.1 Theory of Gender and Power

This theory addresses the wider social issues surrounding women, such as distribution of power and authority, influences and gender-specific norms within heterosexual relationships (Connell, 1987). Women are often unable to practice safer sex when men hold the economic and physical power in the relationship, or when they have been socialized to be sexually passive. The woman's commitment to a relationship and lack of power can influence her risk reduction choices (DiClemente, 1995). The determinants of sexual behaviour can be seen as a function not only of individual and social but of structural and environmental factors as well (Caraël, 1997, Sweat, 1995).

B.2 Social Marketing Theory

Health information is targeted towards consumers, who may adopt new health behaviours if they believe that there is a valuable exchange in which they satisfy their wants and needs with little sacrifice. *Eg: Condom Social Marketing* (Kline,1994).

B.3 Social Identity Theory

Individuals identify themselves based on their membership of social groups. Group memberships can boost an individual's self esteem when one's social group is perceived favourable when compared to another group. *Eg: Positive Peoples Network*

4.2.3. Structural and Environmental Theories

C.1 Empowerment model (Morrell, 2001)

Empowerment increases problem solving in a participatory fashion, and should enable individuals to understand the personal, social, economic and political forces in their lives in order to take action to improve their situations (Israel, 1994). The feelings of powerlessness, which can come from lack of skills and confidence, have to be cast off. Personal empowerment deals with the psychological processes of building up self efficacy and self esteem. Organizational empowerment encompasses both the processes that enable individuals to increase their control within the organization and the organization to influence policies and decisions in the community. An empowered community uses the skills and resources of individuals and organizations to meet respective needs.

C.2 Social Ecological model for health promotion (McLeroy, 1988)

According to this model, patterned behaviour is the outcome of interest and behaviour is viewed as being determined by the following:

1. Intrapersonal factors – characteristics of the individual such as knowledge, attitudes, behaviour, self-concept, skills
2. Interpersonal processes and primary groups formal and informal social network and social support systems, including the family, work group and friendships
3. Institutional factors – social institutions with organizational characteristics and formal and informal rules and regulations for operation
4. Community factors – relationships among organizations, institutions and informal networks within defined boundaries
5. Public policy – local, state and national laws and policies.

C3. Perception of risk construct (Stevens, 1998)

Increasing perception of risk has been shown numerous times to increase HIV protective behaviour. Yet most behavioural models measure risk as individually determined which might not be relevant in many contexts. Many women often perceive themselves at risk not because of their own behaviour, but because of the past or current behaviour of their sexual partner. In addition, perception of risk as a predictor of future behavioural change has further complexities in circumstances where individuals report high perception of risk and high self-reported behavioural change. This situation may demonstrate limited realistic and behavioural change options, or feelings of fatalism.

The above theories certainly reflect the conditions under which human beings may be motivated to change their behaviour. However, in the world of HIV/AIDS the HCP are trained on the ABC model of bringing about behaviour change amongst PLHIV

4.2.4. ABC - Model of Behaviour change

The ABC Model of Behaviour change presented here is adapted from World Health Organisation and is considered as a tool by National AIDS Control Organisation (NACO) and its daughter implementing agencies, in bringing about HIV prevention and behaviour change. This model is well known as the ABC-Model (A- Abstinence, B- Being Faithful, C-Consistent Condom Use) (NACO, 2006). Its theoretical framework is as follows:

1. The Risk Elimination Model: Abstinence is best

This model uses abstinence as a means of eliminating any possible risk of transmission of HIV infection, with the individual no longer engaging in sex. The risk of infection is eliminated because the risk behaviour is eliminated. An example of an educational message for prevention directed at young people would be: 'Just say No'. While this model guarantees full safety from infection, it is very often the least useful of the behaviour change models. Most people find it extremely difficult to suddenly quit certain behaviour, which may be both enjoyable and long-standing. This model does not acknowledge that individuals find pleasure in engaging in certain behaviours. Neither does it allow room for alternatives and turns a blind eye to human behaviour.

2. The Risk Reduction Model: Being Faithful, Use a condom

This model acknowledges that individuals do engage in sex and use substances such as intravenous drugs. Assuming that abstinence is not a viable alternative, the risk reduction model advises individuals to engage in 'safe' sexual acts by using condoms whenever they have sex. However, this model cannot provide total guarantee that individuals will remain uninfected. For example, condom breaks/ slips during intercourse. Since WHO realised that both the above model lacks the humanistic and individualistic approach necessary for behaviour change, they have derived the third model as explained below.

3. The Harm Reduction Model

Promoted by WHO for IDU, harm reduction model challenges the *'all or nothing'* approach to behaviour change characterized by the previous models. This model acknowledges that risk is a part of everyone's life and ranks an individual's risk/s for HIV infection among other life issues such as illness, unemployment and drug use. It also acknowledges the difficulties in effecting behaviour changes, particularly in cases of substance abuse. Harm reduction is designed to acknowledge the meaning attached to risk behaviours. In this model, change takes place over time and is incremental. Any positive change is good and one step closer to safe behaviours.

The counsellor herein has to assist the client to:

- Identify risk behaviours they indulge in
- Understand the reasons for their continuing engagement in them
- Develop strategies for identifying strategies to move toward healthier behaviours
- Facilitate the development of self-efficacy

This model however acknowledges the possibility of relapse after abstinence or other unsuccessful attempts to modify behaviour. Therefore some counsellors may undergo an ethical dilemma because this model does not provide the client with protection from immediate infection, as other models do.

These models are cautioned not to be used as absolutes but as helpful tools in their interaction with clients. Therefore, WHO leaves the decision to the discretion of the counsellor to follow suitable models in the context of the client's lifestyle and differing needs. These 3 models are commonly used by the counsellors/health care workers in addressing problems related to human behaviour. Just as there are variations in sexual behaviour, there are variations in the practice models too. These models respond to various categories of people. Unfortunately the counsellors do not explore the ambiguous areas of the youth's sexuality before selectively imparting appropriate models.

4.3. FACTORS INFLUENCING BEHAVIOUR CHANGE

From the above theories, it is seen that, researchers focused on identifying key variables that would enable the prediction and understanding of individual's behaviour. Researchers claim that these eight variables are: intention; environmental constraints; skills; anticipated outcomes (or attitude); norms; self-standards; emotion; and self-efficacy. The first three variables namely intention, environmental constraints and skills are necessary and sufficient factors for producing behaviour change. Eg. If an Injecting Drug user is committed to using bleach every time he shares injection equipment, has bleach available, and has the necessary skills to use the bleach, the probability is greater that he will use the bleach. The remaining five variables namely, anticipated outcomes, norms, self-standards, emotion and self-efficacy are described as factors influencing the strength and direction of intention. (Catania,1990; Tawil, 1995)

The factors influencing behaviour change are as follows

A. Individual Focused Factors

Perceived Susceptibility: False assumptions about who gets HIV, or false beliefs on how HIV is transmitted. A male may believe he is not at risk because he doesn't have sex with men, even though he engages in risk with multiple female partners. *"I'm not at risk for HIV; only gay men get that disease"* (Tawil, 1995)

Illusion of non-vulnerability: A personal belief that one is immune to risk exists in some. People tend to underestimate their own risk in comparison to others engaging in the same behaviours they are. *"I just don't think it will happen to me because my partner is not a sex worker"* (Tawil, 1995)

Fatalism: A belief that circumstances are beyond one's control. Nothing a person does will change what is destined to happen anyway. *"HIV is gonna get me eventually, might as well enjoy myself while I'm here"* (Tawil, 1995).

Perceived severity: Some people perceive HIV to be less of a threat now that treatment is available. While some may place high value on behaviours associated with HIV (e.g., sex vs. intimacy); because of this, the threat of infection is seen as a less severe outcome. *"Although my husband is infected, we can't cease our sexual relations"* (Tawil, 1995).

Self-Efficacy: The degree of confidence a person has about their ability to perform behaviour. Ideas about self influence one's confidence, but self-efficacy may increase through practice, or by watching others similar to you, perform it. *"I was upfront before, so with a new guy, condoms will be easier to bring up."* (Catania, 1990).

Self-Esteem: Self-esteem is a sense of being a loveable, likeable, and valuable person. People may have different areas of high vs. low esteem, e.g., they may have high esteem about their appearance, but low esteem about other abilities. *"I know she's cheating, but I am so happy she has chosen a loser like me."* (Catania, 1990).

Intentions: Intention is a plan to perform a specific behaviour. When intentions are strong, there is commitment to carry out behaviour. Behaviours tend to follow intentions more closely when it doesn't involve the cooperation of others. *"I've really thought about it. Next time we're gonna use condoms"*. (Catania, 1990).

Expected Outcomes: People perceive the effect that behaviour change will have on their relationships and other's opinions. Some perceived outcomes may be desirable, some not. This balance may tip the scales for or against behaviour change. *"If a rich and hot client wants me, mentioning condoms is the last thing on my mind."* (Catania, 1990).

Ambivalence: Sometimes a person may have plenty of information about a health risk and may see the need for change, but because the change is felt to be difficult, or to involve tough trade-offs, an attitude of ambivalence is adopted. *"I know I need to use condoms, but I love the feeling of bareback so much more"* (Catania, 1990).

Positive and Negative moods: Behaviours are more than the result of purely rational thought. Mood may have a direct, or indirect effect on risk behaviours. A person might be sad or depressed, deal with it by drinking, which can lead to engaging in unsafe sex. *"I feel so lonely sometimes, I just want to go out and get laid."* (Catania, 1990).

Shame and guilt: Two emotions that appear to be especially relevant in the case of sexual behaviours are shame and guilt. Because of cultural or religious stigma about homosexuality, or about sexuality in general, sex can bring up difficult emotions for a person. One way people may cope with feelings of shame or guilt is to participate in sets of high-risk behaviours. (O'Leary, 2001).

Sexual arousal: Arousal, and the desire to continue being aroused, can motivate risk-taking behaviours, even when an awareness of risk exists at other times. Being aroused can also make correct use of condoms or other protection more difficult. Sexual arousal is a powerful motivation. (O'Leary, 2001).

B. Social Factors influencing behaviour change

Communication and negotiation: Comfort levels and communication skills related to talking with a partner about sexual practices or drug use will affect both the likelihood of such conversations taking place and their outcome. While communication enhancement can be an intervention goal, it's important to recognize cultural groups have varying standards about the appropriateness of talking about sex with one's partner or others. *"We've never talked about our sex life. I wouldn't know where to begin."* (Caraël, 1997).

Cultural norms: Every culture has norms for sexual behaviour, especially around the proper behaviour for women and men. Traditionally, men are expected to take charge. Also, within some cultural groups, sex outside marriage may be acceptable for the husband, but not for the wife. Some may involve family or religious ideas and practices. *"I wouldn't dare bring it (condom) up to my husband. He would accuse me of not trusting him and then he'd suspect that I 'd been sleeping around."* (Sweat, 1995).

Interpersonal power dynamics: Sometimes, people pressure their sexual partners to engage in high-risk activities. Unequal power in the relationship, and the stakes involved in not complying, can make refusal difficult. (Sweat, 1995)

Relationship development: To some extent, the relative ease or difficulty in dealing with sexual issues in a relationship will depend on the type of relationship or how long the two people have been together. The challenges of addressing safer sex issues are often different in a new or casual relationship than in established ones. (Sweat, 1995).

Peer pressure: Beginning in adolescence, the attitudes and behaviours of one's peers are an especially important influence on an individual's behaviour (Sweat, 1995).

C. Structural and Environmental Factors

Environmental barriers or facilitators: Physical environment can help or impede adoption of risk reduction behaviours. Availability of transportation and neighbourhood safety are physical environment aspects that can affect health-related behaviours.

Social policies: Social policies, in the form of local regulations as well as legislation on the state and federal level, have an impact on STD prevention.

Social inequalities: Racism, sexism, hetero-sexism, and socioeconomic stratification are deeply embedded in our culture, and they affect the resources available to people. Misinformation may persist among people with less access to education.

Sense of community: People may have a sense of a shared belongingness and identification. There is a shared belief that members can exert some control over what takes place around them, and are influenced, in turn, by the community as a whole.

Skills: The skill at which someone knows how to properly use a condom or with regards to coping ie. the ability of someone to face and deal with specific challenges. Further the ability to assertively state one's position or insist on what one wants without denying the rights of others is important in HIV prevention. (Porche, 2004)

Mental Illness: Medical mental conditions such as bipolar disorder, schizophrenia and other mental illnesses affect the degree to which a person can protect themselves from acquiring HIV/STDs, often treatable with prescription medications. (Porche, 2004)

Substance Use or Abuse: Use of mind-altering substances such as alcohol and drugs affect an individual's ability to change behaviour. Alcohol or drug use can lower inhibitions which may cause an individual to not engage in protective behaviour or affect the proper intake of ART. (Sweat, 1995; Caraël, 1997)

Lack of Knowledge about HIV/AIDS/STDs: An individual who does not know the ways in which HIV is transmitted, or has incorrect information, may engage in unsafe behaviour because they do not know the correct information. Accurate information is a key for an individual to protect themselves.

4.4. PROCESS OF BEHAVIOUR CHANGE – STEPS INVOLVED

Behaviour change is rarely a discrete, single event to which many may not readily comply. The Stages of Change model (adopted from model promoted by Centre for Disease control and Prevention) shows that, for most persons, a change in behaviour occurs gradually, with the patient moving from being uninterested, unaware or unwilling to make a change (pre-contemplation), to considering a change (contemplation), to deciding and preparing to make a change. Genuine, determined action is then taken and over time, attempts to maintain the new behaviour occur. Relapses are almost inevitable and become part of the process of working toward life-long change (Prochaska, 1992).

1. Pre-contemplation Stage

During the pre-contemplation stage, persons do not even consider changing. Smokers who are "in denial", may not see that the advice applies to them personally. Patients with high cholesterol may feel "immune" to the health problems striking others.

2. Contemplation Stage

During the contemplation stage, persons are ambivalent about changing. Giving up an enjoyed behaviour causes them to feel a sense of loss despite the perceived gain. During this stage, patients assess barriers (in terms of time, expense, hassle, fear, etc) as well as the benefits of change.

3. Preparation Stage

During the preparation stage, patients prepare to make a specific change. They may experiment with small changes as their determination to change increases. eg. sampling low-fat foods may be experimentation towards greater dietary modification.

4. Action Stage

This stage is the one that most physicians are eager to see their patients reach. Any action taken should be praised because it demonstrates the desire for lifestyle change.

5. Maintenance and Relapse Prevention

Maintenance and relapse prevention involve incorporating the new behaviour "over the long haul." Discouragement over occasional "slips" may halt the change process and result in the patient giving up. However, most patients find themselves "recycling" through the stages of change several times before the change becomes truly established.

The Stages of Change model encompasses many concepts from previously developed models. The Health Belief model, and other behavioural models fit together well within this framework. The researcher feels that this model suits the scenario of behaviour change in the field of HIV/AIDS too. During the pre-contemplation stage, patients do not consider change. PLHIV may not believe that their high risk behaviour is a problem or that it will negatively affect them (Health Belief Model), or they may be resigned to their unhealthy behaviour because of previous failed efforts and no longer believe that they have control. During the contemplation stage, patients struggle with ambivalence, weighing the pros and cons of their current behaviour and the benefits of and barriers to change. In addition to Interpersonal communication and counselling provided on behaviour change education on the issue needs to be backed by multiple strategic communication interventions at family and community level through Support Group Meetings of infected / affected persons, Peer education, Self Help Groups, General community awareness, Workplace outreach, Hotlines and through mass media. For it is only through follow up counselling an building a support system that behaviour change can be sustained.

Conclusion

The Chapter 2 on sexuality, in this study, threw light on the factors influencing high risk behaviours and the congeniality between HIV and Sexual behaviours. Consecutively, the focus of this chapter was to understand how MLHIV initiates and practices 'safe' sexual behaviours. This chapter provided theoretical framework on various factors, which can influence behaviour changes and also presented various models of behaviour change that could be adopted. This study would explore the behaviour change measures adapted by MLHIV with their spouses and other sexual partners. It will also ascertain the various factors influencing their changed practices.

The next chapter swims through the literatures available in the field of this study and poses the rationale and objectives of this study based on the theoretical framework developed in all these preceding chapters.

Chapter 5
LITERATURE REVIEW, RATIONALE AND OBJECTIVES

Introduction

HIV insinuates itself silently and enters into the blood stream of newer individuals each day. Ever since the last two and half decade, instead of the trend of infection reversing itself, there has been an exponential acceleration in the number of deaths each year. In this context this chapter throws light on the relevance of this research in the context of reversing the epidemic. A lot of advancement has been made in clinical and behavioural research under the paradigm of HIV and the findings are well documented. Ample researches have been conducted with PLHIV and their caregivers to assess their knowledge, attitude, behaviour and practice, in the context of HIV transmission and prevention. Quite a few researchers have also explored the socio-economic problems, stigma and discrimination faced by HIV infected individuals (Acharya, 1992). This chapter attempts to document the secondary data available on sexual behaviours of MLHIV, their HIV status disclosure and behaviour change patterns and highlight the findings of the researches carried out in this context. Based on the literatures reviewed, the rationale and objectives of the study shall be set up towards the end.

5.1. Review of researches on Sexual Behaviour

Sexual Debut

A survey conducted by Nana Chauda on 1000 students in Mumbai the age group 16-20 in urban colleges of Mumbai found that the boys were more sexually active and most of them had their first sexual experience before the age of 20 (Panda, 2002). The salient findings of the Behaviour Sentinel Surveillance (BSS) with youth across India state that the first sexual intercourse was initiated amongst the youth of the country at the age of 20 years in urban areas and 6 percent of youth reported sex with non-regular partners during 12 months preceding the survey. Women in India aged 15-24 who ever had sex were observed to have a sexual partner who was 10 or more years older. Such women they are almost twice as likely to be HIV positive as other women (NFHS, 2005).

Knowledge on HIV

Sex education in India was aimed to reduce the increasing incidence of unintended pregnancy, abortions and STI/ HIV/ AIDS. However, this approach only deals with bio-medical issues and doesn't focus on relationships or responsible sexual behaviour or on values and attitudes within human sexuality. An absence of education on human sexuality leads to 'inappropriate' behaviour and coping skills for making rational and responsible decisions (FPAI, 2005). Lately quite a number of schools in the country have banned 'Sex Education' after an uproar of the political leaders, claiming it to be overtly vulgar and irrelevant for school going children. Such out sightedness places the younger generation at a greater threat to the acquisition of HIV. (Fakir, 2004)

High Risk Behaviours

Men who are away from home frequently or for long periods of time are generally thought to be more exposed to the risk of HIV infection because they may be more likely to adopt high-risk sexual behaviours, when they are away from home. Contrarily it was observed that the men with the highest HIV prevalence are those that have not slept away from their home community at all in the past year (NFHS, 2005). Also, men who had more than two sexual partners in the past 12 months have a much higher HIV prevalence. HIV prevalence was more than six times as high among young men who have had five or more lifetime partners as among men with 1 - 2 lifetime partners (NFHS, 2005).

Cade et al (2002) studied the Predictors of high-risk sexual behaviour among people living with HIV/AIDS in Las Vegas, USA, interviewed 360 PLHIV adults (292 men and 68 women) receiving outpatient medical care for HIV/AIDS-related issues. The results claim 34 percent reported at least one occasion of unprotected anal or vaginal intercourse in the previous 6 months. Consistent with other researches, the correlates with high-risk behaviours included multiple sexual partners, negative attitudes about condoms, lack of risk avoidance strategies, and intravenous drug use prior to sex. However, contrary to other research, no association was found between low self-esteem, depression and anxiety, receipt of skill-based training or use of alcohol with unprotected sex (Tawil, 1995).

Sexual Partners

BSS study of India point out that 3 percent of the sexually active males reported sex with a commercial partner in the last one year preceding the survey. Among the respondents who had sex with any non-regular sex partner in last year nearly three-fifths reported non condom use with non-regular partner. Among the respondents who had sex with a commercial partner during the last year, over four-fifths reported condom usage. The increase in the consistent condom use was reported in almost all the states, except Goa and Daman & Diu, Maharashtra and Himachal Pradesh. Among the male respondents, 3 percent were indulged in MSM activities and only one-fifth of them used condoms during the last occasion of sex. (NACO, 2006)

Podesia (1998) in his research with 100 MLHIV found nearly 80 percent of the men had bisexual orientation and most of the times the respondents involved in sexual relation with no protection at all. The reasons for unprotected sex being stated as 'chronic depression' and 'high intake of alcohol'.

In 2005, 75 MSM who have sex for commercial benefits called Male Sex Workers (MSW), attached to the organisation Humsafar Trust in Mumbai were interviewed to understand the characteristics of MSW and male sex work in India. About 15 percent of the MSW were married to a woman or lived with a male partner. Nearly half of the MSW were HIV infected. About 80 percent identified sex work as their primary occupation. About 77percent of the MSW met their clients at public places and 67percent reported having sex in a private environment (clients home, their home, or hotels). About 13, 87 and 83 percent of the MSW reported having anal insertive, anal receptive and oral sex respectively in the past six months. One third of MSW had 'always' used a condom, 53 percent used it 'sometimes', and 13 percent 'never used'. The most common reason for not using a condom was non-availability (43percent) and refusal of condom use by the partner (20percent). One third of them were diagnosed with STI. (Priyamvada, 2007)

Lurie in her study "Sexual Behaviour and Reproductive Health among PLHIV in Urban and Rural South Africa" surveyed 3819 PLHIV from clinical settings. Urban residents were more likely than rural residents to have current regular sex partners, to have any current sexual indulgences, to report consistent condom use with regular partners and to have sex with casual partners. In multivariate analysis, independent predictors of consistent condom use with regular partners included across gender, urban residence, and higher education levels; for women, disclosure and younger age; and for men, no history of alcohol consumption. Male and female participants with a casual sexual partner were less likely to use a condom consistently with regular partners. Additionally, the predictors of having a regular sexual partner include urban residence, CD_4 count greater than 200 cells/mm, higher household income and a history of non-alcohol consumption. (Lurie et al, 2003)

Sex outside marriage

Although there is widespread disapproval of sex outside of any committed relationship, not everyone engages in monogamy. Some people have sexual relations outside of their primary relationship while still trying to maintain the primary relationship. Early studies in US (Hunt, 1974; Kinsey et al, 1948; Pomeroy, Martin, & Gebhard, 1953), suggested that nearly half of married individuals are involved in extramarital sexual relationships but recent studies, with more representative samples, suggest that the percentages are lower (Greeley, 1991; Laumann, Michael, Gagnon, & Michaels, 1994). Partners in gay couples are more likely than partners in lesbian or heterosexual couples to have sex outside the relationship (Blumstein & Schwartz, 1983; Kurdek, 1991).

A study on Sexual behaviour of PLHIV aged between 21-51 in Yaounde, Cameroon, Africa revealed that more than half of the respondents were single due to their HIV status. However 88 percent of the respondents maintained their sexual activities and half of the married men continued to maintain extra-marital intercourse. Among unmarried respondents, 38 percent had unprotected sex, while only 28 percent of the married respondents had unprotected sex with their sexual partner. (Antagana, 2000)

Van de Velde et al (2004) reviewed the safe sex practices and sexual needs of PLHIV, in Flanders, Belgium, Europe and found that only 17 percent of Flemish men 30 percent of Flemish women had not indulged in sexual relations in the last year.

Sexual behaviours after HIV

PLHIV sexual behaviour in Africa shows that their sexual activities do not almost change even after sero-positivity announcement and is highly unsafe in pre/ extramarital relationships. (Antagana, 2000)

Meystre-Agustoni (2006) in their research 'Sexual life of PLHIV' conducted in Switzerland found that sero-conversion brings with it a loss of self esteem and feeling of guilt leading to profound disturbance in sexual life of PLHIV. They reported painful feelings like an acute sense of the danger about life, feeling responsible for use of protection and of the limitations that their serological status imposes on their partner. The respondent's reduced self-image, due to HIV-positive status, constitutes a major obstacle to establishing relationships. Limitations are imposed on sexual life owing to the reduced possibility for spontaneity and fantasies with regard to sex. The strict use of protection, running contrary to desire for physical intimacy and the need to adopt a behaviour, which does not fit with socially idealized images of sexual togetherness, also proves problematic in long-term relationships.

Strauss (2002) studied the "Intimate partners and sexual risks in PLHIV in the non-urban South Eastern US". His study states that 42 percent of interviewed PLHIV were worried about passing HIV to their sexual partners. About 57 percent chose not to have sex at least 'sometimes' to avoid spreading HIV, while 43 percent of PLHIV had unprotected sex with their main partners, who were not HIV-infected. One fourth had unprotected sex with other partners who were HIV negative or of undetermined sero-status. This study shows how PLHIV although aware about their status are engaging in unprotected sex thus posing a public health threat.

Men who self-identified as gay/bisexual in the 2001 California Health Interview Survey, reported that 86percent knew their primary partner's sero-status, while 62percent knew their most recent secondary partner's HIV sero-status. Knowledge of one's most recent secondary partner's HIV serostatus was inversely related to history of injecting recreational drugs and reporting a primary partner in the past year. Two-fifths of HIV-positive men and three-fifths of HIV-negative men engaged in sero-sorting (serocordant unprotected anal intercourse) with their primary partners, whereas 33percent HIV-positive men and 20 per cent HIV-negative men did so with their most recent secondary partners. This population-based survey documented the extent to which MSM know their partners' serostatus and practice serosorting behaviours. (Xia, 2006)

Desai (2000) recruited 200 PLHIV couples in metropolis of South Mumbai, to study and categorise the challenges faced by them. It was observed that the frequency of sexual relation decreased drastically. The practice of safer sex was denied by majority of couples. Although PLHIV may be aware of the risk of infecting their sexual partners, they deliberately ignore the risk because other considerations, such as wanting a baby, take precedence. Consequently, condom access is inadequate to change risky sexual behaviour that spreads HIV. Condom decreased pleasure, caused irritation, was not believed to be protective and looked upon with suspicion. The prospect of living with HIV cannot be discussed with the spouse as the family infringes on their privacy with personal opinions, taboos & alternative therapies. Most couples were newly married and hence the prospect of remaining infertile or not seeing their children grow into adulthood was frightening. Decreasing economic productivity and increasing health care cost remained a major hurdle.

Sexual behaviours after ART

Over the past 5 years, research on the reproductive intentions of PLHIV has increased. Studies show that considerable number of PLHIV, particularly younger or having few/no children and taking ART, do wish to be biological parents.

The French MANIF cohort study group in Paris found that HAART does not increase sexual risk behaviour among French HIV infected IDUs amidst Hospital departments. GEE multivariate models confirmed that the prescription of HAART was associated with reduced sexual risk. The concern that HAART might result in clinical improvement leading to resumption of high risk activities that could inadvertently result in HIV transmission was not supported by these data. (Bouhnik, 2002)

Unsafe sex between HIV positive concordant people has sometimes been interpreted in terms of "negotiated safety". With the advent of HAART, it has become an important issue to the extent that potential re-infections with viral strains that had already become resistant to antiretroviral drugs may jeopardise the effectiveness of the newly available therapeutic regimens. The availability of HAART certainly calls more attention about the necessity to increase efforts for both primary and secondary prevention among patients who are already HIV infected. But this study, counters the a priori fears that HAART may facilitate risk behaviours among HIV infected IDUs. (Cade et al, 2002)

Baseline data were collected in Cape Town, Africa during 2006 to study if patients on ART experience decreased inhibition to avoid risky sexual behaviour. Out of 924 PLHIV, 520 had been initiated ART. Nearly half of men (40 percent) and women (46 percent) reported having unprotected sex in their last act. Men and women who did not disclose their HIV status to their partner, were twice as likely to have had unprotected sex their last time. Some patients who have just begun HAART may be experiencing symptomatic illness that may decrease interest in sex. Additionally, HAART may produce adverse effects that reduce sexual desire. (Eisele, 2008)

Bunell et al (2004) studied the "Changes in sexual behaviour and risk of HIV transmission after antiretroviral therapy and prevention interventions in rural Uganda, Africa". It assessed the changes in risky sexual behaviour and estimated HIV transmission from HIV-infected adults after 6 months of ART. In this prospective cohort study performed in rural Uganda, between May 2003 and December 2004, a total of 926 HIV-infected adults were enrolled and followed in a home-based ART program that included prevention counselling, voluntary counselling and testing (VCT) for cohabitating partners and condom provision. At baseline and follow-up, participant's HIV plasma viral load and partner-specific sexual behaviours were assessed and it was observed that after 6 months of initiating ART, risky sexual behaviour reduced by 70 percent. Over 85 percent of risky sexual acts occurred within married couples. At baseline, median viral load among those reporting risky sex was 1,22,500 copies/ml, and at follow-up, < 50 copies/ml. Estimated risk of HIV transmission from cohort members declined by 98 percent, from 45.7 to 0.9 per 1000 person years. Thus providing ART, prevention counselling, and partner VCT was associated with reduced sexual risk behaviour and estimated risk of HIV transmission among HIV-infected.

Aloisi et al, analyzed HIV-infected antiretroviral naive persons enrolled in the ICONA cohort in 57 hospital units of Infectious diseases in Italy, Europe in 1997-2000. A self-administered questionnaire was distributed at enrolment to study and repeated 12 months thereafter. In this analysis persons who initiated ART were compared with persons who were on ART for at least a year. The proportion of persons who were sexually active after one year was similar among those starting ART was 75percent. Among those sexually active, reported condom use (79.8percent vs. 71.8percent), proportion of those with at least one new partner (39.7percent vs. 40.3) or with at least one new partner with unknown HIV status (31.9percent vs. 34.6percent) in the last six months did not significantly differ between persons on therapy and those not on therapy. The data however provides no evidence that the initiation of ART therapy has any role, at least in the short term, in increasing sexual risk taking behaviour. (Girardi, 2004)

Sgombich et al (2004) studied the 'Sexual behaviours and condom use among PLHIV in Chile, America', comparing sexual and preventive behaviours of ART patients and non ART persons. A random sample of 800 PLHIV (161 women, 639 men including 435 MSMs), followed up by the Chilean Public Health System have been interviewed in 2001. In the last 12 months, 69percent were sexually active. ART patients (n=548) are less often sexually active than persons not on ART (n=247) (65.5percent vs 76.9 percent, p=0.002) and they have had less frequently more than one partner (16.2 vs 22.2 percent p=3.3, NS). The frequency of sexual relationships was observed to be lower for ART patients than for persons not on ART (more than once a week: 43 percent vs 53 percent, p=0.03). The consistent condom use is higher among persons on ART, significantly for the multi-partners (use of condom in each sexual intercourse: 92 vs 69 percent, p=0.01). Disclosure of sero-status to the regular partner is not significantly different between persons on ART and persons not on ART (84 vs 80 percent, p=0.2). The proportion of persons on ART who report a reduction of the frequency of sexual relationships since the initiation of treatment is higher than those reporting an increase: 50.4 vs 7.8 percent for mono-partners ; 43.8 vs 5.62 percent for multi-partners. Thus in Chile, persons on ART are more often sexually abstinent in the last 12 months than those not on ART. They report less sexual relationships and use condoms more consistently.

Nicole Crepaz et al (2004) conducted a meta analytic review of 25 studies on 'HAART and sexual risk behaviour' conducted between 1996 and 2003. The prevalence of unprotected sex was not higher among PLHIV receiving HAART (median, 33percent) vs those not receiving HAART (median, 44percent; odds ratio [OR], 0.92; 95percent confidence interval [CI], 0.65-1.31) or among HIV-positive persons with an undetectable viral load (range, 10percent-68percent; median, 39percent) vs those with a detectable viral load (range, 14percent-70percent; median, 42percent; OR, 0.99; 95percent CI, 0.82-1.21). The prevalence of unprotected sex was elevated (OR, 1.82; 95percent CI, 1.52-2.17) in HIV-positive, HIV-negative, and unknown serostatus persons who believed that receiving HAART or having an undetectable viral load protects against transmitting HIV or who had reduced concerns about engaging in unsafe sex given the availability of HAART ([median, 49percent] vs [median, 38percent] for counterparts)

In the above researches conducted on ART patients, it was noted that there was a comparative risk reduction, increase in condom use, greater monogamous indulgences and the respondents were less sexually active.

Sexual Satisfaction

Most PLHIV in Belgium, Europe claimed that the factors influencing dissatisfaction included 'very little' or 'no' sex at all, 'loss of libido', 'lesser interest in sex', 'fear of infecting their sex partners', anxiety about disclosure of serostatus to sexual partner. More than half of them were dissatisfied concerning sexuality within marriage (Van de Velde et al, 2004)

Impact of HIV on sexual health

According to a study in America reported in the Journal of the American Medical Association, 43 per cent of women and 31per cent of men under age 60 have some type of sexual dysfunction. And the numbers rise with age. The Massachusetts Male Aging Study found that by age 65, two-thirds of men have some degree of erectile dysfunction and one-sixth are completely impotent. In sharp contrast, of the adults who responded to the AARP sex survey, relatively few —just 28 per cent of men and 10 per cent of women, had ever sought medical advice for sexual problems. Although many adults place a high value on a healthy sex life, most don't know where to turn when sexual problems creep up. Some assume that the loss of sexuality is an inevitable part of aging and resign themselves to a sexless existence. Others are too embarrassed to seek advice, thus intensifying feelings of frustration, anger, and inadequacy. The popularization of Viagra in the late 1990s went a long way toward normalizing the issue of erectile dysfunction. (Parker, 1995)

The AARP sexuality survey found that healthy individuals are more likely to engage in sexual activity. The survey found that 44 percent of people who characterized their health as excellent or very good had intercourse at least once a week. But as health status declined, so did sexual activity. About 33 percent of the people with good health and just 20 percent of those with fair or poor health had intercourse this frequently. And many of the respondents reported that better health for either themselves or their partner would improve their sex lives. (Parker, 1995)

Legal issues in sexual practice

In November 2007, the Delhi High Court has ruled divorce to a HIV discordant couple on the pretext that marriage was "anathema" without sex. Additional district Judge Rajnish Bhatnagar said that a person cannot live "happily" with a spouse who is HIV infected. The judge thus granted divorce to a man whose wife is HIV positive, saying her ailment had prevented him from leading a "happy married life" as the disease is sexually communicable. The court added that sex was an integral part of marriage and in this particular case; the husband was deprived of that enjoyment. "The HIV status of the wife no doubt resulted in non-enjoyment of sexual intercourse between the parties and marriage without sex is anathema," the court said. This judgement arose a debate on whether HIV discordant couples are justified in taking a divorce on the basis of sexual relations. Sexuality within marriage is therefore clearly portrayed by the Judiciary as only a 'carnal relation'. Currently about 27 countries have established criminal penalties for knowingly exposing or transmitting HIV to someone else. In California, the "Wilful Exposure" law, makes exposing someone else to HIV a felony, punishable by up to 8 years in prison. In Alabama, one can be prosecuted for "Conducting oneself in manner likely to transmit the disease". (http://www.lawyerscollective.org/hivaids/activities/legal-services-sc-right-to-marry, last accessed on June 2009)

The results of the above mentioned studies on sexual behaviour, points out a varied indulgence in risky sexual practice after HIV detection. In every study a few PLHIV continue to indulge in risky sexual behaviour with multiple partners and non use of condoms. The frequency of sexual indulgences, kind of partners, number of sexual partners, the sexual desires of the PLHIV who practiced abstinence are some areas which can be further explored amongst PLHIV sampled in this study.

5.2. STUDIES ON DISCLOSURE

Research findings have presented a mixed picture between disclosure, sexual risk behaviours and potential transmission of HIV. Some studies have found that increased disclosure is associated with reduced sexual risk behaviour. Other studies show that disclosure doesn't always alter risk taking behaviours. Even with disclosure, unsafe sex sometimes occurs. Some people engage in safer sex behaviours without any discussion of HIV status. Half of the respondents did not reveal their sero-positivity to their sexual partners particularly respondents who were single (Antagana, 2000).

In most studies from both developing and developed country settings, HIV status disclosure to sexual partners was associated with positive outcomes, including increased social support, acceptance, kindness, decreased anxiety and depression and strengthening of relationships. Negative outcomes included blame, abandonment, anger, violence, stigma, and depression and were less commonly reported among those who disclose than positive outcomes. However, it is important to note that those who choose not to disclose may well be those who are most likely to have negative outcomes.

Disclosure to sex partners is more likely in longer-term relationships than in casual relationships (one-night stands, anonymous partners, group scenes, etc.). Disclosure also varies depending on perceived HIV status of partners, level of HIV risk of sex activities, sense of responsibility to protect partners and alcohol / drug use.

Kalichman (1999) researched the "Self-efficacy and disclosure of HIV-positive sero-status to sex partners", sampled within the Center for AIDS Intervention Research, Medical College of Wisconsin, Milwaukee, USA. HIV status disclosure in 266 sexually active PLHIV recruited from the community was examined. Results showed that 41percent had not disclosed their HIV status to sex partners.

Nachega (2003) studied "HIV status disclosure, gender and socio-economic status of PLHIV from Chris Hani Baragwanath Hospital in, South Africa". Of 105 patients evaluated, the average length of time a participant had known of their status was 3.5 years. Almost 90.5 percent reported having disclosed their HIV status to at least one person. However, of the 73 participants who reported having a spouse or sexual partner, 38 percent had not disclosed their status to their sexual partner. Disclosure was not significantly associated with the length of time known to be HIV-positive, antiretroviral use, age, gender, education or socio-economic status in multivariate regression analysis. When asked who they had disclosed to, the most common response was a sibling (70.5percent). Results show that a significant proportion of PLHIV, do not disclose their status to sexual partners. Status disclosure wasn't associated with gender, education or socio-economic status. The ethical dilemma of HIV status disclosure among sexual partners, the potential role of stigmatization as well as the risk of super-infection with continuing unprotected sex were the observed barriers in disclosure.

Greeff (2008) studied "Disclosure of HIV Status: Experiences and Perceptions of PLHIV and Nurses involved in their care in South Africa". Thirty-nine FGDs were conducted in five countries in both urban and rural settings suggesting that nearly one third of primary sex partners were not disclosed and were at risk of contracting HIV, whereas a pattern of lower disclosure among casual partners was evident. As the number of sex partners increased, the likelihood of disclosure to all sex partners decreased. Interpersonal factors that positively influenced self-disclosure included spousal support, emotional investment, and communication about safe sex, including asking about a partner's status. Voluntary disclosure was also not consistently associated with safer sex.

Lurie in her study "Sexual Behaviour and Reproductive Health Among PLHIV in Urban and Rural South Africa" surveyed 3819 PLHIV and found that the average rate of disclosure to current or steady partners was reported to be 49 percent, considerably less than the average rate reported from studies conducted in developed countries (79 percent). The lowest disclosure rates were among pregnant women tested in antenatal care (ANC) in sub-Saharan Africa (Range: 16-32percent). In addition, larger proportions of studies from developing countries report that women do not share their HIV test results with anyone (10-78percent) as compared to women in developed country studies (3-10 percent). Studies from both developed and developing country settings found that disclosure rates to sexual partners tend to increase over time. Results from both settings also found discrepancies between intention to disclose and actual disclosure behaviour, with actual disclosure rates lower than intended disclosure rates. (Lurie et al, 2003)

Among studies in the developed world, rates of HIV status disclosure to sexual partners is ranged between 42 to 90 percent, depending largely, on the type of partner to whom the person disclosed. The lowest rates of disclosure were reported among past partners or current 'casual' partners. The rates of disclosure in studies from developing countries were notably lower than rates reported from the developed world. Among the studies that reported disclosure rates to current or 'steady' partners the average rate of disclosure was 49 percent, considerably less than the average rate reported from studies conducted in developed countries (79 percent). The lowest rates were among pregnant women tested in antenatal care (ANC) in sub-Saharan Africa (16-32 percent). In addition, larger proportions of studies from developing countries reported that women did not share their HIV test results with anyone (10 – 78 percent) as compared to women in developed country studies (3 – 10 percent). (Naidoo, 2007)

Impact of Disclosure

A study of Latino gay men in America found that disclosure was related to greater quality of social support, greater self-esteem, and lower levels of depression. Disclosure also can lead to support that facilitates initiation of, and adherence to, HIV treatment and medications. A survey by Shari Margolese July 2003 of HIV+ persons found that 42percent of gay men, in USA, 19percent of heterosexual men and 17percent of women had sex without disclosing their HIV status. (Zea, 2007)

David et al (2002) researched on 'Disclosure as a tool in combating discrimination, stigma and social exclusion in Atlanta, America', found that disclosure has been an effective means in combating stigma, discrimination and in creating an enabling environment for PLHIV. Disclosure has effected a change in the attitudes of many people in the society thus gaining an acceptance for people living with HIV.

Kalichman (1992) found that men who had not disclosed to partners indicated lower rates of condom use during anal intercourse and scored significantly lower on a measure of self-efficacy for condom use compared to individuals who had disclosed. Emotional distress was also high among persons who had not recently disclosed. Having not disclosed to sex partners was closely associated with lower self-efficacy for disclosing.

Leickness (1999) conducted anonymous surveys with 413 HIV positive men and 641 HIV positive women in Cape Town, South Africa, conveniently sampled from HIV/AIDS service providers. Half of the respondents were on ART and most participants were currently sexually active. About 42 percent indicated that they had sex with a person that they had not disclosed their HIV status to in the previous 3-months. Participants who had not disclosed to all of their sex partners were significantly more likely to have multiple sex partners, HIV negative partners, partners of unknown HIV status, and unprotected intercourse with discordant partners. Having not disclosed HIV status to partners was also independently associated with having lost a job or a place to stay because of being HIV positive and feeling less able to disclose to partners. HIV-related stigma and discrimination were associated with not disclosing HIV status to sex partners and non-disclosure is closely associated with HIV transmission risk behaviours

Klitzman (2005) examined "Intricacies and inter-relationships between HIV disclosure and HAART" through a qualitative study, in order to study the impact on PLHIV peer educators public disclosure. In-depth interviews were conducted with 75 Peer Educators involved in community education through Public Disclosure, from 20 countries in Africa and the Asia-Pacific region. Decreasing stigma and stopping new infections were equally strong motivators in becoming community AIDS educators. Most respondents had good support from peers and family. Public disclosure was extremely rewarding and led to a diminution of discrimination. Disclosure led to a less stressful, more productive life and improved wellbeing. Virtually all 'Positive Speakers' had no regret and they saw only the benefits of public disclosure of their HIV status. The paradox of coming out openly as an HIV-positive person is that one finds psychological release—liberation from the burden of secrecy and shame. (AIDS Care, 2004)

As seen in the above researches, disclosure seems to result in greater psycho-social benefits. Disclosure has generally been noticed only amongst partners who share a log term intimate relationship. Many researches show that PLHIV who disclosed their status, experienced increased intimacy with partners and reaffirmation of their sense of self and the act of sex much more comfortable and relaxed. However, focus on disclosure to sexual partner, the time and process of disclosure, the factors influencing such disclosure and the impact of disclosure on sexual relations are some lacunae in the literatures.

5.3. STUDIES ON BEHAVIOUR CHANGE

Matovu (2007) examined the effects of "Repeat Voluntary HIV counselling and testing on sexual risk behaviours and HIV incidence in Rakai, Uganda" in 6,377 initially HIV-negative subjects enrolled in a prospective STD control for HIV prevention trial. Two thirds who regularly underwent counselling accepted VCT services and were more consistent in condom use and reported a decline in the number of sexual partners, suggesting the success of risk-reduction counselling interventions among MLHIV.

In rural south western Uganda, Africa, a setting with high HIV prevalence, the majority of respondents reported that they had already made behavioural changes because of HIV epidemic, but making further changes to protect themselves was contingent on knowing their HIV sero-status (Bunnell, 1996). Trinidad showed that couples receiving intense counselling and testing reduced unprotected intercourse among their spouses, especially among sero-discordant and sero-positive concordant couples. However, results specifically found that VCT produced significant changes in reducing high-risk sexual practices with non-primary partners. Same findings have been elicited by a study done by Moore (1991) in San Francisco, USA (Coates, 1998).

A study, "Sexuality at Midlife and Beyond," conducted by AARP, illustrates that five out of six of the respondents disagreed with the statement that "Sex is only for younger people." Six out of 10 people stated that sexual activity was a crucial part of a good relationship. Only 10percent of adults reported that they don't particularly enjoy sex, and just 12 percent agreed that they would be quite happy never having sex again. According to the AARP sexuality survey, 64 percent of men with partners and 62 percent of women with partners are primarily satisfied with their sex lives. This is in sharp contrast to the small proportion of those without partners (19 percent of men and 28 percent of women) who are pleased with their sex lives. The partner gap is a particular problem for American women because their average life span (80 years) is about five years longer than that of men. Because American women marry men who are on average three years older, that can mean even more time alone. Should a woman want to remarry, her chance of finding a new mate in her age bracket dwindles yearly; there is an average of only 7 men for every 10 women ages 65 and above. (AARP, 2004)

Rao (India) assessed the 'Behaviour change in HIV infected subjects following health education' with 85 new PLHIV registrants in the STD Department in India, who were given health education measures directed at avoiding high risk behaviours. The emphasis was on use of condoms, discontinuing promiscuous behaviour, abstaining from homosexual acts, avoiding pregnancy, and advice against marriage for those contemplating it. The Health Education Program was delivered individually to each subject over 2-3 sessions, each lasting for 30-45 minutes. At the time of follow-up (1-24 months), 42percent of subjects had become non-promiscuous. There was good compliance on the advice against marriage and that of avoiding pregnancy. The 7 infants born during follow-up were sero-negative. The use of the condom was not found to be acceptable. The prostitutes comprised the most resistant group to education. Among the factors that influenced the behaviour change favourably showed absence of STI or a short duration of the current STI. Literacy, marital status, or awareness of AIDS did not influence the outcome of education. The study demonstrated the feasibility of health education at the individual level in the clinical setting. (Rao, 1991)

Contraceptive use

Most PLHIV in Belgium, Europe practiced safe sex. Perceived peer norms, which reflect community assumptions about whether anal sex should (or should not) involve condoms, have been shown in numerous studies to be associated with sexual risk among MSM (Van de Velde et al, 2004). The main reason for denying condom use was the refusal by sexual partners and desire to procreate (Antagana, 2000). Studies undertaken in USA with HIV infected men concluded that they were sexually less active, less likely to engage in unprotected sex and more likely to use a condom. (Fakir, 2004)

Adam Carr (1991) studied behaviour change in response to the HIV epidemic amidst gay communities show few gays enjoy using condoms. The use of condoms for anal intercourse was a compromise between fear of HIV infection and fear of giving up sexual gratification which most gay men were prepared to accept and able to implement. Many younger people are likely to be under the influence of alcohol and "soft" drugs while having sex. Many gays were of the opinion that nothing bad can happen to them, although many of their friends were HIV positive. The gay organisations have succeeded to the extent that they have in bringing about rapid and sustained change in the sexual behaviours of gay men, without resort to any kind of coercive mechanism, offers hope that changing the sexual behaviours of heterosexual men is not beyond the scope of human ingenuity.

Kerr (1991) reviewed the 'Behaviour change in a cohort of discordant heterosexual couples' from the records of 256 HIV positive clients who visited three community health centres in high sero-prevalence areas of South Africa between March and September 1990. Respondents indicated substantial short-term changes in the following behaviours: 67 percent said they had fewer sex partners, 65 percent stated they had adopted condoms more frequently and 61percent said they are using contraceptives more regularly. Only 20 percent yet continued high risk practices, although all of them integrated themselves to primary prevention and access to primary health care setting.

Simon in his report associated 'Decline in HIV prevalence within Eastern Zimbabwe with sexual Behavior Change' between 1998 and 2003. HIV prevalence fell most steeply at young ages, ie. by 23 percent among men aged 17 to 29 years and in more educated groups. Of the men in risky sexual behaviour, 49 percent reported reductions in casual sex. Smokers reported higher rates of high-risk behaviours, including more lifetime sexual partners ($p<0.001$), being less likely to be married ($p<0.01$), and being more likely to have visited folk healers ($p<0.01$). Other factors included having more than 2 lifetime sexual partners (OR 3.4; 95percent CI, 1.7-6.8) and lower socioeconomic status (OR 8.6; 95percent CI 3.3-22.0). Thus indicating that behavior change is easier practiced in people who have lower drug dependence. (Gregson, 2006)

A review of researches conducted with young people in Canada on 'Impediments to safer heterosexual sex' state that verbal communication prior to intercourse is rare. A silence that protects the self-esteem of the partners and precludes a discussion of their sexual histories, but which also prevents discussion of condom use. Condom use is also limited by the embarrassment of buying, carrying, or using a one. Condoms still appear to be the most widely used contraceptive during young people's first intercourse, but if a sexual relationship is perceived as long term, the woman is likely to go on the pill. Economic needs and the expectation that a man's sexual gratification is paramount constrain women's choices. Most studies highlight that safer sex is easier with one's non-primary partner than with the primary partner. (Wight, 1992)

Content analysis and descriptive statistics were used to examine 'Factors that influence adolescents to engage in sexual activity without adequate contraception'. The non-random purposive sample of 24 pregnant adolescents in the age group 14-19 years was drawn from a maternity home in Los Angles, California, USA. Those who were more knowledgeable about sex, contraception and had parents who spoke to them about sex used contraception more frequently. The mean age at first intercourse was 14.3 years, with no differences between blacks and whites on initiation of coitus. Interestingly contraceptive usage was not related to age, religion, and type of relationship with the father of the baby. The reasons given for non-use of contraceptives were unplanned coitus or no thoughts about birth control or pregnancy. (Petosa, 1991)

The results of NFHS conducted in 2005 amidst the general population of India, show that the knowledge of contraceptive methods is practically universal; at least 98 percent of women and men age 15-49 know one or more methods of contraception, of which modern methods like female sterilization, male sterilization, emergency pills, IUD, and condoms are more widely known. The use of condom is most widely known among men. Among traditional methods, the rhythm method, withdrawal etc are less known. Married women were found to be more knowledgeable on contraception than unmarried. Adolescent men were found to be more knowledgeable about contraceptive methods than women. Almost two-thirds of women who do not intend to use contraception in the future cited fertility-related reasons for their decision. In particular, one fourth does not intend to use contraception because they feel that contraception is in-fecund. Young men who use condoms have an elevated prevalence of HIV (NFHS, 2005).

A few literatures on 'Choosing Contraceptive Methods', point out that men with intelligence, discipline, religious conviction and the ability to tolerate frustration may choose periodic abstinence and have better control over their own bodies or desire avoidance of intimacy. Risk taking and spontaneity are compatible with 'withdrawal method' in sex. Advance preparation i.e., planned use of condom and diaphragm, may decrease spontaneity in sex. 'Condom use' appeals to those with an obsessive compulsive nature, and to protect the female from semen and *'being soiled by the ejaculate'*, which she may construe as dirty. Choosing Condoms may be a badge of masculinity. However, agents such as 'Foams' are considered messy. 'Douching' is generally not condoned as a contraceptive method, but it washes away the tattle of feeling guilty. The Pill, IUDs, and Implants may appeal to those sexually inhibited and less self-confident. (Prochaska, 1992)

Factors influencing Behaviour Change

Populations at risk of HIV infection which have been subjected only to information-based mass media campaigns have failed to show any significant change in behaviour. Research shows that people do not change deeply-entrenched behaviour, such as sexual practices, simply on the basis of an induced awareness that the behaviour may be dangerous to them. A study of gay men in Los Angeles showed that those who were continuing to engage in unsafe sexual practices had exactly the same level of knowledge about HIV and safe sex as those who adopted and maintained safe practices (Steiner, 1994). The factors which have influenced behaviour change attempts amongst men living with HIV have been little explored and various studies have only shown the implied behaviour changes.

Impact on Women

Researches show that the reasons for 'unwanted pregnancy' in HIV infected women are the same as that of HIV negative women. HIV infected women have rejected their pregnancy for the following reasons: high viral loads, restricted income to access medication and treatment, other family members also being HIV infected, fear of HIV infected child and his long term support. Researches on 'HIV and Abortion' claims that the reasons for termination of pregnancy are fear of miscarriage or still birth and in most cases abortion is influenced by the husband's decision.

Ogilvie (2004) surveyed 230 women living with HIV in British Columbia, Canada, of whom 80percent were of reproductive age (<45 years). Of women living with HIV, 26 percent indicated an intention to have children. In multivariate modelling, non-aboriginal ethnicity, younger age and having a regular partner were associated with an increased likelihood of reporting the intention to have children in the future. Other studies in United States have shown that 70 percent of women with HIV infection are sexually active, effective contraception use amongst them is variable, and unplanned pregnancies are common. Further with increasing access of women to ART, the risk to unwanted pregnancy, conception needs, and reduced contraceptive methods were observed.

HIV infected women often report marked decreases in sexual functioning and quality of life. It was found that depressive symptoms, intrusive thoughts and sleep quality individually predicted poorer sexual life (Berer, 2003). Medical researches show that HIV interaction affects the sexual and reproductive health in a complex manner leading to several negative outcomes like, decreased sexual desire or satisfaction, feelings of guilt or shame, a negative association of sex with HIV, resentment towards a sexual partner, ill health or mental stress interfering with sexual function, vulnerability to sexual violence and STI, reduced ability to become pregnant (Manjar, 2007).

5.4. FINDINGS OF PRECURSOR QUALITATIVE RESEARCH

The researcher himself conducted a precursor qualitative study in Oct. 2007 to understand the sexual behaviour of people living with HIV/AIDS using a Biographical Narrative research design. Eight HIV infected men on ART from ART Centre, Sir J. J. Hospital, Mumbai, were interviewed on this regard (Thomas, 2008).

The findings pointed out that sexual fantasies emerged right from the age of 12 and it gradually shaped into initiating actual penetrative sexual intercourse between the age of 14 and 22. Although the sexual debut happens at such a young age, a significant postponement in the age of marriage (i.e. between 16 and 32) was observed. This gap between the age of desires and that of marriage was bridged by initiating pre-marital sexual relations. In the initial stages, the respondent's elder peer led them into discussion on sex and in reading porn literatures or viewing porn in a group. On some occasions the porn films were brought home and watched all alone individually. Masturbation happened in the peer group, while watching the porn films or 'after sexual discussions for educative purposes'. In a few years it was practiced by the respondents privately. In a couple of years, the respondents indulged in penetrative sex with varied commercial partners with a frequency of 1 to 6 intercourses a week. The frequency of relations and the number of partners reduced after the knowledge of HIV status and in particular after the onset of ART.

The study observations suggest a possible co-relation of risky sexual behaviour influenced by lower education status, higher income levels/ savings, exposure to porn media, alcohol addiction, peer culture, rising age of marriage, loss of lover and disharmony with spouse or family, which needs to be further ascertained in this study.

An interesting observation of the male sexuality is that, men, while selecting mates during their earlier sexual expeditions, look at younger age, physical appearance and variegated females. But with growing age and experience they prefer to settle down few selected women, who are generally of the same age, hospitable personality, women with whom, long term relationship can be built, burdens can be shared. Non brothel based women are generally preferred in this stage.

A couple of respondents started their sexual relations with the same sex individuals but ended up being a heterosexual, in fear of isolation by the family/ society. The use of condoms was seen to increase after the knowledge of HIV and particularly after the onset of ART. Apart from a reported increase in condom use, HIV prevention messages have had little impact on the sexual activity of PLHIV.

None of the respondents ever revealed their HIV status to any of their sexual partners outside marriage. Disclosure to spouse was seen in a few cases during their medical illness or during spouse's insistence on procreation. It was informed that disclosure of the man's status did not create a hostile environment within marriage or have any negative repercussion whatsoever. The respondents mentioned to have changed their sexual behaviours post ART and they claim that this 'transformation' is a chosen lifestyle and not as the side-effect of ARV drugs.

Review of documented literature on aspects of sexual behaviour, disclosure pattern and behaviour change practices amidst PLHIV's; points out that sufficient exploration have been well conducted in American and African continents. However, not as much studies have been conducted in India on this issue in particular. This lacuna in the precedent literatures enhances the need to venture in the said areas.

5.5 RATIONALE OF THE STUDY

The mammoth spread of HIV is mainly attributed to the sexual route of transmission, specifically, by the practices of unsafe sex. The sexual behaviour of men involved in high risk activities is what puts them at risk to HIV and also puts those in sexual contact with them at risk too. Disclosure of one's HIV status helps both the sexual partners to negotiate safer sexual practices and to indulge into lower risky behaviours. Hence HIV status disclosure is believed to be cornerstone firstly in prevention of the infection from PLHIV to the uninfected population and secondly to help prevent PLHIVs from acquisition of super-infection. Behaviour change post the knowledge of one's HIV status is the only vaccine to curb the spread of HIV from infected populations into the general community and also behaviour change strategies are quintessential for the PLHIV to regain health and live longer. This is why all intervening organizations working in the field of HIV address the issue of sexual behaviour change through various models.

The rationale for choosing the study topic and the sample, the study objectives and assumed hypotheses are highlighted herein.

Need for studying Sexual Behaviours of MLHIV

The presence of HIV takes toll on the individual's food, hygiene, exercise, recreation, rest, medical care, housing, sexuality and spiritual aspects. Intervening organizations have been addressing varied socio-economic issues of PLHIV without doubt. But how many activists or organizations have shown the interest to investigate or advocate for the sexual well being of PLHIV? People with HIV are at a risk of being denied their right to control their fertility, occasionally by coercive efforts with the intention of preventing transmission to sex partners and to the new born. (Kelly, 1998)

Sexual well being is a very personal choice for PLHIV and it comes from doing a self assessment of risk behaviours. For a concordant couple deciding to have unprotected sex, obviously the risk of transmitting HIV is not an issue, so the worry here is related to transmission of other STDs or "re-infection". Sexual entity is a fundamental basis of human existence. Hence many PLHIV couples have become 'fatalistic' and chose to practice unprotected sex within the context of a monogamous relationship as evident from the pre-cursor study. Whether or not a couple practices safer sex is not the issue at hand. What is most relevant is that they have established a line of communication regarding HIV. The fact that they have disclosed their status to each other before engaging in sex, and educated themselves about their options, is what is most important. (Mane, 2002)

The purpose of sexual union is procreation and pleasure but such messages on limiting sexual activity bars the freedom of HIV infected persons and leaves them unable to comply with sexual desires in order to live a sexually healthy and satisfied life. A few studies show that some PLHIV perceive pain in practicing sexual abstinence and feel responsible to use condoms out of choice (Kelly, 1998). Sexuality is a natural urge, which needs to be channelized either through fantasies, foreplay or through actual sexual intercourse. There is a social sanction for this only within marriage. A loving, passionate, emotionally and physically satisfying sex life is not something that can be denied to PLHIV (Ortner, 1989). Moreover, knowledge on fidelity and gratifying one's own sexuality are stories untold in the counselling process. Isn't the exponential spread of HIV a strong indicator that such a moral policing on human behaviour is ineffective?

Documentation in India regarding the indigenous sexual practices has been increasing ever since the discovery of HIV epidemic, due to the close association between HIV and sexual transmission. However, sexuality issues in the society continue to be shrouded in secrecy and ignorance. Moreover, the sexual needs and concerns of PLHIV are sidelined even by the intervening organizations, as they hasten to cater to their psycho-social needs. Even the counsellors seem to blanket discussions on sex due to one's own embarrassment in discussing and inadequate skills in handling such concerns. Since many HIV service professionals enter the field with little or no focused training in human sexuality other than a review of strategies for sexual risk reduction of HIV infection, discussions about sexuality are often cursory, and focus almost exclusively on disease prevention. A large section of the society continues to believe that *"the sinner (HIV infected person) has to pay the price of the sin (illicit behaviour)"* (Gregorio, 2005). This approach however ignores many complex dimensions of human sexuality impacting sexual behaviour.

This study therefore explores of the various dimensions and the constructs of sexuality, as practiced by PLHIV, over a period of time, right from their detection of HIV to the onset of ART adherence. It seeks to compare the sexual experiences and practices of the respondents within the three phases of infection namely, before HIV, after HIV but before ART and after ART. The findings made herein shall open doors to understand the influencing factors of disclosure and the process of behaviour change in order to design appropriate intervention strategies.

Need for studying Disclosure

Self Disclosure is not just a vital component for timely health seeking behaviour like testing and treatment but also a ground for behaviour change to happen ie. to enable the practice of safer sex in an attempt to prevention of the epidemic. Research findings have presented a mixed picture between PLHIV's risky sexual behaviour and their HIV status disclosure. The behaviour of disclosure of status by male PLHIV to their sexual partners will certainly increase the dependency of people affected by HIV on safer sexual practices. Some studies points out a correlation between non disclosure and a likelihood of having multiple sex partners and risky sexual practices. HIV infected men's disclosure with spouse was not a commonly observed phenomenon due to the fear of perceived stigma. Disclosure and Behaviour Change are thus significant tools in maintaining a healthy relationship and in preventing the spread of the epidemic.

Need for studying Behaviour Change

HIV prevention, care and support programmes have been rigorously up-scaled since the last decade in order to curb the spread of further infection. But in an attempt to curb the infection, HIV infected persons are generally educated to abstain from illicit sexual behaviour, abstain from homosexual acts, avoid pregnancy, advised against marriage for those contemplating it and lastly are forced to repress their sexual thoughts or to practice safer sex, with the use of condoms (Nyblade, 2000). Counselling on sexuality for PLHIV is all too often mainly centred on complete abstinence or the use of protection. Furthermore advices to PLHIV has mainly been in the form of prohibitive recommendations, which reinforce a sense of decreased self-esteem, leading to negative repercussions on all aspects of sexual life (Matovu, 2004). The counsellors training module also promotes abstinence and monogamy as the only 'Harm Reduction Strategies' for the disease (NACO, 2006). It is silent on biological details of reproduction and information related to safer sex. For many years now, the focus of prevention has been on trying to get society as a whole to adopt condom use as a way of life.

Contrarily, condom use is highly debated by PLHIV networks and MSM groups as an unworkable long term strategy. Safer sex practices seem to have been denied by PLHIV due to their priorities of procreation, intimacy needs in new wed-locks, and inaccessibility of condoms. AIDS is no longer perceived by the general public as a "crisis," and many people in the HIV community after decades of being ultra-conscious in their safer-sex practices, PLHIV have become more relaxed as well (Kelly, 1998). The effort to prevent HIV has to be connected with a vision of a better world rather than the goal of universal condom use. A world has to be envisioned, where every PLHIV, lives with respect and satisfactory sexual life. As people live longer with this disease, the focus should be on improving quality of life.

Need for studying men

It has been pointed out that, biologically, HIV in women is a disease of fidelity, not of promiscuity, since most women who contract HIV infection sexually do so from repeated exposure to a single infected man, usually their husband, rather than from single exposures to many infected men (Dandona, 2005). As mentioned in earlier chapters, it is known that HIV infected men start their sexual carriers early in adolescence and generally before the age of marriage (Dandona, 2005). Reproductive health issues and Family planning techniques are little known at this stage of life. High risk sexual indulgences and multiple sexual partners are experimented in this stage for curiosity and experimentation. All this factors puts them at a risk to unwanted pregnancies and STI/HIV. Furthermore, the infidelity practiced in their sexual behaviour make those vectors in the spread of HIV epidemic. Hence the prevention of the epidemic focuses on bringing about a behaviour change amongst men. This study will explore the sexual behaviours which put men to risk and then study the impact of behaviour change interventions in their lives. Moreover, the Researcher himself being a male will elicit comfort amongst the male respondents to freely ventilate their sexual practices.

Need for focussing the study in Mumbai

Mumbai is coined to be the AIDS capital of India with over 5 lakh PLHIV, 60 percent of who are men. Mumbai also being a modernized metropolitan has non interference and liberal attitudes towards the practice of alternate sexualities. Various high risk groups of men inclusive of, gays and bisexuals, clients of sex workers, male sex workers, prisoners, transgenders, drug users and mobile men (migrants and truckers) are all flag points of the incidence of HIV infection. About 20,000 men are claimed to be registered on free ART roll out under the National AIDS Control Programme-3 (MDACS, 2008). The precursor qualitative study undertaken by the researcher, the experiences shared by HIV counsellors and through informal discussions with men on ART through the CHIRAG project, there is substantive evidence that most male with HIV have a story to tell about their illicit sexual lives. The researcher is concerned of this assumption that if every HIV infected man infects at least one person in his lifespan, the toll of PLHIV is going to be two-fold. In this commercial hub of Mumbai, where avenues for dating and casual sex is not a herculean task and in the city where a high proportion of married men are already infected, it needs to be ascertained if 'Behaviour Change Campaigns', which seek to promote monogamous relationships and marital fidelity is appropriately reflected in sexual practices of HIV infected men.

Need for studying MLHIV on ART

Highly active antiretroviral therapies (HAART) including protease inhibitors (PIs) have been proved to be effective for decreasing HIV viral loads to undetectable levels thus significantly reducing the incidence of HIV related OIs, and thereby restoring a decent quality of life for a good number of PLHIV. The upscale of ART has led to a significant decline in the number of deaths due to AIDS and helped PLHIV regain health and increase their CD4 count. Some literatures in India, point out that the frequency of sexual relations initiated by men on ART has reduced drastically and so has the practice of multiple partners (Dandona,2005). Recurring symptomatic illness has further barred PLHIVs interest in sexual indulgence. Sexual and erectile dysfunctions have been observed in aging men who were on ART, needs to be ascertained. Little is known about the modification of sexual behaviour in response to new therapies among PLHIV.

In opposition, concerns have also been raised that these treatment improvements may increase the opportunities for continued or relapse to risk behaviours among male PLHIV, and that they may create a new threat for public health through transmission of HIV viral strains that have already acquired genetic resistance characteristics against actual treatments (Elford, 2000). Such concerns may even be more pronounced for high risk groups, who are often confined to unsupportive social environments and squalid physical living conditions that create additional barriers for HIV secondary prevention. A possible unintended consequence of ART, emerging in western researches is that the onset of ART leads to resumption of high-risk behaviours that facilitate transmission of HIV, including drug-resistant isolates. (Wainberg, 1998)

Most researches target newly enrolled ART clients to study the impact of behaviour change counselling. The researcher feels that the behaviour change seen in newly enrolled ART patients may not be sustained in the long run. Further, the practice of unprotected sex between concordant couples under the assumption of no further harm is not adequately recorded. Factors influencing behaviour change and retarding it needs to be further explored in order to have systematic intervention with such patients.

The substantive rationale for choosing men on ART as sample for this study is to assess their sexual histories in a biographical fashion, which will serve as a point of reference to study behaviour changes over a period of time at these three main periods, namely, Sexual behaviour before the HIV infection, sexual behaviour after the HIV test but before the onset of ART and sexual behaviour after the onset of ART. Comparative analysis, which is aimed to be 'within cases', will provide better indicator of conceptualising the individual's behaviour change over a period of time than that of 'across cases'.

5.6 STUDY RELEVANCE FOR SOCIAL WORK PRACTICE

The above particularities in the spread of HIV, amply justify the need of contending with the virus by a change in sexual behaviour of HIV infected men, until a medical solution is found. For if the indulgences in unsafe sexual practices of

PLHIV does not cease the spread of the epidemic amidst the general population and the chances of re-infection and STI amidst PLHIV will continue to mount. The greater incidences of infection will impact the availability and access to the already miniscule treatment options. The acquisition of a drug resistant virus will increase the dependency on second line treatment and in most cases; people may become resistant to the commonly available line of ART. Furthermore, researcher feels that any attempt to methodically document the issues regarding sexuality would give visibility to this issue and help explore and understand its dimensions.

The sexual needs and behaviour of PLHIV thus documented will provide better prospects for undertaking appropriate counselling. The outcome of this research shall therefore attempt to prepare a module on sexuality related counselling for people living with HIV/AIDS, which will be recommended to National AIDS Control Organisation (NACO) in training its counsellors and shall be disseminated to other intervening agencies in the field of HIV counselling.

5.7 STUDY OBJECTIVES

This research has been framed into 3 phases based on its sampling methodology and aims to address the following objectives:

PHASE 1: Hospital Based Counsellors

1. To study the counsellors understanding about their MLHIV clients in areas pertaining to sexual behaviour, disclosure and behaviour change

PHASE 2: MLHIV on ART

Sexual Behaviour

2. To study the socio economic profile, health and sexual practices of the HIV infected respondents and their spouses
3. To understand the respondents perception of male sexuality

Disclosure

4. To trace the process and consequences of disclosure
5. Ascertain factors influencing disclosure and the barriers in disclosure

Behaviour Change

6. To study the affect of the 'HIV +ve status' and 'ART' on sexual behaviour
7. Ascertain the factors influencing sexual behaviour change

PHASE 3: Spouses of MLHIV

8. *To study the spousal perception on their husband's towards disclosure and behaviour change initiatives.*

The next chapter will surface the methodology of this study and identify various variables on which the study findings shall revolve upon.

Chapter 6

RESEARCH METHODOLOGY

INTRODUCTION

A Research Design is a logical and systematic plan that directs the research and Research Methodology is a framework that provides an explanation on the utilization of various procedures and techniques involved in the study along with the rationale for selecting the Research Design (Das, 2000). The chapter begins by explaining the rationale of the selected Research design and the Phases of Data Collection. The Sources of data, Tools of data collection, Sampling techniques and the Researcher's Experiences involved therein are described. It further enlists the important Concepts and Variables identified for the study and its Operational definitions. This chapter, in conclusion, speaks of the procedures followed in Data Processing and Analysis, the scope and limitations of this study and the expected results and policy outcome.

HIV being a chronic and a long-term illness, a broad range of knowledge and understanding must be brought together to support both the quality of the life of PLHIV. Chronic diseases like HIV, by their very nature, require the complementary use of qualitative and quantitative research methods in order to quantify the effectiveness of treatments and qualify the illness experience as it progresses over time.

The purpose of **Applied Research** is to improve a phenomenon or a process and testing theoretical concepts, in actual problem situations. Applied Researches are directed towards solution of immediate specific and practical problems and places importance in problem solving (Srivasatava, 1994). Applied Researches in the field of HIV, helps extend our understanding of how best to manage the illness through a broad range of perspectives and skills. It is imperative that researchers move beyond traditional adherence to particular methods of inquiry and study an issue from a combination of perspectives, using both qualitative and quantitative methods. Holman states *"good social research recognizes the complementarity and interpretation of quantitative and qualitative methods of inquiry"* (Michael, 2004).

Unfortunately, the ability to combine research expertise across traditional methodological boundaries is often thwarted. Qualitative and quantitative researchers often operate with a different set of assumptions about the world and the ways of learning more about it. These assumptions may be seen as mutually and inevitably irreconcilable (Das, 2000). Researchers are often taught to master only one type of method. The result is that the two major approaches (qualitative and quantitative) are seldom combined and their respective strengths are ignored by adherents of each approach. The inherent danger in this strict separation of research perspectives is the likely production of incomplete results regarding the health problem being studied.

Applied Research is classified into two major methodologies namely Qualitative and Quantitative as explained below:

Qualitative Methodology: Qualitative research is described as "the non-numerical examination and interpretation of observations, for the purpose of discovering underlying meanings and patterns of relationships" (Das, 2000). The word qualitative implies an emphasis on processes and meanings that are not rigorously examined or measured, in terms of quantity, amount, intensity, or frequency. Qualitative researchers stress the socially constructed nature of reality, the intimate relationship between the researcher and what is studied, and the situational constraints that shape inquiry.

***Quantitative Methodology*:** Quantitative research is defined as "the numerical representation of observations for the purpose of describing and explaining the phenomena that those observations reflect" (Das, 2000). Quantitative studies emphasize the measurement and analysis of causal relationships between variables, not processes. Inquiry is aimed to be within a value-free framework. It is thought that in gaining, analyzing and interpreting data, the researcher can remain detached and 'objective'. Quantitative research is inclined to test theory *(deductive process)* and tend to produce results that can be generalized.

The dichotomy of quantitative, deductive analysis under standardized, objective conditions versus qualitative, inductive inquiry aimed at understanding phenomena in uncontrolled, natural contexts remains a barrier between researchers from different analytical disciplines, particularly those studying the etiology and consequences of disease (Michael, 2004). Instead of either ignoring or defending a particular research paradigm, it is possible and more instructive to see qualitative and quantitative methods as part of a continuum of research techniques, all of which are appropriate depending on the research objective. The point here is not to understand the specific differences of these techniques, but to highlight the existence of a range of options under both the qualitative and quantitative paradigms. This study is an attempt to adapt the conduct of both methods of analyses in order to help identify relevant phenomena of sexual behavior, disclosure and behavior change and to gain equal value from both types of data.

6.1 RESEARCH DESIGN

Background

As a precursor to this research, the researcher had carried out a qualitative study on 'Sexual behaviour, Disclosure and Behaviour Change of men on ART', in Mumbai, with an urge to understand the existing sexual behaviour and its patterns amidst male PLHIV on ART. As explained in the literature review, this study used a *'Biographical Method'* to capture the 'mosaic' nature of sexual histories of the male PLHIV and through triangulation using FGD with the ORWs in the field, various variables were coined for the purpose of this study. The findings of this pioneer initiative pushed the researcher to explore further the behaviours of PLHIV and the insights gathered from it, also helped conceptualise the design this study.

Study Design

Based on the objectives of this study and the research areas for probing, the researcher divided the collection of primary data of this study into three phases as under. Each phase has been arranged in a linear fashion and the information gathered and variables identified in each phase helped snowball the paradigm of exploration for the next phase. The table below summarises the Research Design for the study.

Table 3: Sampling Method in Phases

Phases	Sample	Method	Vision
Phase 1	Hospital based Counsellors	Quantitative	Understand counsellor's perception of MLHIV and areas of counselling
Phase 2	MLHIV on ART	Quantitative	Record dimensions and extent of behaviours
Phase 3	Spouses of MLHIV	Qualitative	Affirm the MLHIV behaviours

6.2 SAMPLING DESIGN

Sampling Technique

The topic of the study is an exploration of the behaviours of HIV infected men. The nature of this study is highly sensitive and comes within the purview of the individuals' right to confidentiality. This creates difficulty to obtain a scientific random sampling. In consideration of the magnanimous number of MLHIV in the country and the counsellors working in hospital based settings, it was considered appropriate to use a **Non Random Sampling technique** in identification of primary sources for data collection. To further homogenise the primary data, the researcher considered MLHIV in Mumbai and Counsellors in Maharashtra as the Sampling Universe. In the 3 phases of this study the following considerations were also made in deciding the sampling method:

Sampling Design Phase 1: Hospital based Counsellors

The counsellors are the entry points of HIV detection and are considered primary change agents in the life of PLHIV. The findings of this study on MLHIV behaviours have primary implication on the counselling component and the education given by counsellors to MLHIV. The findings are indicators to prepare a road map for developing a curriculum for training counsellors. The researcher's experience in working with counsellors did indicate that the counsellors would not be willing to speak freely in their work settings and that they perceive any research, involving them as a sample, as a further threat to their insecure working conditions. In consideration of this, the researcher chose to collect samples of counsellors who attended Counselling training programs at the Institute where the researcher worked. The researcher's rapport with the counsellors during the training and the counsellor's choice for voluntary participation, made it convenient for the researcher to decide on a **non random purposive** sampling method.

Sampling Design Phase 2: MLHIV on ART

The official records of the MLHIV are considered confidential and non transferable, as per the guidelines of the Ministry of Health and hence under ethical considerations MLHIV cannot be approached, through a probability sampling, by any agencies external to the system. The areas of exploration with MLHIV for this study include their sexual behaviour, disclosure and their behaviour change aspects. The explored areas are considered a very private affair of an individual and it is presumed from past researches that MLHIV would not wish to discuss these issues in public domain. Hence the convenience and availability of the sample was a major concern.

The researcher through the data collection, of his precursor study, observed that the hospital environment from where the MLHIV take medications was not considered conducive to such a sensitive research interview, due to various onlookers and fear of recognition. The sampling units of MLHIV are also distributed sparsely across Mumbai and hence it was convenient for the researcher, to collect data from consenting individuals, within the safe and non threatening environment of the project CHIRAG they were associated to. The MLHIV who were voluntarily associated with the project, where they sought care and support was considered as an entry point for this research purpose. This consideration encouraged the researcher to find convenient and interested MLHIV samples from the community, who were invited to a drop in centre of this project, for interviews. Some MLHIV chose not to disclose their sexual behaviours, when they were oriented to the study content and these MLHIV were conveniently permitted to leave respectfully during the course of the interview process. Thus the **purposive** sampling was the best alternative to be implemented.

Sampling Design Phase 3: Spouses of MLHIV

Given the limitations as above, the spouses could not be directly approached to be interviewed on their spouses for triangulation of data. The spouses of the MLHIV, who were interviewed, could not be directly informed about the interview of their male counterparts for reasons of maintaining confidentiality of the MLHIV behaviours assessed. Most of the spouses of these MLHIV were a part of the Self Help Groups of project CHIRAG. It was thus more convenient for the researcher to reach the spouses through the SHG forum. Thereby two such FGDs were arranged with the women who were part of the SHG, within the project. It was confirmed by the project that most of the women in these SHG were spouses of the interviewed MLHIV respondents.

Thus the researcher had to conduct an FGD during the monthly SHG meeting of the project based on convenience of both parties. The women's participation in FGD and their co-operation on the subject of research was non-threatening for the women, since all the women were associated with the project and knew each other well. Thus non random **purposive** sampling method had to be used in this phase too. The anonymity of the responses raised in the FGD, was also assured and maintained by the researcher.

A female moderator appointed for the FGD was introduced to the subject of study and the areas of data gathered in in-depth interviews gathered from the MLHIV. A checklist of areas to be explored with the spouses of those MLHIV was prepared and the discussion flow that needs to be conducted with the women was rehearsed. It was decided that the researcher would play a passive role in this process by only taking notes and would hint the Moderator if further exploration needs to be done on emerging issues, in the context of the study.

Since the researcher also served as the Project Coordinator of CHIRAG and had known many of the interviewed PLHIV, who used to come for counselling, it was easy to obtain Informed consent from all the respondents in this phase.

Sample Size

The Universe of study and the sample size, selected through a purposive non random design, across the three phases of this study have been summarised in the table below:

Table 4: Sample Size in Phases

Phases	Study Population	Study Universe	Sample Size
Phase 1	Hospital based Counsellors in Maharashtra	ICTC and ART Counsellors in Maharashtra	85 counsellors from Maharashtra
Phase 2	MLHIV on ART in Mumbai	MLHIV registered on ART in Mumbai	152 MLHIV on ART in Mumbai
Phase 3	Spouses of MLHIV residing in Mumbai	No data available	21 spouses of MLHIV in Mumbai

Sampling Criteria

In order to provide homogeneity in the data collected across study subjects and also from the perspective of the study rationale of the sample selection, the following prerequisite inclusion and exclusion criteria have been developed. These inclusion and exclusion criteria have also been formulated to minimise the known external variables skewing the research findings, in consideration of experiences from the past researches documented in the Literature Review chapter.

Table 5: Inclusive Criteria for Study

Phases	Study Population	Inclusive Criteria for Respondent
Phase 1	Hospital based Counsellors in Maharashtra	Willingness to participate in the
Phase 2	MLHIV on ART in Mumbai	Have been on ART for at least 6 months Aged more than 24 years but less than 50 years Resident of Mumbai research and discuss on the concerned issue
Phase 3	Spouses of MLHIV	Willingness to participate in the research and discuss on the concerned issue

Exclusion criteria

The respondent has been considered excluded from the study if s/he

- demonstrated physical or mental disability
- was physically ill or hospitalized for clinical care
- verbally refusing before or during the course of the interview

6.3. TOOLS FOR DATA COLLECTION

Primary Data : In order to triangulate the data and to consolidate a holistic understanding on the researched subject of Sexual Behaviour, Disclosure and Behaviour Change, the researcher identified three different tools, as mentioned below, for data collection. Each tool was prepared based on the data gathered from precursor phases. Informed Consent has been recorded from each of these respondents, in the administration of the tools, as deemed necessary by International Research Ethics.

Table 6: Tools used for Study

Phases	Study Population	Tool Used
Phase 1	Hospital based counsellors	Questionnaire
Phase 2	MLHIV on ART	Interview Schedule
Phase 3	Spouses of MLHIV	FGD Interview Guide

Secondary Data was gathered from past researches, books, journals, magazines, International and National Conference reports and websites that were relevant to the study. The researcher also gleaned valuable information form informal conversations with the Out Reach Workers of CHIRAG and Counsellors from other states, which was of great help in formulating the interview schedule.

6.4. DATA PROCESSING AND ANALYSIS

Each schedule was checked for consistency and completeness. The open-ended questions were initially categorized explicitly and exhaustively and then coded. Quantitative data has been summarized numerically using frequency tables, percentages and cross tabulations and analyzed using the statistical package (SPSS) and multi-variate tables. Statistical methods have been computed to find the measures of central tendency, measures of dispersion and variable relationships. Qualitative data was subjected to content and narrative analysis. Cross case and within case analysis to highlight similarities and differences have been used to see the trends and patterns in data within group and also to triangulate and compare inter sample data.

6.5 OPERATIONAL DEFINITIONS

A. Operational Definition - MAJOR CONCEPTS

A concept is an abstraction representing an object, property of an object, or a certain phenomenon (Wilkinson, 1997). The following are the major concepts discussed in the context of this research.

Sexuality refers to the expression of who we are. It involves a person's thoughts, feelings, and sexual expression and relationships, as well as the biology of the sexual response system. This study attempts to classify MLHIV into 3 broad categories of sexual orientation based on their reported behaviours:

1. **Homosexual** is a person whose sexual orientation refers to having sexual and romantic attraction primarily or exclusively to members of one's own sex. In this study, *homosexuality* refers to the sexual behaviours practiced between men.
2. **Heterosexual** is a person whose sexual orientation refers to sexual behaviour with, or attraction to, people of the opposite gender, or to a heterosexual orientation.
3. **Bisexual** refers to a person whose sexual orientation sexual behaviour with or physical, emotional, and affectionate attraction, to both, their own sex and the opposite sex. Men who were termed to have a bisexual orientation in this study are the ones who have reported sexual intercourse with both male and female partners.

Sexual intercourse, also known as **copulation/coitus**, in this study refers to the act, which involves penetration of the male reproductive organ into another individual.

Vaginal sex refers to the penetration of the male sexual organ into the female reproductive organ.

Oral sex refers to sexual activities involving the use of the mouth, and may include use of the tongue, teeth and throat, in order to stimulate the genitalia. 'Cunnilingus' refers to oral sex performed on a woman while 'Fellatio' refers to oral sex performed on a man. 'Analingus' refers to oral stimulation of a person's anus. Oral stimulation of other parts of the body (as in kissing and licking) is usually not considered oral sex. Oral sex may be practiced in both heterosexual and homosexual sexual contexts.

Anal sex in this study refers to the sex act involving insertion of the penis into the anus. It is a form of sexual behaviour considered to be comparatively high in risk, due to the vulnerability of the tissues and the septic nature of the anus. As the rectal mucosa provides little natural lubrication, a lubricant is most often preferred when penetrating the anus.

Sexual partners outside marriage refer to the male respondents sexual indulgences with partners other than spouse. These are classified for analysis as pre and extramarital partners.

1. **Premarital sex** refers to the sexual intercourse engaged in by the MLHIV, who is not yet married. The individual/s with whom the MLHIV has engaged in this activity is referred to as pre-marital partner/s.
2. **Extramarital sex** refers to the sexual intercourse engaged in by the MLHIV with an individual who is not their spouse. The individual/s with whom the MLHIV has engaged in this activity is referred to as extra-marital partner/s.

Sexually transmitted Infection/ Disease (STI/ STD), is an illness that has a significant probability of transmission between humans or animals by means of sexual contact, including vaginal intercourse, oral sex, and anal sex. A person may be *infected (STI)*, and may potentially infect others, without showing signs of *disease (STD).*

Sexual Behaviour is the outward manifestation of one's sexuality. It encompasses a wide range of activities such as sexual thoughts, feelings and expressions, the search for partner/s, interactions between individuals comprising of physical or emotional intimacy and sexual contact.

Disclosure implies giving out of information about one's own HIV status, either voluntarily or to be in compliance with legal regulations. The intent of disclosure is to help adopt safer sexual practices. It is both the conscious and unconscious act of revealing more about oneself to others. Disclosure in this study pertains to the act of MLHIV revealing their HIV status to their spouse or sexual partners.

Human immunodeficiency virus (HIV) is a lentivirus (a member of the retrovirus family) that can lead to *acquired immunodeficiency syndrome* (AIDS). Infection with HIV occurs by the transfer of blood, pre-ejaculate, semen, vaginal fluid, or breast milk.

People living with HIV (PLHIV) are people who have acquired HIV infection, the agent of the currently incurable disease AIDS. This is an umbrella term which involves HIV infected persons along with the corresponding HIV affected populations. Males' Living with HIV (MLHIV) refers to the male sex within this HIV infected population.

Acquired Immune Deficiency Syndrome (AIDS) is a condition in humans, characterized by a set of symptoms and infections, resulting from the damage to the human immune system caused by HIV. This condition progressively reduces the effectiveness of the immune system and leaves individuals susceptible to opportunistic infections and tumours. Most of these conditions are infections caused by bacteria, viruses, fungi and parasites that are normally controlled by the elements of the immune system that HIV damages.

Opportunistic infection (OI) is an infection caused by pathogens that usually do not cause disease in a healthy immune system. A compromised immune system, however, presents an "opportunity" for the pathogen to infect.

Anti Retroviral Therapy (ART) are medications for the treatment of infection by retroviruses, primarily HIV. When several such drugs, are taken in combination, the approach is known as Highly Active Antiretroviral Therapy (HAART). The American National Institutes of Health and other organizations recommend offering antiretroviral treatment to all patients with AIDS. But because of the complexity of selecting and following a regimen, the severity of the side effects and the importance of compliance to prevent viral resistance, various organizations emphasize the importance of involving patients in therapy choices and recommend analyzing the risks and the potential benefits to patients without symptoms. The current guidelines for ART from the World Health Organization (WHO) recommend that in resource-limited settings (i.e. India), PLHIV can register for ART when HIV infection has been confirmed and one of the following conditions is present:

1. Clinically advanced HIV disease;
2. WHO Stage IV HIV disease, irrespective of the CD4 cell count;
3. WHO Stage III disease with consideration of using CD4 cell counts less than 350/µl to assist decision making;
4. WHO Stage I or II HIV disease with CD4 cell counts less than 200/µl.

Counselling is defined as the process of providing information, education, problem-solving, therapeutic interventions and support through a safe, confidential, non-sexual, professional relationship aimed at increasing the capacity of individuals to cope with, understand or overcome difficulties they are experiencing in their lives.

Counsellor in the context of this document is defined as any service provider who is conducting either pre- and/or post-test HIV counselling and/or ART counselling to HIV-positive people.

Spouse in the context of this document refers to the individual who is currently married to the MLHIV

Health status of the MLHIVs for this study is considered to be an accumulation of variables like CD4 status, ART status, Body Weight, frequency of STIs and Opportunistic Infections

Condom is a device most commonly used during sexual intercourse. Condoms, most frequently made of latex, cover the penis during sexual activity so as to avoid contact with blood, vaginal fluid, and semen during sexual activity (oral, vaginal or anal). Female condoms are inserted into the vagina prior to intercourse. Condoms are used to prevent pregnancy and transmission of sexually transmitted diseases.

6.5. B. Operational Definition - MAJOR VARIABLES

A variable is a measurable characteristic that varies. An important distinction having to do with the term 'variable' is the distinction between an independent and dependent variable. This distinction is particularly relevant when investigating cause-effect relationships.

Independent variables are those that the researcher has control over. This "control" may involve manipulating existing variables or introducing new variables in the research setting. The Independent variables for this study are to be understood as explained:

Age Chronology includes age of onset of sexual feelings, sexual intercourse, HIV test, HIV awareness, Disclosure to spouse, Onset of ART medication.

Profile of the respondents comprises the respondent's marital status, educational qualification, occupation, income and current age

Health status of both the respondent and his spouse measured as a cumulative of HIV stage, CD4 stage, ART stage, Body Weight, frequency of STI and Opportunistic Infections

Period before HIV refers to the lifespan of activities performed by the MLHIV before the HIV positive test.

Period between HIV and ART refers to the lifespan of activities performed by the MLHIV after the detection of HIV but before the onset of ART

Period after ART onset refers to the lifespan of activities performed by the MLHIV after the initiation of lifelong ART treatment.

Sexual partner is a person with whom one engages in sex acts. The partner can be commercial or otherwise and this pattern may change throughout life

Brothel based partner refers to the sexual partners specifically identified from the brothels for commercial purposes

Non brothel based partner refers to the sexual partners identified by the MLHIV within the community (excluding brothels) who may or may not indulge in a commercial relationship.

CD4 levels are another predictor of MLHIVs health. The CD4 levels are the amount of HIV-susceptible white blood cells per millimeter cubed (cells/mm3); uninfected men will have a range between 400 and 1200, uninfected women, between 500 and 1600 (Aldrich et al., 2000).

Dependent variables are the ones that show the effect of manipulating or introducing the independent variables. The variation in the dependent variable depends on the variation in the independent variable. The Dependent variables for this study are to be understood as explained below:

Frequency of Sexual desires is calculated to be the number of sexual thoughts arising in the MLHIV in a period of a month

Frequency of sexual intercourse is calculated to be the number of penetrative sexual acts that the MLHIV indulged in with his partner in a period of a month.

Initiator of sex within marriage refers to the individual who initiated the sexual intercourse

Number of sexual partners refers to the total number of individuals with whom the MLHIV has indulged in sexual intercourse

Level of sexual satisfaction refers to the extent of pleasure achieved within an act of penetrative sexual intercourse

Time period of disclosure refers to the time taken by the MLHIV from the day of HIV test detection as 'positive/ reactive' to the day when the spouse was informed about the MLHIV's HIV positive status.

Disclosure to other sexual partners refers to the non spousal sexual partners of the MLHIVs with whom sexual contacts are established.

Impact of ART refers to the kind of routine behaviours that have changed after the onset of ART and its consequences.

Safe sex is the practice of sexual activity in a manner that reduces the risk of infection with STIs. From the viewpoint of society, safe sex in this study is regarded as a harm reduction measures initiated by the MLHIV.

Sexual abstinence is the practice of voluntarily refraining from some or all aspects of sexual activity. Common reasons for practicing sexual abstinence may include: religious or philosophical reasons (e.g., chastity); material reasons (to prevent conception [undesired pregnancy] or STI transmission); psycho-sociological reasons (e.g., clinical depression, social anxiety disorder, or even just negative past experiences); or, legal injunctions requiring conformity.

Masturbation is an act of stimulating one's own genitalia towards eroticising and is considered safe so long as contact is not made with discharged body fluids of others.

Non-penetrative sex (Outercourse) refers to range of sex acts which restrains fluid exchange, can be enjoyed by partners with significantly reduced risks of infection and pregnancy.

Sexual pleasure is derived from any kind of sexual activity, most commonly masturbation and sexual intercourse. Though orgasm (sexual climax) is generally known as sexual pleasure, it includes erotic pleasure during foreplay and pleasure due to fetish.

Impact of Disclosure is cited either positively in terms of care and support received by the MLHIV or as a degree of fear of rejection, stigmatisation or abandonment by loved ones as a consequence of disclosure.

Behaviour change within the paradigm of sexual behaviour is an alteration in individual's behavioural patterns, such that it reduces the harm of infection to oneself and others, thus promoting healthy lifestyle. The influencers of behaviour change could either be environmental or personal.

6.6. SCOPE AND LIMITATIONS OF THE STUDY

The researcher did not have adequate time or access to resources to cover a greater number of respondents in the 3 phases and had to rely on the conveniences of the respondent in participation. Furthermore, the subject of sex being associated with cultural taboos, there is an apprehension that the accuracy of information provided by the respondents, may not be complete and may be influenced by the respondent's personal, social and moral concerns. The researcher's outlook therefore, is not to resolve these inconsistencies or contradictions in the information shared, but to capture the entire gamut of their experiences and practices in the context of the study themes.

The study sampling technique of 'non random purposive sampling', maintain a possibility for likelihood of deviations from the experiences and practices of the 'Sampling Universe'. Hence, the results of the study would thus need to be understood, specifically in the context of the sample. The objective of this research is therefore not generalisation of the study findings but to understand the dimensions, extent and processes involved in sexual practices, disclosure and behaviour change amongst MLHIV on ART. The opinions and experiences shared by all the respondents in the 3 phases of this study are strictly limited to the sample, and as such do not constitute a representative sample contextually. The behaviours are also to be considered in the context of socio-cultural environment of Mumbai.

Table 7: Scope and Limitations of the study

Phase	Sample	Scope for estimations of results	Limitations
Phase 1	Hospital based counsellors	- The counsellors participating were from ICTC and ART Centres giving a holistic understanding of the counsellors perspective	- These views expressed by counsellors in 2009 may perhaps have changed over a period of time
		- Most of the counsellors interviewed were from the ART background and hence would have had a greater understanding of their male clients due to greater number of follow-up encounters	- The counsellors undertaking induction training may not have interacted with all their clients and their statements may reflect their generalisation for their clients
		- The interview with counsellors helped conceive the framework for devising variables in assessing the interview with MLHIV - The perceptions of counsellors identified from this study can be used as a building block to educate the counsellors on the issue further	- All counsellors were interviewed when they came for their training. These interviews were a part of the training need assessment of counsellors towards curriculum building needs identified at CSWNN
		- The aim of this exploration was to assess the content of knowledge and skill level of counsellors when dealing with issues pertaining to sexuality and not to rate the counsellors.	- When saturation was obtained with 85 counsellors, the sample size was freezed. Hence this sample may not be representative of the population.

Contd...

Phase	Sample	Scope for estimations of results	Limitations
Phase 2	MLHIV on ART	The researcher feels that his prior association with the interviewed MLHIV was a factor influencing their frank responses. Most of the respondents at the end of the interview have stated that they have never ever talked about their sexual behaviours so explicitly to anyone before this.	- Refers to the MLHIV practices and behaviour change attempts until May 2010 - There is also a fair possibility that the researcher may have missed a certain aspects of their experiences if they had wilfully kept some information undisclosed or even understated their actual sexual behaviours in fear of being identified as overtly sexual.
Phase 3	Spouses of MLHIV	Efforts have been made to capture the basis on which they have stated their opinions and perceptions Women feel more comfortable to open up in their peer group	- Findings cannot be generalized to the observations of Phase 1,2- Findings restricted to behaviours amongst their husband- Refers MLHIV husband's practices and behaviour change attempts made until May 2010.

This research will be of utmost assistance for all organizations working with PLHIV on care and support issues. The findings of this study would benefit NACO/ other HIV-organizations to design suitable programmes and appropriate strategies of communication in reaching out to PLHIV. Those wanting to study sexual behaviour or disclosure in future can frame their questionnaires based on the questions or the salient findings of this study, for they are exhaustive and have been intensely researched on. The 14 point scale for attitude developed herein was calculated to be highly internally reliable with a value of 0.758 for the 14 items taken together.

A word of caution is established herein for all the readers against any generalisations. The counsellors interviews were to elicit their perceptions about MLHIV's sexual practices and the knowledge of its dimensions. The counsellor's interviews were terminated on reaching saturation of their responses on dimensions of MLHIV practices. FGD with spouses was facilitated by a female investigator, keeping in mind the gender comfort levels of the sample. The sample size for FGD was decided on the availability and consent of spouses.

6.7. RESEARCH AREAS & HYPOTHESIS

This research has been framed on the following objectives, to explore with the sample:

PHASE 1: Hospital Based Counsellors

Objective 1: To study the counsellors understanding about their MLHIV clients in areas pertaining to sexual behaviour, disclosure and behaviour change

PHASE 2: MLHIV on ART

Sexual Behaviour

Objective 2: To study the socio economic profile, health and sexual practices of the HIV infected respondents and their spouses

Research Questions :

- ☆ *HIV related Health profile of self , spouse (CD4, HIV/ART status, Weight, STI/OI)*
- ☆ *Socio Economic profile of respondent*
- ☆ *Age chronology of sexual behaviour, HIV infection and ART onset*
- ☆ *Frequency of sexual desires and sexual indulgences, sexual preferences and types, satisfaction*
- ☆ *Pre marital and Extra marital sexual indulgences*
- ☆ *Factors influencing high risk behaviour among men*

Hypothesis

1. Earlier the sexual initiation greater is the multiple sexual partners
2. Men have multiple sexual partners before the knowledge of their HIV status
3. The HIV test would be the first exposure to their education on HIV
4. Men would have rarely ascertained the STI or HIV status of their sexual partners before sexual intercourse

Objective 3: To understand the respondent's perception of male sexuality

Research Questions :

- ☆ *Perceptions about factors like gender, power and morality influencing Male sexuality*
- ☆ *Influence of alcohol consumption on sexual performance*
- ☆ *Risk taking behaviour*

Disclosure

Objective 4: To trace the process and consequences of disclosure

Research Questions :

- ☆ *Age of HIV discovery and time period for disclosure*
- ☆ *Need of disclosure, Process of disclosure to spouse, Consequences of disclosure and its benefits*
- ☆ *Process of disclosure to sexual partners, felt need of disclosure, its Consequences and benefits*
- ☆ *Content of disclosure*
- ☆ *Reaction of spouse and other sexual partners*
- ☆ *Frequency of Indulgence in risky sexual practices with disclosure and without disclosure*

Hypothesis

1. Longer the duration of living with HIV, greater the comfort level of HIV status disclosure to spouse
2. HIV status Disclosure to spouse will be more prevalent after ART onset
3. HIV status Disclosure to other sexual partners will be minimal

Objective 5: Ascertain factors influencing disclosure and the barriers in disclosure

Research Questions:

- ☆ *Role of counselling support in influencing disclosure,*
- ☆ *Influence of alcohol/drugs on disclosure*
- ☆ *Safe sex practices after disclosure*
- ☆ *Reasons for discomfort in disclosure and help required*

Behaviour Change

Objective 6: To study the affect of the 'HIV positive status' and 'ART' on sexual behaviour

Research Questions:

- ☆ *Respondents perception of one's own behaviour change*
- ☆ *Methods (A-B-C) followed in prevention of sexual transmission of HIV*
- ☆ *Frequency and nature of high risk behaviour after the knowledge of HIV status*
- ☆ *Frequency and nature of high risk behaviour after the onset of ART*
- ☆ *Consequences of ART on sexual behaviour,*

Hypothesis

4. Frequency of Sexual indulgences would have comparatively decreased after the onset of ART.
5. Condom use with sexual partners would have increased after ART

Objective 7: Ascertain the factors influencing sexual behaviour change

Research Questions:

- ☆ *Behaviour change strategies advised to the respondents in counselling sessions*
- ☆ *Role of individual's HIV status, Counselling, Condoms, Religiosity, Family, and psycho-social support in influencing behaviour change*
- ☆ *Reasons for resorting to high risk behaviour*
- ☆ *Problems faced in sustaining of safe practices in sexual behaviour*

PHASE 3: Spouses of MLHIV

Objective 8: To study the spousal perception on their husband's to disclosure and behaviour change initiatives.

Thus the process of selection of a research design and methodology has been rationalised in this chapter. The chapters following this will describe at length, the study findings under themes of Sexual Behaviour, Disclosure and Behaviour change.

Chapter 7

PHASE 1 - FINDINGS COUNSELORS PERCEPTION ON MLHIV BEHAVIOURS

Introduction

The College of Social Work, Nirmala Niketan, trains hospital based counsellors supported by the National AIDS Control Program. The researcher has been associated with these HIV Counselling trainings of counsellors since 2007. The existing training curriculum has laid sufficient emphasis on counselling PLHIV on safe sexual behaviours. The researcher's interest was to ascertain the counsellor's awareness on sexuality related issues of their clients, who come to them for counselling. The information gathered herein would help the researcher sharpen his enquiry with the MLHIV, which was scheduled in the second phase of the study. With this intention a semi structured questionnaire was administered to the counsellors as seen in Annexure 1. This chapter compiles the data gathered from the counsellors along with its cursory analysis. The findings of this analysis would be later triangulated with the findings from the MLHIV in order to identify their counselling need areas related to sexuality issues which may require further strengthening. It is important to draw the attention of the reader here that the data compiled here has been collected on the basis of counsellors' recollection of the information and the inferences are only indicative. They need to be understood along with the findings of the next chapter where the information was directly solicited from the MLHIV.

These counsellors in Maharashtra interact with at least a hundred MLHIV in a month and hence would have rich experiences to share about the MLHIV sexual behaviour. The variables thus identified in this Phase-1 of data collection are structured to be the ground for designing the tool for data collection with MLHIV in its Phase-2.

Research Design

Counsellors from Maharashtra (either ART or ICTC), who attended trainings at the CSWNN Institute, were conveniently selected by the researcher using the Non Random Sampling design. The sample was purposively designed such that more ART counsellors could be included in the study, since the researcher was interested in understanding the behaviour changes of MLHIV, in the aftermath of ART onset.

A **'Questionnaire'** was circulated among the consenting counsellors to elicit their perceptions on Sexual Behaviour and Disclosure patterns of their MLHIV clients. Efforts have been made in the tool to validate the perceptions of the counsellors, by asking them to state substantial evidences backing their claims. The evidences may range from their direct observation of MLHIV behaviours to their interactions with the affected family members. In the absence of any hard data the researcher had to rely on these perceptions of counsellors. The inference generated from this Phase-1, is therefore not sufficient to establish significance of variables but will certainly help to understand and explore the dimensions of the researched subject and the counselling experiences therein.

Findings

The findings have been collated and analyzed on SPSS and has been reported in tabular and graphical manner as seen below in the following sequence:

1. Profile of Counsellors
2. Sexual Behaviour of their PLHIV clients
3. Disclosure patterns amongst their PLHIV clients
4. Training Intervention areas on Sexuality Counselling

7.1 Findings on Profile of Counsellors

This segment introduces the reader to the profile of the counsellors, which includes the nature of training they undertook, the type of centre, their years of experience in HIV Counselling etc apart from their personal background in terms of their gender, age, religion and educational background. The findings of the profile of counsellors have been summarised as under:

Employed with: The counsellors from Maharashtra interviewed in the sample were employed either under the supervision of MDACS (20 percent) or under MSACS (80 percent).

Training status: More than half of the counsellors were partaking the Refresher training (58 percent), while the other 42 percent were attending the Induction training, organised at CSWNN.

Type of Centre: About one fifth (21.2 percent) of the counsellors were from ICTC centres while four fifths (78.8 percent) were purposively sampled from the ART centres.

Sex: It is interesting to note that only around one third of the counsellors (31.8 percent) were females and more (68.2 percent) were males. This is in line with the database of counsellors in Maharashtra, where one third of the counsellors are females (MSACS, 2007). This is an interesting observation in comparison to the studies of the West, which shows that more number of females opts for counselling as a profession.

Years of experience: The mean and median years of experience of the counsellors was observed to be 2 years. All those who attended the Induction training were fresh appointees and had less than a year's experience, while those who came for the refreshers training were found to have more than a year's experience. As seen in the graph below, 55 *(29+25)* respondents (64.7 percent) had less than 2 years of experience in counselling.

Figure 4 Gender wise frequency of years of experience of the respondents

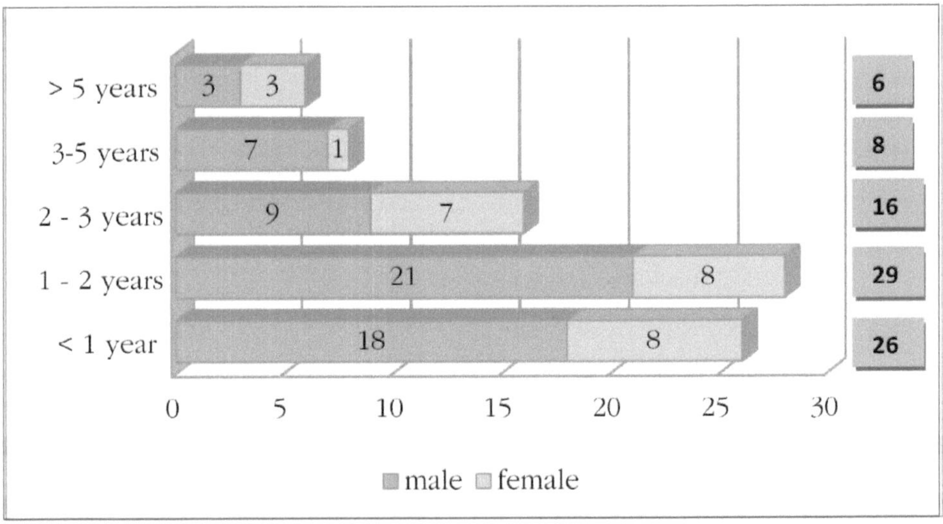

Age: Thirteen (15.3 percent) of the respondents were fresh graduates and were new in the field of counselling with less than 25 years of age. Over half of the respondents (51.76 percent) were in the age group 26 – 30 years and only 4 of the respondents (4.7 percent) were older than 36 years. The mean age of the counsellors was observed to be 29 years with a standard deviation of 3.7 years. The gender wise age distribution graph also depict that this profession of counselling is sought by men and women at more or less the same age.

Figure 5: Gender wise distribution of the age of the respondent

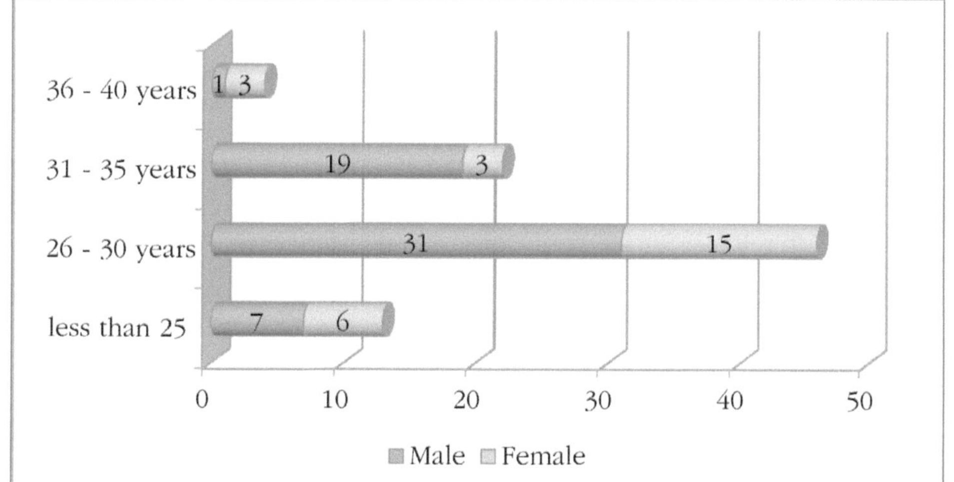

Educational Background: Most counsellors (72.9 percent) were post graduates in Social Work discipline as shown in the table below. It is interesting to note that although the nature of the job demands a psychological understanding, not many psychology graduates apply for this profession. This finding is also similar to the study done on MDACS counsellors alone by the College of Social Work in 2010 (Alphonse et al, 2010).

Table 8

Educational Background	Frequency	Percent
Masters in Social Work	62	72.9
Masters in Psychology	17	20.0
Masters in Arts/ Sociology	5	7.1
Total	**85**	**100.0**

7. 2 Perceptions on Sexual Behaviours of MLHIV

The counsellors perception on the sexual behaviour of their MLHIV clients were explored which include, their frequency of discussions on sex, concerns raised by the clients related to sex, barriers faced by MLHIV in asking questions related to sex, frequency of sexual acts, frequency of safe indulgences, MSM behaviour of MLHIV, questions asked in relation to homosexuality and their responses given. The knowledge of counsellors about the sexual orientation of the MLHIV clients and their sexual behaviours was also elicited. The detailed analyses on these aspects are presented below:

7.3 MLHIV's Questions related to sex

The counsellors were inquired to recollect, the percentage of their MLHIV clients, who ask them their queries related to sex and sexuality. It was calculated that on an average, 43.59 percent of MLHIV clients (standard deviation of 26.8 percent) asked their counsellors questions related to sex. The responses of the counsellors were classified into percentiles of 25 as demonstrated graphically.

Figure 6 Percentile of clients asking questions related to sex to the counsellor (Y axis) vs Percentage of Counsellors to whom questions were asked (X axis)

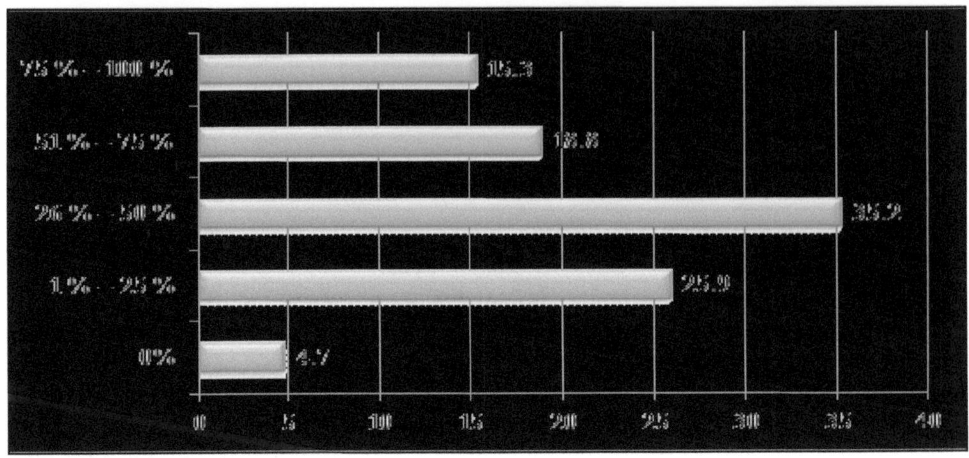

Figure 7 Percentage of MLHIV asking questions related to sex vs. Counsellor's experience

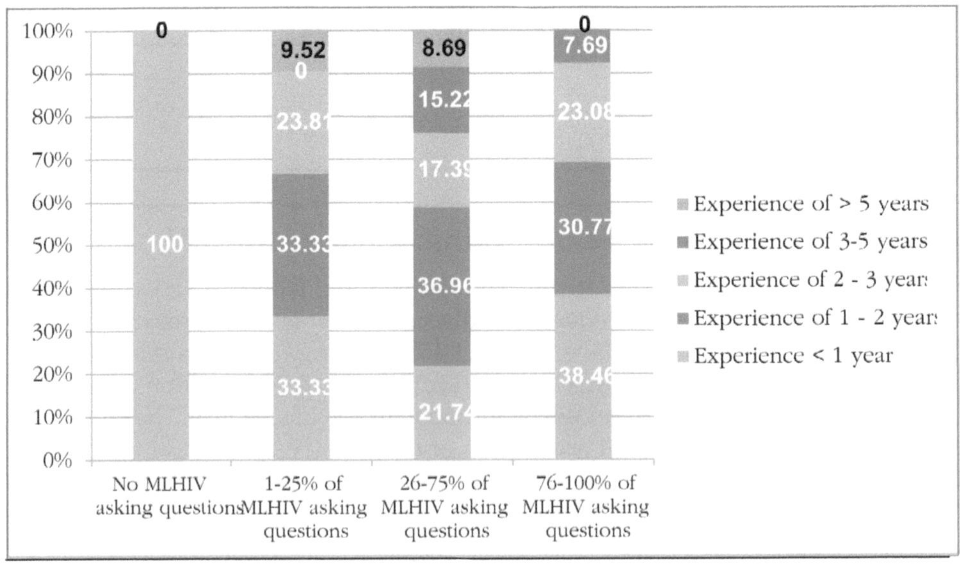

As seen above, the 4.7 percent of the counsellors admitted that they were not asked any questions related to sex by MLHIV. Some of the counsellors explained this further by mentioning that they were new to the ART Centre, which was in the process of establishment and that ART counselling had not started there in a full-fledged manner. These 4 counsellors were attending the Induction Training at CSWNN immediately after their selection. Moreover, it is interesting to observe that over one third of the counsellors (18.8 + 15.3 = 34.1 percent) reported that more than 51 percent of the MLHIV have asked them queries related to sex.

An attempt was made to observe the relation between the percentages of MLHIV asking their counsellors questions regarding sex, in correlation with the counsellor's years of experience in counselling. The findings of this correlation have been demonstrated below:

Figure 8 Gender of Counselor vs. Percentage of clients asking queries related to sex

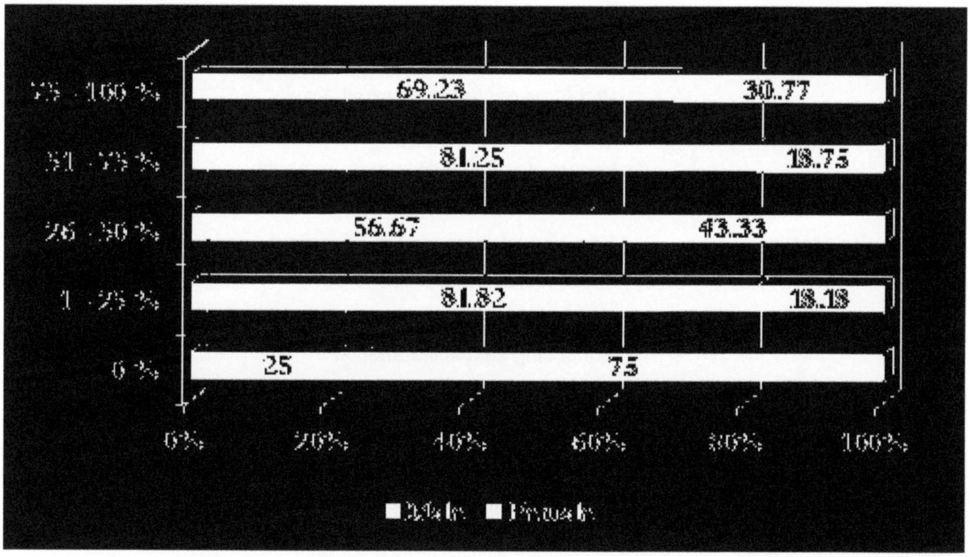

As seen graphically, it was observed that all male counsellors were asked questions related to sex irrespective of their years of experience (Pearson Chi-Square value = .025 with a degree of freedom = 6). Further, it was also observed that the female counsellors who were newly recruited (having less than a year's experience) were rarely asked any queries related to sex. Moreover, the senior female counsellors reported more males asking them questions pertaining to their sexuality (Pearson Chi-Square value = .007 with a degree of freedom = 6). However, the age of the counsellor did not show any significance with the number of MLHIV asking them questions related to sex.

7.4 Queries related to sex

The counsellors who reported that their MLHIV clients discussed with them, questions pertaining to sex, were probed further on recollecting the concerns raised by the MLHIV. Thus common concerns of their MLHIV clients derived from the counsellors have been thematically collated and briefed in the table below:

Table 9 Queries related to sex

#	Areas of concern		Specific Issues/ Concerns
1	Concerns related to knowledge on Sexual Practices	-	Types of sexual practices
		-	Coping with sexual desires
		-	Methods of sexual satisfaction
		-	Clarifying myths about sexual behaviours
		-	Family planning methods
		-	Natural period of having sex without pregnancy
		-	Sexual relations during pregnancy
		-	Frequency of having sex, which will not affect the health
		-	Impact of sex on CD_4
		-	Problems encountered in the last sexual act
		-	Problems related to bisexual activity
		-	Oral and anal sex related discussions
		-	Impact of seminal discharge on health
2	Concerns related to Safe sex practices	-	Safe sex methods
		-	Safe sexual methods for discordant partners
		-	Precautionary measures to be taken
		-	Level of risk in lip kissing, foreplay, oral sex, multiple partners
		-	Enhancing sexual life after ART
		-	Reducing fears about transmission to other partners
		-	Masturbation related discussions
		-	Contraceptives that prevent the spread of HIV
3	Concerns related to Condom use	-	Ensuring safety in condom use
		-	Risks in having sex without condoms
		-	Rationale for condom use among concordant
		-	Condom breakage issues
		-	Condom dissatisfaction related discussions
		-	Negotiation skills if partner denies condom use
4	Concerns related to Relationship with non spousal partner	-	Communication skills on safe sex negotiation
		-	Denial of discordant partners to use condoms
		-	Skills to proceed with sex, when spouse denies
		-	Meeting mutual sexual desires within relationship
		-	Lack/ loss of sexual interest among spouse
		-	Continuing extramarital sexual relationships
		-	Remarriage & marriage intentions
		-	Partner disclosure

Contd...

5	Concerns related to Procreation	-	Procreation need issues amongst concordant couples
		-	Pregnancy related issues of spouses
		-	Vertical transmission precautions
6	Concerns related to addressing Sexual problems	-	Prevention of STI,
		-	Safe sexual behaviour during STI
		-	Issues of white discharge in sexual partners
		-	Problems in private parts
		-	Wounds due to sexual relations
		-	Sex during menstruation,
		-	Blood flow after intercourse
		-	Night falls
		-	Sexual impotency feelings after HIV infection
		-	Early discharge,
		-	Penile erection issues,
		-	Concerns on size of penis,
		-	Increasing the duration of sexual act
		-	How to perform sex during old age

7.5 Barriers faced by MLHIV in asking questions related to sex

The counsellors were asked to state on what could be the barriers or the possible reasons on why the male PLHIV did not discuss sex related concerns with them.

Table 10

#	Barriers		Reason for MLHIV not discussing about sex
1	Personal	-	MLHIV's priority concern is on getting well
		-	PLHIV's questions focuses on treatment, medication and other infections as those are their primary concerns.
		-	Sense of shame and discomfort to ask in hospital setting
		-	Client feel that they are not prepared to ask
		-	Lack of self confidence and fear of asking questions on sex
		-	MLHIV's disinterest to talk about taboo things
		-	They don't remember to ask
		-	Their depressed state of mind
		-	Guilt feeling does not encourage them to discuss about sex
		-	Most MLHIV want to distance themselves from sex as they abstain from sex or rarely perform an intercourse
		-	MLHIV become more religious after ART
		-	MLHIV have greater comfort to discuss this with their peers
		-	Sense of distrust in sharing with counsellors
		-	Male ego won't allow them to ask questions related to sex to female counsellors

Contd...

2	Social	- Comparatively lower age of the counsellors
		- Discomfort due to counsellor being of opposite gender
		- MLHIV feel that counsellor will think bad about them and are fearful on how the counsellor will react
		- MLHIV fear that others in the centre/ hospital will eventually know of their behaviour
		- Social stigma about HIV and sex doesn't allow
		- Cultural inhibitions, rural area culture doesn't allow such discussions on sex
		- MLHIV have reduced social interactions after HIV+ve status, don't want to open up
3	Structural	- Time constraints at the Centre for such discussion with the counsellors
		- ART counsellors have no time for individual counselling
		- Counsellors being involved in hospital paper work don't find quality time themselves for such discussion
		- Men perceive that their knowledge on the subject of sex is sufficient
		- Low education of clients does not encourage information seeking behaviour on sex.
		- Non-availability of a confidential room for one to one counselling
		- Presence of more than one person in the counselling room
		- Presence of spouse or other family members during counselling
		- Mostly only group counselling occurs, due to patient load at the ART and no individual sessions happen at the Centre

7.6 Frequency of MLHIV indulging in penetrative sex

The counsellors were inquired on their perception on how often did most of their MLHIV clients indulge in sexual relations, after their detection of HIV positive status. A few counsellors (5 percent) admitted that they never probed their MLHIV clients pertaining to the frequency of sexual indulgences and had no clue on this. The other counsellors who had probed into MLHIV's sexual behaviour state as below

Figure 9 Perceived frequency of MLHIV clients having sex after HIV detection

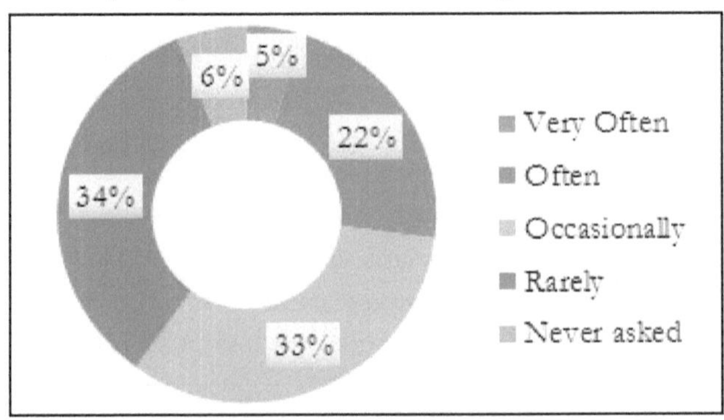

As seen in the graph above only 5 percent of the counsellors felt that their clients could be having sexual relations 'very often' *(more than 10 acts a month)* and 22 percent of the counsellors mentioned that most clients would be having sex 'often' *(4-10 acts a month)*, as they usually used to have before the HIV infection. Interestingly, two thirds of the counsellors (67 percent) were of the view that their MLHIV clients would possibly be having sex 'Occasionally' *(2-3 acts a month)* or 'Rarely' *(2-3 acts in a quarter)*. It is thus observed that 89 percent of the counsellors perceive that most of their clients have sex at least occasionally or more, even though they are HIV infected. This finding is triangulated with the data directly collected from the MLHIV in the next chapter.

Evidence which depicts the perception on frequency of sex

In order to ensure that the responses of the counsellors are not a notional perceptions but a result of active probing, the counsellors who perceived that their MLHIV's are having sex at least occasionally were asked to state the evidences on which they could base their perceptions. Thus the supportive evidences as provided by the counsellors on the frequency of MLHIV having sex are as follows.

Table 11 Evidence which depicts the perception on frequency of sex

#	Evidence base		Explanation
1	Spouses of MLHIV	-	MLHIV's spouses have asked the counsellor on the acceptable frequencies of having sexual
		-	intercourseSpouses have shared about their husband's sexual behaviours
		-	Many spouses confessed during their HIV counselling that they were not informed of their partners HIV status and hence they frequently allowed unsafe sex
		-	Spouses mention that MLHIV continue to have sex and they cannot refuse
2	MLHIV confessions during counselling	-	"ART medication has regained MLHIV health and hence the urge to have sex has increased"
		-	MLHIV have shared that sex being a basic human need cannot be withheld
		-	MLHIV confess that they have to meet the sexual demands of spouse
3	MLHIV's queries/ concerns	-	MLHIV clients asking for condoms/ picking up condoms from ART Centre.
		-	MLHIV raising queries on condom use and sharing their experiences in condom use
		-	MLHIV seeking information on safe sex methods
		-	Queries about their sexual performances
4	Probing skills of the counsellors	-	Risk assessment done by counsellor
		-	Risk reduction and behaviour change discussions with MLHIV
		-	Follow up visit reports of NGO outreach workers
		-	Experience sharing by peer educators

7.7 Frequency of safe sex indulgence

The counsellors were asked to perceive how frequently their MLHIV clients would be practising safe sex methods, based on the above evidences that they have explored. As observed in the graph below, most of the counsellors (89percent) iterated that their clients were having unsafe sex even after being detected HIV positive. About 11 percent of the counsellors confessed that they had no idea on the safe sex practices of their MLHIV clients.

Figure 10 Frequency of safe sex indulgence by MLHIV

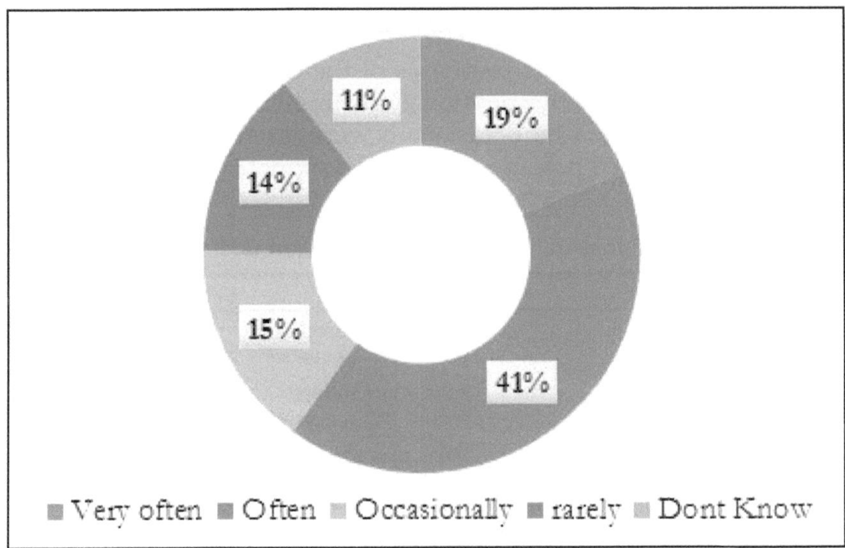

As seen in the figure above, only 19 percent of the counsellors felt that their MLHIV clients indulged in safe sex 'Very Often/ Always'. It is surprising to note that there is a major chunk of MLHIV who practice safe sex, not on every occasion, which is no doubt an enormous threat in the spread of the infection. It is also interesting to note that 14 percent counsellors felt that their clients 'Rarely' practiced safe sex, in spite of regular counselling and MLHIV being aware of the risks. This could be a matter of debate and therefore it further ascertained with the MLHIV data in the next chapter.

7.8 MLHIV who have sex with men

When probed on the counsellor's knowledge about their MLHIV clients who indulge in sex with men, it was observed about fifth of the counsellors (20 percent) did not know how many of their clients have sex with men. The other four-fifths of the counsellors substantiated that their clients are involved in MSM behaviour, either based on the risk indulgences, as explained by the clients or based on the clarifications sought by them on MSM behaviours.

The male female ratio of the counsellors, who reported that more than 5 percent of their MLHIV clients indulged in MSM behaviour was found to be 1:1. This implies that homosexual behaviour of MLHIV clients is shared with the counsellors irrespective of their gender. It was also observed that out of the 8 counsellors who stated that more than 5 percent of their MLHIV clients indulge in MSM behaviours, 7 counsellors were from MSACS and 1 from MDACS, implying the scope to understand that the MSM behaviour is also as pertinent in other districts of Maharashtra, as that in Mumbai.

The graph below shows the percentage of MLHIV clients who are MSM, as per the knowledge of the counsellors.

Figure 11 Percentage of MLHIV who had sex with men

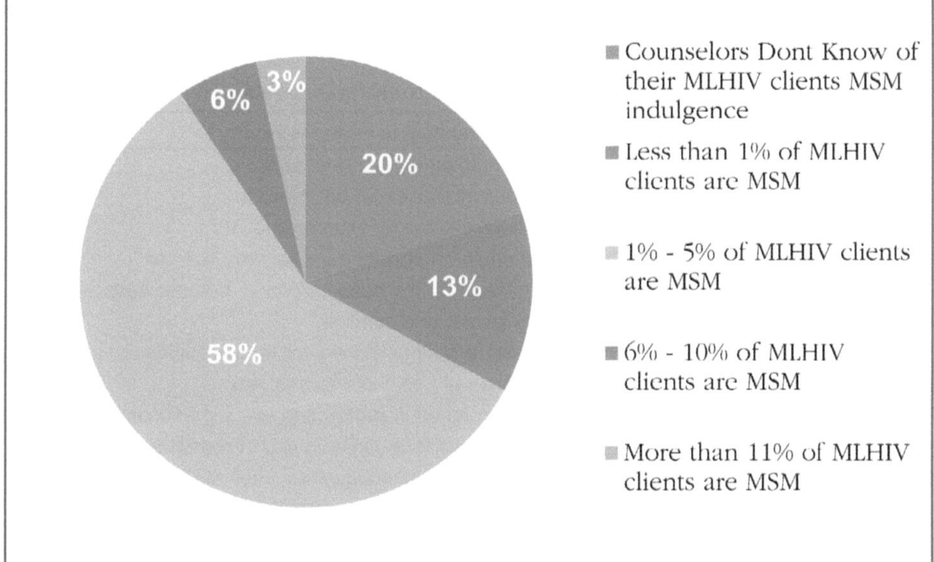

Safe sex measures practiced by MSM:

The counsellors were further enquired if the above mentioned clients indulging in MSM behaviour practiced safe sex. A few (15.3 percent) of the counsellors admitted that they never probed with their MSM clients if they practiced safe sex or not. However, half of the counsellors (50.6 percent) answered in negative stating that their MLHIV clients would sadly be practicing unsafe sex with men. Only less than one third of the counsellors (30.6 percent) felt assured that their MLHIV clients, who are MSM, practiced safe sex.

7.9 MLHIV asking questions pertaining to homosexuality

In an attempt to understand the homosexual practices amongst MLHIV, the counsellors were further probed on how many of the MLHIV counselled by them had ever asked them questions related to homosexuality. Around half (45.8 percent) of the counsellors reported that none of their MLHIV clients had ever asked them any query with regards to homosexuality. While 41.2 percent of counsellors reported that around 1 to 5 percent of their MLHIV clients, whom they had counselled, had ever asked questions pertaining to homosexuality.

On comparing the percentage of MLHIV who indulge in MSM behaviour, with the percentage of MLHIV asking counsellors questions pertaining to homosexuality, it is observed that there are comparatively greater number of MLHIV clients are practicing homosexuality than those asking questions related to homosexuality. This finding is in contrast to what is logically expected out of the MLHIV clients. Thus the MLHIV who are MSM seem to be placing themselves at greater risks, by not eliciting proper/ adequate information from the counsellors. The reasons for this have been explored in the MLHIV interviews.

MLHIV's Queries related to homosexuality

In order to get more insight into the concerns of MSM, the counsellors further persuaded to explain the kind of questions asked by the MLHIV with relation to homosexuality, which have been tabulated as under:

Table 12: Queries related to homosexuality

#	Themes	- Queries related to homosexuality
1	Seeking knowledge on understanding concepts of MSM	- Understanding the concept of MSM - Common homosexual behaviours - Link between homosexuality and HIV - Information on performing anal sex, oral sex - Percentage of HIV susceptibility in homosexuals - Moral issues and conflicts - Process to adopt children, for MSM couples
2	Addressing Sexual Problems	- Weakness of penis due to anal sex - Problems faced in performing sex with discordant partners - Handling partner's denial in use of condoms - Scope for sexual indulgences after ART - Anxiety of HIV infection bothering sexual relations
3	MLHIV assessing risk behaviours amidst MSM	- Risk behaviours for HIV transmission to partner - Safety precautions while performing anal sex - Risk involved in oral sex - Is oral sex safer than anal sex? - Chances of STI in anal sex - What to do in case of an STI? - Risk reduction practices
4	Safe sex related queries amidst MSM	- Precautions to be taken while performing safe sex - Techniques & issues in masturbation, mutual masturbation - Use of condoms designed for anal sex - Impact of condom use and condom related issues - More information on jelly use, other lubricants - Other methods of safe sex besides condoms
5	Seeking skills in handling situations arising amongst MSM partners	- Addressing relationship issues among discordant MSM - Skills related to ascertaining partners HIV status - Convincing partner for HIV testing - How to play safe if partners are coercive - Issues related to heterosexual marriage pressures - Maintaining MSM partners and relationships - Maintaining confidentiality on one's sexuality

Counsellor's response on queries pertaining to homosexuality

In view of the above questions asked by MLHIV in relation to homosexuality, the counsellors were asked to mention their responses to these queries. During analysis, the responses of the counsellors were classified into those which were in favour (70 percent) or not in favour (30 percent) of homosexuality as seen below:

Table 13 Counsellor's responses to queries related to MSM behaviours

In favour Responses 70 percent counsellors	Not in favour Responses 30 percent counsellors
- Being faithful to one MSM partner	- Abstain male partners
- Correct and consistent condom use	- Focus on having sex only with the spouse
- Condom demonstration	- Homosexuality exposes greater risks to HIV than heterosexuals and should be avoided
- Emphasizing that anal sex is safe	- MSM behaviour is not natural and has to be changed
- Promotion of oral sex	- MSM activity has scientific problems hence should not be practiced
- Use condoms for oral sex too	- Masturbate instead of having oral sex
- Treat MSM inclinations as normal	
- Safe sex methods explained	
- Explained high risk behaviours	
- Risk reduction plans discussed	
- Referrals to STI counsellor	
- Partner reduction	
- Partner notification	
- Importance of Consent	

The responses of counsellors who were in favour of MSM counselling did not seem adequate and there is certainly more scope for further harm reduction inputs on counselling MSM. The 'Not in favour' responses of the counsellors in the above table, also provides a scope to understand the attitudes of the counsellors towards the issue and this area that has to be considered for further inputs during counselling training.

MLHIV clients who are bisexual

In this context of MSM behaviour, the counsellors knowledge was further sought on how many of their MLHIV clients seem to be bisexual. It is observed that more than half (57.6 percent) of the counsellors believe that 1 to 5 percent of their clients are bisexual. Interestingly, one-tenth of the counsellors (9.4 percent) believe that more than 6 percent of their clients were bisexual. The remaining one - third of the counsellors had no clue if their MLHIV clients practiced bisexual behaviour or not. The correctness of this perception of the counsellor will need to be ascertained and understood in detail in the MLHIV interviews.

The need for identifying and counselling bisexuals are also an area that needs due attention in Counselling Trainings.

7.10 Types of penetrative sexual behaviours by practiced by MLHIV

The type of penetrative indulgences of the MLHIV clients that were shared with the counsellors was probed into. The counsellors reported the MLHIV indulge in

Anal, Oral or Vaginal sex, as penetrative practices. The counsellor's perception on the frequencies of MLHIV's penetrative indulgences is discretely recorded as below.

Figure 12 Penetrative Sexual Behaviour: Anal vs Oral vs Vaginal

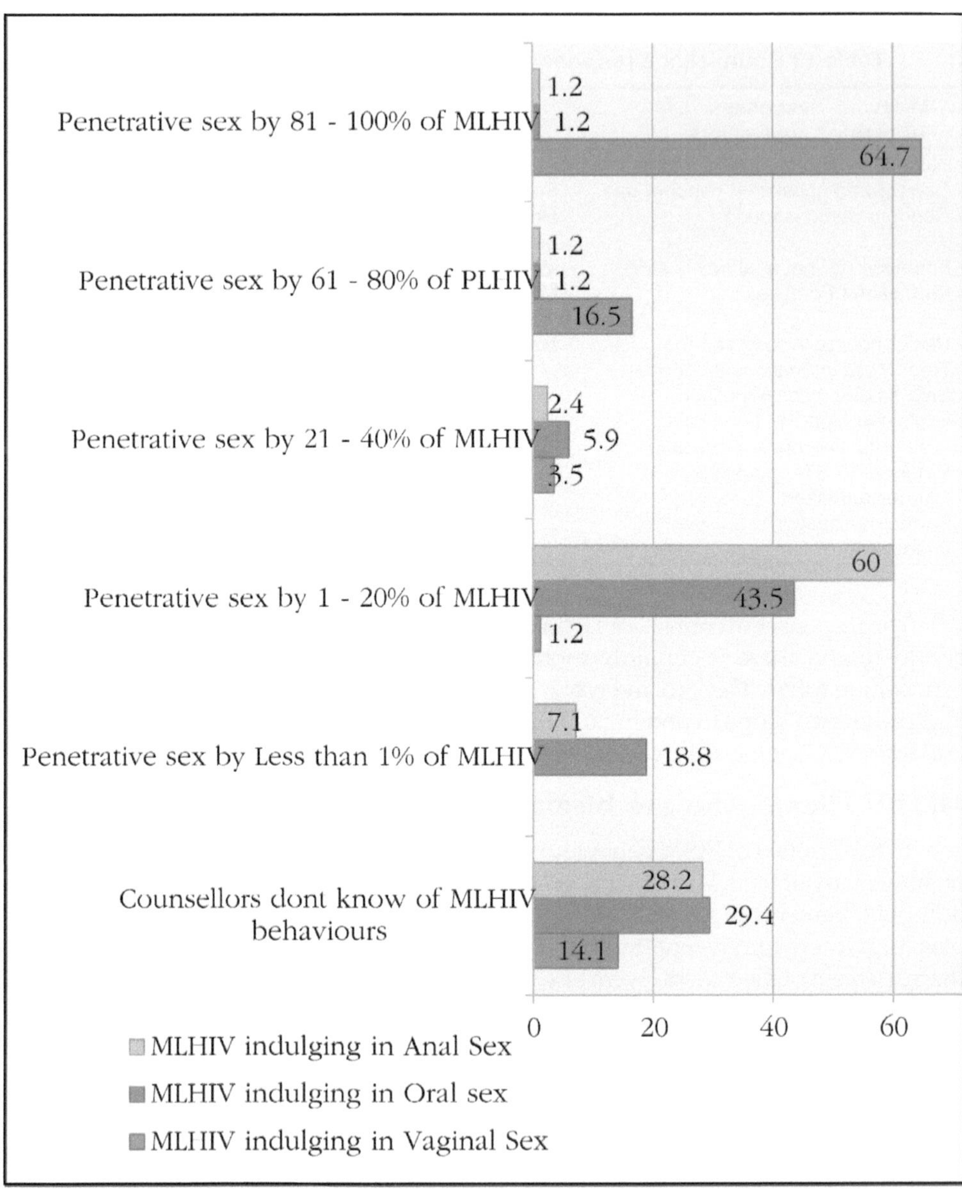

The bars in the graphs above indicate the percentile of MLHIV indulging in each of the penetrative practices. It is observed that about three in every ten of the counsellors (28.2 & 29.4 percent) did not know whether their MLHIV clients indulged in oral and anal sexual behaviour respectively, while 14.1 percent did not know if their clients had vaginal sex. Most of the counsellors (60 percent) report that 1-20 percent of their MLHIV clients indulge in Anal Sex. According to the counsellors, it is interesting to note that oral sex is not commonly practices by the MLHIV clients.

The percentage of MLHIV's penetrative sexual behaviour as perceived by the counsellors reveal the following statistics about MLHIV penetrative sexual behaviour:

Table 14 Counsellor's perception on Penetrative practices of MLHIV

Penetrative practices of MLHIV	Mean% of MLHIV	Standard Deviation	Median
Anal Sex	8.06 %	15.37 %	3 %
Oral Sex	8.79 %	17.23 %	2 %
Vaginal Sex	86.68 %	17.04 %	90 %

Couple of counsellors working for 2 years with ART-MSACS mentioned that 70 and 100 percent of their MLHIV clients respectively indulge in Anal and Oral sex. Due to these 2 outliers the mean value seems to be skewed to a higher value, the Median value therefore has been considered to understand the central tendency in this discussion. In conclusion, an average of 3 percent of MLHIV clients indulge in anal sex, while 2 percent indulge in Oral sex and 90 percent indulge in Vaginal Sex.

The knowledge of counsellors on MLHIV's 'Type of penetrative sexual behaviour' was correlated with 'Years of experience of the counsellor', also with the 'Type of Centre' and with the 'Age group of counsellors'. However none of these variables seemed to be significantly correlated. It can thus be stated that the counsellor's knowledge of their MLHIV behaviours is not dependent on their age, years of experience or even the type of centre that they are working with.

However, when the number of counsellors who did not know of the types of MLHIV sexual behaviour practiced, were correlated with their gender, it was interesting to observe that at least double the number of female counsellors did not know about the MLHIV client's sexual behaviour. This indicates that gender of the counsellor seems to play a role in their knowledge of MLHIV client's penetrative sexual behaviour.

7.11 Counsellor's Response in addressing sexual concerns of MLHIV

The counsellors were asked of their focus in counselling, when an MLHIV client expresses his need to have sex with his partner. The counsellor's response provided to the MLHIV is as recorded Table 15.

Table 15 Behaviour Change input by Counsellors

#	Themes	Behaviour change inputs of counsellors for MLHIV wanting to indulge in sexual relations
1	Focus on Abstinence	Abstinence from sex as much as possible
		Stress on abstinence messages for discordant couples
		Avoid vaginal sex (in case of heterosexual)
		Avoid anal/oral sex (in case of homosexual)
		Disadvantages in having sex
2	Focus on Risk reduction	Being faithful
		Correct and consistent condom use
		Education on disadvantages of not using condoms
		Provision of condoms
		Avoid visiting risky places and getting further infected
		Have sex only 'occasionally'
		Reduction in number of sexual partner
3	Harm Reduction messages	Education on sex and safe sex practices
		Positive prevention techniques
		Contraceptive use education
		Inputs on non-penetrative sex include masturbation, hugging, kissing, oral sex
		Risk education
		Inputs on chances of acquiring resistant virus
		Inputs on viral load increase
		STI information
4	Partner focused messages	Need for consent of both partners in sex emphasised
		Need for regular partner check up
		Condom use for discordant couple
		Encouraging safe sex with non PLHIV
		Discussions on choosing partners for sex
		Express your interest of having sex with spouse
		Training partners on condom negotiation skills

The focus on abstinence and risk reduction education by the counsellors as mentioned in the table above indicate that counsellors tend to be moral policing their MLHIV clients. It will be interesting to observe the acceptance of these by MLHIV as steps towards behaviour change in the next chapter.

7.12 Prevention strategies used by MLHIV

In continuation to counsellors education on behaviour change, the counsellors perception on its implementation by the MLHIV clients were solicited. The percentage of MLHIV clients implementing behaviour change strategies in the areas of Abstinence, Being Faithful or Condom Use were discretely investigated with the counsellors. There were about 15 percent of the counsellors, who did not have any knowledge about their MLHIV client's preventive behaviours. A consolidated view of each strategy used by the MLHIV in prevention of HIV transmission through sexual route, is graphically represented Figure 13

Figure 13 Counsellors Perception of MLHIV using the 'A – B – C' prevention strategies

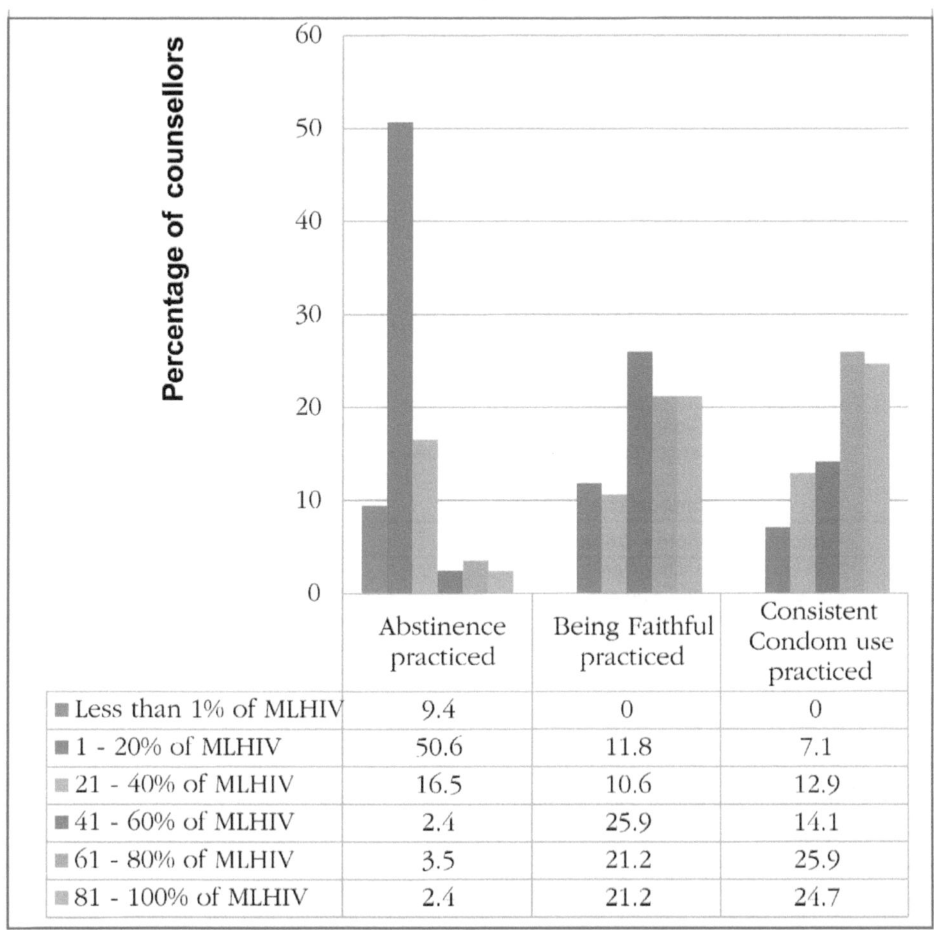

	Abstinence practiced	Being Faithful practiced	Consistent Condom use practiced
Less than 1% of MLHIV	9.4	0	0
1 - 20% of MLHIV	50.6	11.8	7.1
21 - 40% of MLHIV	16.5	10.6	12.9
41 - 60% of MLHIV	2.4	25.9	14.1
61 - 80% of MLHIV	3.5	21.2	25.9
81 - 100% of MLHIV	2.4	21.2	24.7

The tallest bars in the graph represent the perceptions of most number of counsellors on the percentile of MLHIV on each of the prevention strategies adopted by the MLHIV. The skewing on abstinence is on the lower end (1-20 percent of the MLHIV), which grows into plateau in use of the strategy of 'Being Faithful'. As expected the strategy of consistent condom use is skewed at the higher end (60-100 percent of MLHIV). Thus the increasing order of the use of strategies A-B-C is clear.

7.13 Factors influencing the use of Prevention Strategies

The counsellors were asked to explain further on the factors that influence the MLHIV clients in choosing appropriate prevention strategies after the onset of HIV infection. This would help provide insight into understanding various intervening variables, which influence the decisions taken by the MLHIV in regard to prevention. According to counsellor's responses, the factors influencing A-B-C were collated under 4 broad themes namely factors related to Self, Partner, Social and Structural.

Table 16

Areas	Factors Influencing Behaviour Change	Abstinence	Being Faithful	Consistent Condom use
	Hopelessness about their situation	Yes		
	Guilt feeling	Yes	Yes	
	State of depression	Yes		
	As repentance for illicit behaviour	Yes	Yes	
	Fear of death/ Wants to live longer	Yes	Yes	
	Fear about acquiring OI	Yes	Yes	Yes
	Fear of STI acquisition	Yes	Yes	Yes
Individual	Hate for sex after HIV infection	Yes		
	Lack/decrease in sexual desire	Yes		
	Feeling of impotence	Yes		
	To prevent any further increase in viral load	Yes	Yes	Yes
	Fear of re-infection	Yes	Yes	Yes
	Focus on medication and improving health	Yes		Yes
	Bed ridden nature of clients	Yes		
	Poor physical health	Yes		
	Fear loss of strength due to indulgence in sex	Yes		
	Window period	Yes		
	Fear of ART complications / failure		Yes	Yes
	Factors Influencing Behaviour Change	**A**	**B**	**C**
	Prevent HIV transmission to partner	Yes		Yes
	Protect discordant spouse	Yes		Yes
	Reduce viral load of partner	Yes		
	Demonstrate love/ commitment to partner	Yes	Yes	
Partner focused	Re-build trust in spouse	Yes	Yes	
	Death of spouse	Yes		
	Dislike for spouse	Yes		
	Divorce or separation of spouse	Yes		
	Fear of separation of spouse		Yes	
	Issues in relationship with spouse	Yes		
	Greater level of sexual satisfaction with spouse		Yes	
	Under sexual partners insistence			Yes
	Factors Influencing Behaviour Change	**A**	**B**	**C**
	Protect others	Yes		
	Save family from the disease	Yes		
	Focus is on planning future of children	Yes		
Social	Family responsibilities, addressing family problems are priority	Yes		
	Concern for future of child and family	Yes	Yes	
	To keep up with social norms		Yes	
	Interactions with the society is lost after HIV		Yes	
	Factors Influencing Behaviour Change	**A**	**B**	**C**
	Can't have sex since children have grown up	Yes		
	Small home *(no private space for having sex)*	Yes		
	Joint family values	Yes		
Structural	Religious involvement	Yes	Yes	
	Disinterest in sex due to aging	Yes		
	Developed understanding of ethics and morality		Yes	
	Developed understanding of HIV		Yes	Yes
	Influence of counselling education on safe sex		Yes	Yes
	Family planning / contraception needs			Yes

It is observed that the counsellors focus more on the abstinence messages addressing the individual rather than focus on social and structural factors.

7.14 Counsellors perception on DISCLOSURE amongst MLHIV

The counsellors were inquired of their knowledge of MLHIV client's status disclosure to their spouse as well as their non-spousal partners. Their responses have been graphically represented as below:

Figure 14 Counsellor's knowledge on their client's level of disclosure

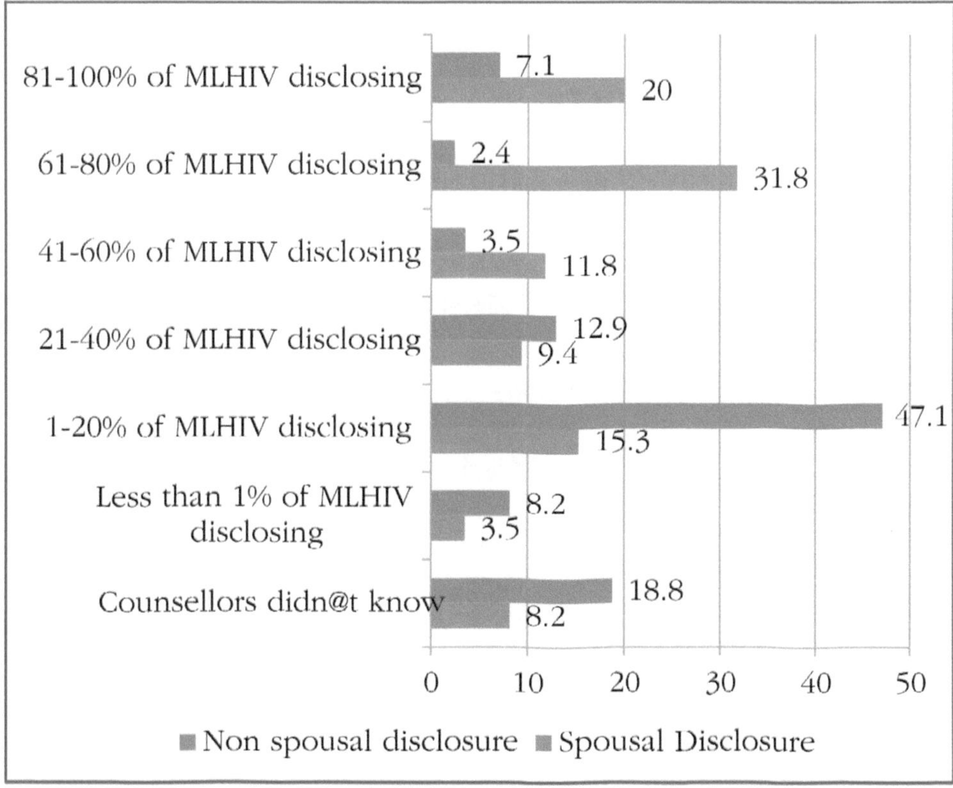

As seen in the graph above, the longest bar represents the maximum number of counsellors who opine about the percentile of 'MLHIV status disclosure'. The skewing of the Non spousal disclosure bars *(red coloured)* towards the lower end (1-20 percent MLHIV) and spousal disclosure bars *(blue coloured)* to the higher end (60-100 percent MLHIV), speaks volumes about the contrast in MLHIV's disclosure patterns.

Spousal Disclosure: As seen above, 8.2 percent of the counsellors admitted that they had no idea if their MLHIV clients had discussed their HIV status with their spouses. As reported by the counsellors, 58.3 percent (Average Mean with a standard deviation of 30.9 percent) {Average median = 70 percent}, of their MLHIV clients seems to have disclosed their status with their spouses. Concealment of HIV status between couples could be problematic because on one hand it may prevent the MLHIV in seeking support from the spouse and on the other hand, it may become a barrier to accepting behavioural interventions for prevention of HIV transmission. The data also shows that some counsellors are not paying adequate attention to the 'spouse disclosure' issue of the clients. The reasons did not feature in the study and should be further explored.

Non Spousal Disclosure: Similarly, 18.8 percent of the counsellors admitted that they had no idea if their MLHIV clients had discussed their HIV status with their non spousal partners. On an average, 24.3 percent (mean value with a standard deviation of 27.8 percent) {Average median = 20 percent}, of the MLHIV would have disclosed their status to non spousal partners. This indicates that the counsellors may probably have to also look into the importance of disclosure to non spousal sexual partners.

7.15 Conditions of HIV Disclosure to Spouse

The counsellors were asked to choose *(multiple responses allowed)*, the conditions under which their MLHIV clients would be influenced to disclose their HIV status to their sexual partner.

Figure 15 Conditions under which MLHIV disclose their HIV status

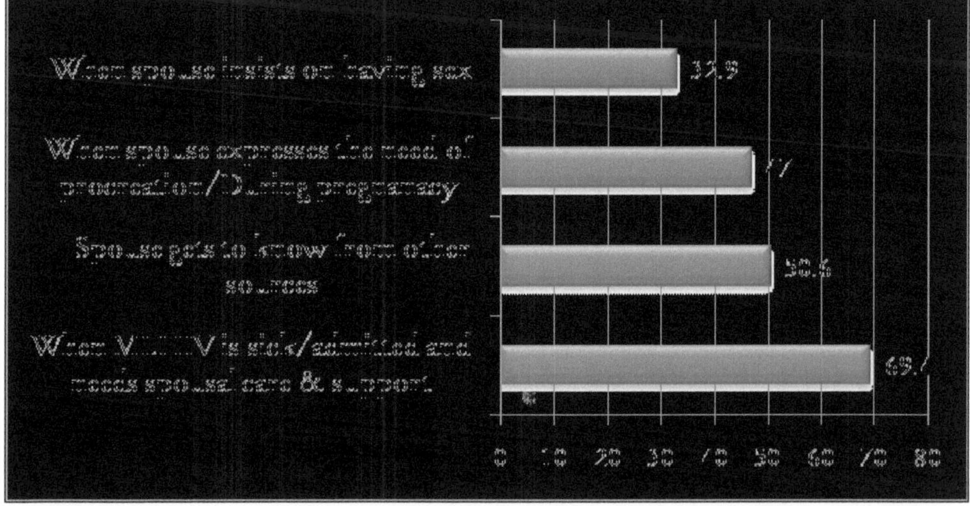

Most counsellors (69.4 percent) agreed that MLHIV disclose their HIV status to their spouse only when they are admitted in the hospital and when in dire need of spousal care and support. Sadly more than half of the counsellors (50.6 percent) were of the view that the MLHIV do not disclose their status and that the spouse gets to know from other sources. This is a serious condition that may cause ruptures in spousal relationship and MLHIV need to be encouraged to address this gap in period of disclosure.

Besides the above mentioned reasons, the counsellors added that the MLHIV clients also disclose their HIV status under these conditions:

1. Immediately after the HIV test of spouse
2. When couple have come to hospital for routine check up or blood tests
3. When the spouse has to tested HIV positive during pregnancy

7.16 Impact of Disclosure on spousal sexual relations

The counsellors were inquired on what according to them was impact of MLHIV's status disclosure to spouse on their sexual relationship. The responses of counsellors have been graphically depicted below

Figure 16 Impact of spousal disclosure on sexual relations

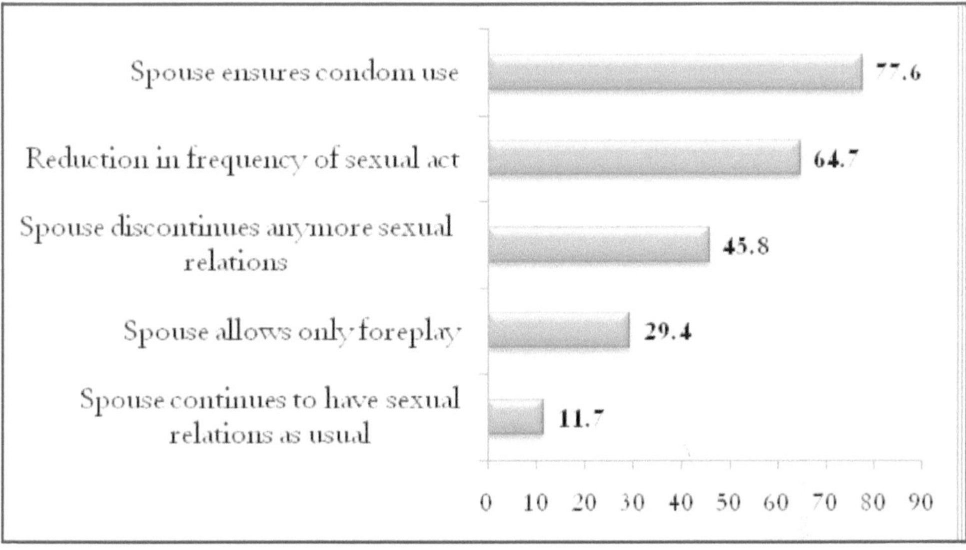

Accordingly, most counsellors were of the view that after MLHIV's disclosure, the spouses would ensure condoms use (77.6 percent) and that there was a reduction in the frequency sexual activity (64.7 percent).

Interestingly, over a tenth of the counsellors (11.7 percent) report the naive attitude of the spouses, who continue to have sexual relations with their male counterparts' as usual in spite of the knowledge of the HIV status. This aspect was investigated further, on what could be the reason why the spouses of MLHIV, continue to have sex, although the spouse knew of their male counterparts HIV infection.

As seen figure-16, most counsellors attribute the sexual partners high risk indulgence with the MLHIV, to their lack of negotiation skills (78.8 percent). Further, over one third of the counsellors (36.4 percent) add that their MLHIV clients have coerced their partners into sex in spite of the knowledge of their own status. Coercion into sex is a violation of human rights and the spouses need to be conscientised on their rights.

Additionally, some other reasons of spousal indulgence in sexual relations with MLHIV, as stated by the counsellors include:

- In a patriarchal society, only the man has a say in sexual relations
- Spousal belief and trust in husband cannot be defeated
- Spouse treats MLHIV husband as God in our culture
- Sex is considered an part of marriage, whether partner is infected or not
- Spouse does not want the MLHIV to have sex with anyone outside
- Spouse fears rupture of interpersonal relationship by denying sex
- Spouse lack knowledge on seriousness of HIV infection
- Non availability of better options for sex for the spouse to meet their desires
- Spouse is fatalistic and not afraid of death

Figure 17 Reasons for the spouses engage in sex knowing MLHIV status

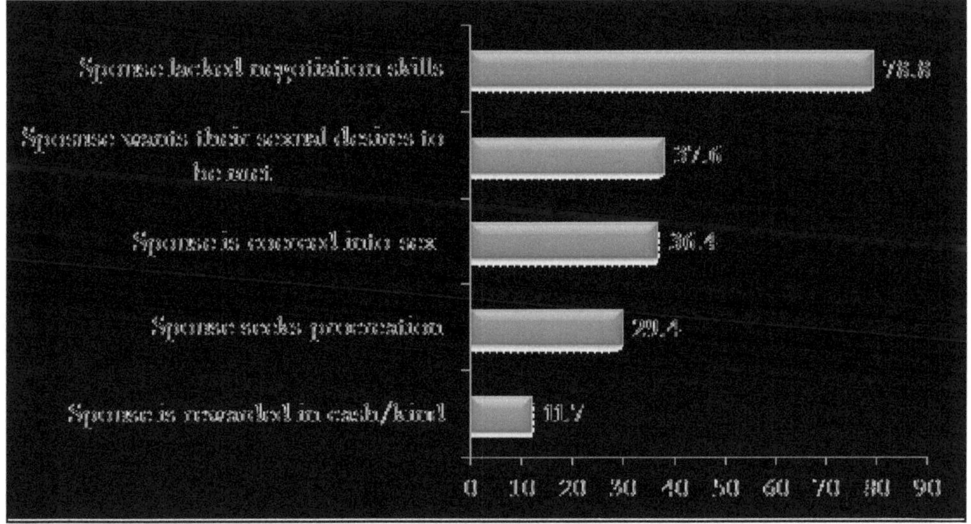

(N = 85, Multiple response)

As seen above, most counsellors attribute the sexual partners high risk indulgence with the MLHIV, to their lack of negotiation skills (78.8 percent). Further, over one third of the counsellors (36.4 percent) add that their MLHIV clients have coerced their partners into sex in spite of the knowledge of their own status. Coercion into sex is a violation of human rights and the spouses need to be conscientised on their rights.

Additionally, some other reasons of spousal indulgence in sexual relations with MLHIV, as stated by the counsellors include:

- In a patriarchal society, only the man has a say in sexual relations
- Spousal belief and trust in husband cannot be defeated
- Spouse treats MLHIV husband as God in our culture
- Sex is considered an part of marriage, whether partner is infected or not

- Spouse does not want the MLHIV to have sex with anyone outside
- Spouse fears rupture of interpersonal relationship by denying sex
- Spouse lack knowledge on seriousness of HIV infection
- Non availability of better options for sex for the spouse to meet their desires
- Spouse is fatalistic and not afraid of death

7.17 TRAINING NEEDS *expressed by counsellors*

The need to develop a curriculum on sex and sexuality in counselling training was rated important by the counsellors and their inputs for the suggested content of the curriculum has been accounted as under.

Table 17 Training needs identified by the counsellors

#	Training Themes	Content to be covered in Trainings
1	Reproductive Health	- Sexual health/hygiene - Male - female anatomy and its functions - Impact of sexual behaviour on physiology - Sexual behaviour during menstruation - Contraceptive methods
2	Sex, Sexuality and Sexual Behaviours	- Basics of sex - Impact of gender on sexuality - Misconceptions on sex - Theories on sex and sexuality - Sexual orientations - Types of sexualities - Types of having sex - Good and bad practices regarding sex - Risky behaviours and non risky practices - Content of sex education for educating PLHIV - How to question clients on their sexual practices - How to educate MLHIV on controlling sexual behaviour
3	Sexual Minorities	- How to identify TG/ homosexual, - TG/MSM counselling on safe sex practices How sex amongst transsexuals happen - Sexual behaviour research findings of PLHA, MSM, TG - Psychology of bisexuals
4	Safe sex methods	- Difference between safe sex and unsafe sex - Benefits in safe sex/ why have safe sex - Stages of safe sex - Attaining orgasm without intercourse - Counselling content on safe sexual practices - Sex for concordant couples - Sex for discordant couples - condom negotiation skills, demonstration of condoms, female condoms, - how to convince women for methods of safe sex - Use of foreplay for orgasm - Abstinence education - Ways to masturbate in males and females, - Thigh sex, breast sex, Afterplay

Contd...

5	Issues and Skills in Counselling	- Building mutual understanding amongst partners to indulge in safe sex - Handling queries of adolescence and children - Whether to promote sex or not - How to reduce extramarital sexual relations - Addressing problems related to sex faced by PLHIV - Communicating with illiterate persons about sex
6	General Areas	- Behaviour change - Behaviour change techniques - Handling impact of disclosure on sexual relation - Risk reduction strategies - How to encourage being faithful - Life of virus in the body fluids - Disclosure pattern with sex partners - Micro skills required in sexuality counselling - Role plays on sexuality counselling
7	Frequently asked questions by MLHIV	- How to increase pleasure - How to prolong sexual act/ penile errection - Choosing partners for sex - Prepare male partner for safe sex, - Disadvantages in having sex

7.18 Major Findings of Phase 1

Out of the 85 counsellors interviewed most were ART counsellors and the findings of this phase are summarised below:

Major Findings: Counsellors Profile

- Two thirds of the counsellors were males
- Only 7 percent of the counsellors retained for five years with more females continuing in this job
- 95 percent of the counsellors were 35 years or lesser in age
- Only one fifths had a psychology background for their Masters Degree

Major Findings: Counsellors perception of Sexual Behaviours of MLHIV

- An average 43 percent of the clients ask counsellors questions related to sex.
- Counsellors with an experience of less than a year were not asked such questions
- Male counsellors are approached by MLHIV with questions related to sex.
- The MLHIV have asked more queries pertaining to sexual behaviours, safe practices, concerns about their sexual problems and about maintaining sexual relationship with non-spousal partners
- The counsellors felt that the MLHIV do not open up in discussing their sexual concerns at the centre mostly due to their personal barriers in communicating freely (like taboo, shame, bias, depression, guilt, perceived threat of being misunderstood) or due to structural limitations of the centre (like time, superiority complex, opposite gender of counsellor, non availability of space for confidentiality.

- One third counsellors never asked their MLHIV about their sexual behaviours post HIV detection. While the other counsellors perceived that the frequency of penetrative sex by MLHIV, were rare or occasional. The counsellors elicited this information not just through confessions of their MLHIV client but also through direct and indirect probing with MLHIV and spouses.
- About 41 percent of the counsellors did not know how often their MLHIV clients practiced safe sex. Of the remaining more counsellors felt that safe sex is rarely practiced by MLHIV.
- One fifth of the counsellors did not have any clue if their MLHIV clients indulged in sexual relations with men. More than half of the counsellors perceived that 1-5 percent of their MLHIV clients indulged in MSM.
- Nearly half of the counsellors were never asked any queries related to sex with men, by their MLHIV clients. While the others claimed that not more than 5 percent of their clients would ask such queries. The queries related to MSM asked to the counsellors include: understanding MSM, addressing problems in practicing homosexuality, ascertaining whether their behaviours were risky, discussions on safe sex and skills in addressing relationship issues within the MSM couple.
- About one third of the counsellors through their responses to MSM clients showed that they were not in favour of MSM behaviour.
- One third of the counsellors did not know if any of their MLHIV clients were bisexual, while more than half of the counsellors claimed that 1-5 percent of their male clients would be bisexual.
- Around one fourth of the counsellors did not know of the types of penetrative sex practiced by their MLHIV clients. One fifth of the counsellors felt that less than 1 percent of the clients would have indulged in Oral sex. About 60 percent of the counsellors felt that about 20 percent of their clients indulged in Anal sex. 65 percent of the counsellors stated that more than 80 percent of their clients would be indulging in vaginal sex.

Major Findings: Counsellors perception of Behaviour change amidst MLHIV

- Counselling on behaviour change of MLHIV varies from counsellor to counsellor and covers the aspects of abstinence from penetrative sex, being faithful, condom and contraceptive use, reduction in number of partners, education on safe sex practices, non-penetrative sex, STI information, steps to reduce viral load and partner focused relationship building messages.
- A Sixth of the counsellors felt that less than 20 percent of their MLHIV clients would be practicing complete abstinence as a prevention strategy. Only two-tenth of the counsellors felt that more than 80 percent of their MLHIV clients would be monogamous. And only one fourth of the counsellors felt that more than 80 percent of their clients would be consistently using condoms.

- The counsellors felt that most of the MLHIV who practiced abstinence would be doing so to protect the health of themselves as well as their partner. Also because abstinence was socially desirable to prevent the spread of infection, or as a family planning tool or as an aspect of demonstrating responsibility to needs of family and children. Structural factors like space limitations at home, religious involvement and growing age have also influenced abstinence.
- Monogamy was practiced since MLHIV felt guilty and repented or in the fear of OI/ STI/ increasing viral load/ ART failure. It was also practiced as to re-build trust in spouse or for the fear of separation or since they found their spouses to be more sexually satisfying than other partners.
- The practice of Consistent Condom use was initiated as a protection from OI/ STI or from fear of re-infection/ super-infection or fearing complications of ART. The partner's discordant status, concern for HIV infection or their insistence of safe sex influenced the MLHIV to use condoms. Other influencing factors include HIV education, safe sex counselling and family planning needs.

Major Findings: Counsellors perception of Disclosure amidst MLHIV

- Two tenths of the counsellors did not know of whether their clients would have undertaken spousal disclosure, while only a fifth of the counsellors felt that more than 80 percent of their MLHIV would have disclosed their status to the spouses.
- With regards to non-spousal disclosure, a tenth of the counsellor did not have any clue if their MLHIV would have done so and nearly half of them feel that only less than 20 percent of their MLHIV clients would have ever disclosed their status to non spousal partners.
- More than half of the counsellors feel that disclosure to spouses would have been during the sickness of MLHIV or the spouse would have got to know from other sources or during their pregnancy.
- More than half of the counsellors perceived that as an impact of disclosure the spouses would have ensured condom use or reduced the frequency of sexual relations or abstained completely.
- The counsellors stated that spouses give in to sexual relations with MLHIV since they lack negotiation skills (79 percent) or in want of their sexual desires to be met (38 percent) or are coerced into sex (36 percent) or because they seek procreation (30 percent).

Conclusion

The data captured in Phase-1 thus illustrate the importance of examining relational factors in order to better understand MLHIV behaviours. The design of the study limits the interpretation of these findings to associations, not causations.

Findings from this chapter have important implications for developing training curriculum targeting counsellors. There seems a need especially for the experienced counsellors have to make proactive attempts to solicit sexuality related counselling with MLHIV. The counsellors need to stress more on harm reduction approaches. Greater efforts need to be taken toward assisting spousal disclosure. The attitudes of the counsellors towards sexuality related discussions with the MLHIV have also come out very strongly, which needs to be dealt with appropriately, in the training programs. The explorations on disclosure and factors influencing behaviour change are potential variables to be studied at length in the Phase-2 interviews with MLHIV.

Chapter 8

PHASE 2: MLHIV INTERVIEWS FINDINGS ON SEXUAL BEHAVIOR OF MLHIV

INTRODUCTION

The Phase-2 of this study elicits data from MLHIV in Mumbai, who are on ART, on aspects of their Sexual Behaviours, Disclosure and Behaviour Change. The MLHIV were selected from the community through non-governmental organisations working in the community. The MLHIV who could give time for this interview, was open to talking about their sexual histories and was willing to give written consent, were purposefully chosen using a non random sampling method. Interviews were conducted with 152 MLHIV respondents in Mumbai using an Interview Schedule with closed and open ended questions. The findings of Phase 1 have been recorded in three different chapters for the convenience of the reader namely Sexual behaviour, Disclosure and Behaviour Change, as bifurcated in the theoretical chapters.

The layout of chapter focuses specifically on the findings derived on the sexual behaviour aspects of MLHIV and covers the following broad areas

1. Socio Economic and health Profile of MLHIV and their spouses
2. Pre and Extra marital sexual relations of MLHIV
3. Dimensions of Sexual practices
4. Attitudes of MLHIV towards male sexuality

Keeping these boundaries in mind a detailed analysis on each of these areas has been presented below:

8.1 SOCIO ECONOMIC PROFILE of MLHIV AND THEIR SPOUSES

The respondents profile was explored before understanding their sexual behaviour. As a part of the profile, respondents were inquired about their age, period of residence in Mumbai, educational achievement, occupation, and marital status, personal and family income. Further, their self and spousal health status inclusive of CD4 count, ART, STI, OI and the subsequent phases of infection were explored too.

Age : The minimum age of the respondent, who participated in this study was 23 years and the maximum age of 56 years. The mean age of the respondent was 38.09 years with a standard deviation of 6 years. Most respondents (88.8 percent) were in age bracket of 30 to 50 years.

Years of stay in Mumbai: In comparison with other researches it will be interesting to assess if the acquisition of HIV infection in Mumbai is influenced by the high risk exposures of the metropolitan hub. One of the inclusive criterions for this study was that the respondents should have resided in Mumbai for at least 10 years. This inclusive criterion was used to achieve homogeneity of the sample. Further, literatures on sexual behaviours point out that duration of stay in Mumbai is an intrinsic variable in contextually understanding the sexual behaviours of men. It is thus noted that about half of the respondents were born in Mumbai and about one fourth of the respondents came to Mumbai before the age of 18 years. The average age of stay in Mumbai was 29.18 years with a standard deviation of 10.4 years. Most respondents (59.9 percent) have spent 20 to 40 years in Mumbai.

The data indicates that greater the respondents age, the greater their years of their stay in Mumbai. Since the respondents were purposefully selected to be residents in Mumbai, the age of the respondent shows significant positive correlation with the duration of stay in Mumbai with a Pearson's asymptomatic significance of 0.000 (with r value=0.349).

Educational Achievement: As seen in the pie below, about 45 percent of the respondents have not completed their secondary education and only one fifth of the respondents (23 percent) had completed at least Higher secondary education (i.e., std 12th and above).

Secondary and Higher secondary education are key stages of education on health, hygiene and prevention of various illness. Would the respondents know of HIV, STI and the significance for use of condoms? Does the level of education have an impact on the health status of the respondent, the level of indulgence in high risk behaviours, their attitude towards sexuality, initiatives towards disclosure and behaviour change, are some question that need further exploration.

Figure 18 Educational Achievement of MLHIV

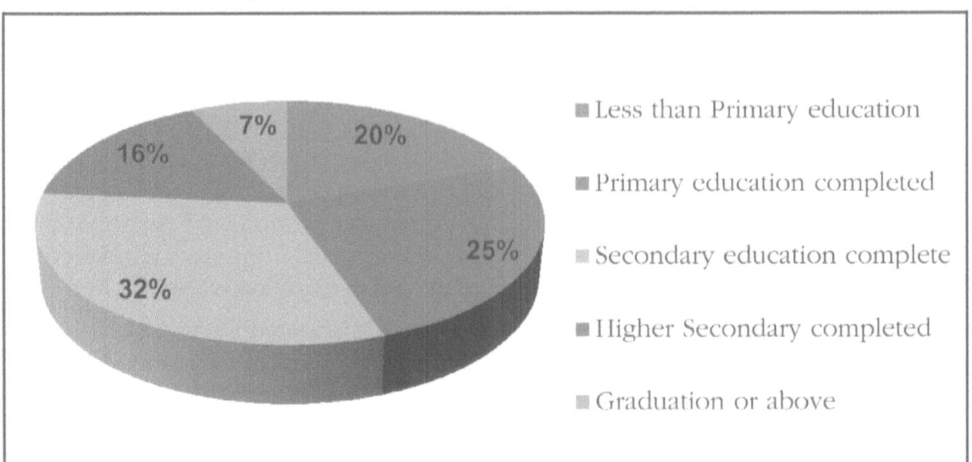

Occupation: Except for about one tenth (9 percent) of the respondents all others were employed. Only one third of the respondents (35 percent), were into service (like printing press, security, company staff, etc.) which offers them a steady income and appropriate leave and health policies. The rest of the respondents were daily wage labourers (28 percent), one fifth of the respondents (20 percent) run their own business and 8 percent of them did home based work (like data entry, papad/ pickle making, tailoring, beading, ornament business). Thus a major chunk of the respondents are seen to be a part of the unorganized sector, which puts them at a risk of job security.

Figure 19 Occupation of MLHIV

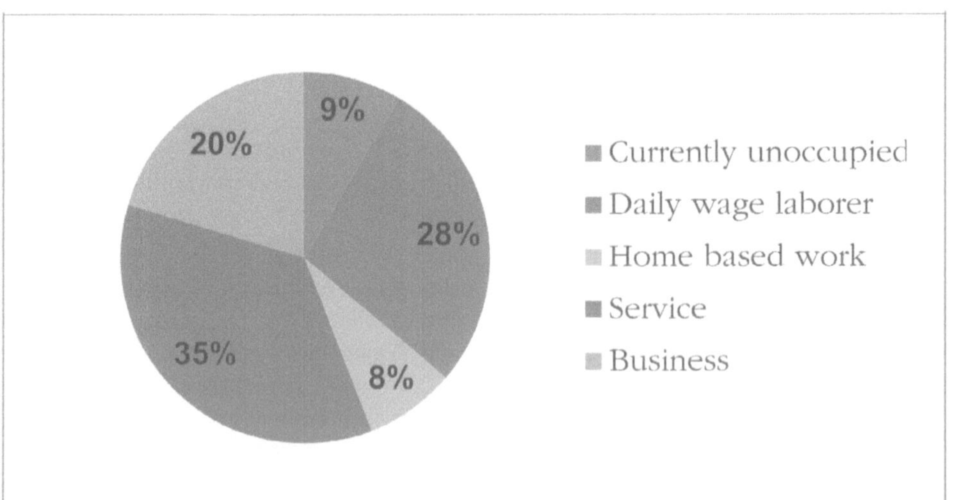

The variables educational achievement and occupation of the respondent were observed to be strongly dependent with chi square significance p value= 0.000 at df=16. The cross tabulation indicates that the respondents who were less educated were either unemployed or did home based work or were daily wage labourers, while those respondents with higher level of education were occupied into service or business. The reader may want to know if the occupation of the respondents has anything to do with their health status, or their frequency of alcoholic indulgence or the reasons for indulgence in sex outside marriage, which will be explored further in this study.

Personal Income : It was observed that 10.5 percent of the MLHIV respondents did not have a personal income of which 7 percent were unemployed and the others who did home based work supplemented their spouses and hence did not have an income. More than half of the respondents earned less than Rs.5000 a month. The mean income of the respondents was found to be Rs. 4,987 with a standard deviation of Rs. 3,634.

Family Income : In most cases (88.8 percent), the respondent's total family income was less than Rs.10,000. This reflects the poor quality of life that the infected and affected family members were reduced to live in the context of access to good health, nutrition and ART treatment. It was calculated that only 44 respondent's (28.9 percent) personal income was supplemented by additional family income, while all other respondents were the only source of income in their family.

Thus majority of the respondents being breadwinners is certainly a concern for their family members, who are entirely dependent on the respondent for their sustenance. The possibility of the respondent's income being affected due to incidence of opportunistic infections or other ailments will severely take a toll on the economic situation of the family. Thus the respondent goes through a major distress of economic crunch in the family, if they stand to lose their income. The following is the frequency of the family members who contribute to the family income:

Table 18 Family members contributing to family income

Type of Family member	Frequency
Spouse	34
Siblings	7
Children	7
Parents	4

(N=44 respondents)

As seen in the table above the brunt of sustaining the family income is also shared by the children of the respondents or their aging parents, which are a cause of concern.

On comparing the occupation of the respondent with their personal income, these variables were observed to be highly significant on chi square with p value= 0.000 at df=12 indicating that the MLHIV's Occupation and their Income are mutually dependent on each other. Thus implying that the respondent's occupational background decide their (personal) income.

Similarly on comparing the educational background of the respondent with their personal income, these variables were observed to be highly significant on chi square with p value= 0.000 at df=12 indicating that greater the educational achievement, greater the income of the respondent. Thus implying that the respondent's educational background have been instrumental in deciding their personal income

Age of Marriage: Seven of the respondents had not married until the time of the interview. The mean age of marriage amongst the male respondents was calculated to be 26 years with a standard deviation of 5 years. It is a matter of concern, to note that 24 MLHIV respondents (15.8 percent) had married before the legal age of marriage ie. 21 years. It can be very well understood that the age of their spouses would have been even lesser, given our cultural practice of marrying a woman, who is younger in age.

Culturally, in India as in many other parts of the developing nations, a girl is ready for marriage when she attains puberty. Early marriages are recommended for girls as it is felt that once married, a girl would have some security and safety for her future, in that she would be cared for both emotionally and financially by her husband. This practice in society exposes the girls to a great risk However, young married girls are more exposed to risk especially when their spouses are infected with HIV and the girl is unaware of his status. A study from sub-Saharan Africa concludes that early marriages increase coital frequency, decreases condom use and virtually eliminates girl's ability to abstain from sex (Thomas et al, 2007).

On cross tabulating the age of marriage of the male respondents with their spousal infection status, it is observed that the association between these two variables tested on chi square is weak with a p=0.109 with df=4. However, on cross tabulating with the STI infection amongst the spouse, the study result mentioned above holds true in the case of this sample. Thus the age of marriage holds strong significance of association with the spousal STI incidence on using chi square test with p=0.001 at df=8, indicating that earlier the age of marriage, greater the incidence of STI. The below table demonstrates this significance, showing that spouses in the early marriage face greater incidences of STI than those compared to those who got married at an older age posing questions on ignorance about STI among those who get married at an earlier age.

Table 19: Age of Marriage of respondents vs Spousal frequency of STI

Age of Marriage of respondents	Spousal frequency of STI			Total
	Often	Sometimes	Never	
Less than 21years	13	5	6	24
21 - 25 years	8	9	16	33
26 - 30 years	6	26	32	64
31 - 35 years	2	6	13	21
Above 35 years	0	1	2	3
Total	29	47	69	145

This finding shall be triangulated in Phase-3, when discussing with the spouses of MLHIV respondents on their incidences of STI and HIV infection.

***Remarriage* :** Of these 145 married respondents, 11 respondents (7.6 percent) have remarried after they have lost their spouses due to AIDS. In most cases the respondents have remarried after the age of 30 years and the marriages have been with widows who were also HIV infected. The respondents stated that their re-marriages have been arranged by the initiatives of the ORWs of the NGOs from where data was collected.

Living with spouse: Amongst the 145 respondents who were married, 78.6 percent are currently living with their spouses, while one fifth (21.4 percent) are not living with their spouses. The reasons for not living with their spouses are mentioned below:

Table 20 MLHIV not living with Spouse

Reasons	Frequency	Percent
Spouse staying in village	17	54.8
Spouse expired	11	35.5
Spouse divorced	3	9.7
Total	**31**	**100.0**

The cases of 17 respondents where the spouse is staying in village indicates mostly that the respondent is a single migrant in Mumbai and their family stays back in village. It is seen in the analysis in Chapter 10: Disclosure, that 14 of these 17 respondents have disclosed their status to their spouses. In a few cases, the spouse has gone back to their village after knowledge of the respondents HIV status, although not separated legally.

Number of Children: The 145 married respondents were also inquired about their number of children, which is as demonstrated below. However, in this study, no effort was made to inquire the HIV status of these children.

Figure 20 Number of children

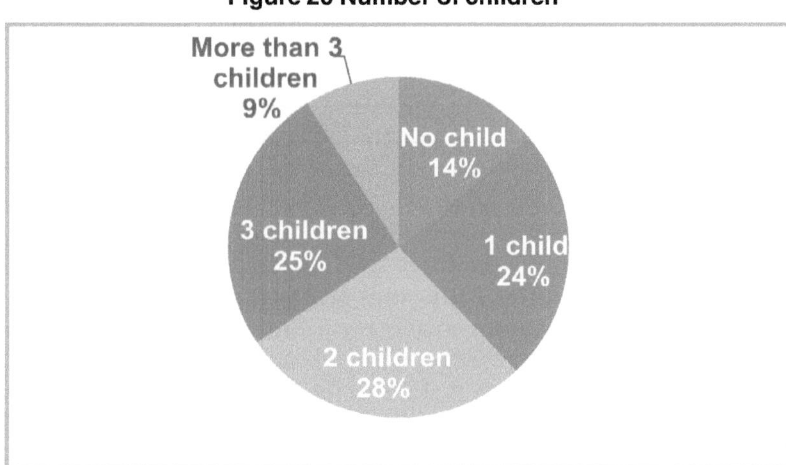

It is seen that 14 percent of the respondents, decided not to have children till the time interview. They mentioned that this decision was influenced by their HIV status and that they did not want to risk the future of the child. The trauma these couples would be undergoing of not wanting to have children, along with the suspicion of the society on why they do not have children, is certainly a concern that the couples would need counselling assistance to cope with. While the other 86 percent of the respondents, who had 1 or more children, constituted to a sum of 287 children altogether. It is to be noted that it is these children who fall under the bracket of 'orphan vulnerable children (OVC) in the context of HIV and would need special attention in counselling, care and support in the days to come.

Also as discussed in the context of family income of the respondent, it is to be noted that in case of any financial crisis or the MLHIV losing their job/income, the responsibility of supplementing the livelihood and survival of the family may fall on these children. Disclosure and treatment are therefore important areas that these children need to be educated on. During the time of this interview, four respondents additionally stated that they were emotionally disturbed about the future of their children, who will be orphaned due to the parents' deteriorating health conditions.

8.2. HEALTH PROFILE OF MLHIV RESPONDENT

The physical health status of the respondent was assessed on the grounds of these health variables, namely the respondent's CD_4 count, ART line, body weight, observed healthiness and their frequency of STI and OI. The findings of each of these variables are discussed in this segment.

CD4 Count *(Health Variable 1):* The CD_4 count of the MLHIV respondents as tested within 6 months prior to data collection was inquired and their CD_4 counts as stated verbally have been categorized as below:

Table 21 MLHIV's CD_4 Count

CD4 count (within last 6 months)	Frequency	Percent
Not tested	9	5.9
Less than 350 (cells/mm^3)	83	54.6
350 to 700 (cells/mm^3)	51	33.6
Above 700 (cells/mm^3)	9	5.9
Total	**152**	**100.0**

Except for 9 respondents (5.9 percent), the others were well aware that they had to be tested biannually for their CD_4 count, as per NACO's operational guidelines for patients on ART (NACO, 2007). More than half of the respondents (54.6 percent) were observed to have a low CD_4 count in spite of being on ART, indicating that they are susceptible to OIs. Studies show that less infectious people on ART, live considerably longer and thereby increasing the duration of potential exposure. At the urban sites, younger age and higher CD_4 cell count is associated positively with increased sexual indulgence (Lurie et al, 2008). These co-relations shall be verified in the report further.

ART Status ***(Health Variable 2):*** Mathematic models of past researches predict that although high levels of ART coverage could potentially reduce HIV incidence, its benefits could be overshadowed by simultaneous increases in risky sexual behaviour. Among men and women at the rural and urban sites, a higher CD4 cell count after the onset of ART was strongly associated with having a sexual partner. If these relations persist, patients returning to health after ART initiation may re-engage in risky sexual relationships (Lurie et al, 2008). In this study, the MLHIV respondents chosen, were purposefully sampled with the inclusive criteria that the respondents should have initiated ART, at least 6 months prior to data collection. This attempt was made to homogenize the sample so as to assess the history of their sexual behaviours and disclosure patterns in the period before and after the onset of ART. The respondents were also inquired about their line of treatment, which is also considered an indicator of their health.

Majority of the respondents (85.5 percent) were found to be on first line ART. Three of the four respondents who discontinued ART mentioned that they did so as to start the treatment for TB, while one respondent had problems in reaching the ART Centre due to his health status and hence discontinued. The line of ART *(as seen in the table below)* is found to be a variable influencing the sexual behaviours of MLHIV (Lurie et al, 2008) which shall be explored further.

Table 22 MLHIV's line of ART

ART Line of respondent	Frequency	Percent
First line	130	85.5
Second line	18	11.8
Discontinued ART	4	2.6
Total	**152**	**100.0**

On cross tabulating the 'Age' of the respondent with their line of ART treatment, a strong significant association has been observed between both these variables on chi square with a p value of 0.004 and df=6, indicating that the line of treatment also depends on their age. This finding reveals that at lower age the respondents started on first line and at moderate age bracket they moved on to second line and then at a higher age bracket the MLHIV have discontinued ART.

Body weight ***(Health Variable 3):*** The MLHIV respondents were inquired about their body weight and as reported by them it is observed that about one fourth (25.7 percent) of the adult MLHIV respondent's body weight was less than 50 kilos.

Table 23 MLHIVs Body Weight

Respondent's Body Weight	Frequency	Percent
Less than 50 kilos	39	25.7
50 - 60 kilos	54	35.5
60 - 70 kilos	38	25.0
70 - 80 kilos	21	13.8
Total	152	100.0

On cross tabulating the Body weight of the respondent with their line of ART treatment, a moderate significance has been observed between these variables on chi square with a p value of 0.016 and df=6. The cross tabulation indicates that most of the respondents on first line treatment show a lower body weight and most of those who are on second line and all of them, who have discontinued ART, show a higher body weight. It is to be further probed if the increase in the body weight is the reason for dis-continual of ART treatment regime in the cases of these 4 respondents.

Observed healthiness: The appearance of the respondents was observed for any apparent conditions of ill-health during the data collection. This helped to understand the current health condition of the respondent and decide whether the respondent looked healthy or weak. This attempt was made to further substantiate the normalcy of body weight of the respondent. It was observed that more than half of the respondents (59 percent) seemed to be healthy.

The variable 'observed healthiness' was cross tabulated with the above 3 health variables and it was found that there is

1. Strong association with respondent's CD4 count, (p-value of 0.001 and df=2)
2. Strong association with respondent's line of ART (p-value of 0.000 and df=3)
3. Strong association with respondent's body weight (p-value of 0.000 and df=2)

In other words most of the MLHIV in seemingly good health had better CD4 count, were on the first line of ART and with higher body weight.

Incidence of STI *(Health Variable 4):* STIs are a marker for unsafe sexual practices and are associated with intrinsic morbidity. There is good evidence that symptomatic STIs are associated with enhanced efficiency of HIV transmission (Gunter Rieg, 2008). Thus the presence of STI is a significant indication of the health status amongst MLHIV and affects their sexual health too. Hence the incidence of STI is studied here to better understand the context of risky sexual relations.

Table 24 STI amongst MLHIV

Incidence of STI	Frequency	Percent
Very Often (infected 6 times or more)	17	11.2
Often (infected 4-5 times)	24	15.8
Sometimes (infected 2-3 times)	36	23.7
Rarely (infected only once infected)	23	15.1
Never Infected	52	34.2
Total	**152**	**100.0**

The above table shows that about one third of the respondents (34.2 percent) never suffered from a STI.

On cross tabulating the respondent's incidence of STI infection with their ART status, a significant negative relationship was observed between these 2 variables with a Pearsons significance value of 0.01, indicating greater the incidence of STI, higher the line of ART treatment. A strong positive correlation was also observed between the frequency of STI and the body weight of the respondent, with a Pearsons significance value of 0.002, indicating that frequent incidence of STI reduced the body weight of the respondent.

Incidence of OI *(Health Variable 5):* The incidence of OIs is an indicator of the stage of HIV infection, affecting not just the physical but also the sexual health of the respondent (Mark Lurie et al, 2008).

Table 25 OI amongst MLHIV

Incidence of Opportunistic Infections	Frequency	Percent
Very Often (infected 6 times or more)	16	10.5
Often (infected 4-5 times)	27	17.8
Sometimes (infected 2-3 times)	61	40.1
Rarely (infected only once infected)	29	19.1
Never Infected	19	12.5
Total	152	100.0

As seen in the table above, over one tenth of the respondents (12.5 percent) mentioned that they never had an OI and is yet initiated on ART. This indicates that PLHIV can have lower level of CD_4 counts without significant symptomatic OIs. While cumulatively, about 104 respondents (68.4 percent) complained to have suffered from OIs at least twice.

The respondent's incidence of OIs was cross tabulated with all the above interval level health variables and following observations are made:

1. High positive correlation was found with CD4 count, when using a Pearsons test (asymptomatic significance=0.002, value =0.244), indicating that people with lower CD4 count suffer from higher frequency (very often or often) of OI.
2. Highly significant association was found with line of ART treatment, when using a chisquare test p-value of 0.007 at df=4, indicating that greater the incidence of OI, higher the line (drug regime) of ART
3. High positive correlation was found with Incidence of STI, a Pearson's test (asymptomatic significance=0.000, value =0.515), indicating that respondents having a greater incidence of STI, also showed a greater incidence of OIs.

Of the 133 respondents, who complained of having suffered from OIs, the different types of OI that they have been infected with have been tabulated below:

Table 26 (a) Types of OIs MLHIV have suffered from

Types of OIs	Frequency	Percent
TB	94	70.7
Herpes Zoster	48	30.1
Diahorrea	26	19.5
Oral Candidiasis	17	12.7
Pneumonia	11	8.3

Contd...

Types of OIs	Frequency	Percent
Jaundice	6	4.5
Malaria	3	2.3
Typhoid	4	3.0
Hepatitis B	2	1.5
Scabies	1	0.7

(N=133)

Many medical researchers have established a connection between TB and ART (Elford, 2001). In trying to correlate the incidence of TB along with the line of ART for this study, it is found that out of the 18 respondents, who are on second line ART majority (78 percent) of them suffered from TB disease and out of the 4 who discontinued ART, 3 discontinued only because of initiating TB treatment.

8.2.2 Consolidated Health Status

It is important to understand the health conditions of the MLHIV respondents in order to better understand their sexual behaviours. Hence the need to derive a consolidated heath score of the respondent was felt, so as to concise the analysis of respondent's health with the other variables on sexual behaviour and disclosure.

As implicit from the findings above, it is clear that the health variables considered for this study were closely associated with each other. Hence a consolidated health status score of MLHIV respondent was prepared (with the five variables namely CD4 count + ART Line + Body Weight + Incidence of STI + Incidence of OI) considering the response values of these 5 variables. The closed ended response values to each of the above health indicators were classified and recoded on 3 broad areas namely Poor, Moderate and Good as demonstrated in the table below.

Table 26: Consolidation of Health Status

	Health Indicators	Poor	Moderate	Good
1	CD4 Count	Less than 350	350 – 700	More than 700
2	ART Line	Discontinued	Second line	First line
3	Body weight	Less than 50 kg	50 – 60 kg	More than 60 kg
4	Sexually Transmitted Infections	Very Often & Often	Sometimes & Rarely	Never
5	Opportunistic Infections	Very Often & Often	Sometimes & Rarely	Never

The 5 health indicators were thus scored on the following points: Poor = 1, Moderate = 2, Good =3. Thus summing up the 5 indicators, the minimum score that can be achieved is 5 points *(ie Poor on all indicators)* and the maximum score that can be achieved is 15 points *(ie Good on all indicators)*. Thus the consolidated health's score range of 5 – 15 points was categorized as follows:

Poor = 5 – 8 points

Moderate = 9 – 12 points

Good = 13 – 15 points

Based on this understanding, the health variables were recoded and the results are as below :

Table 27 Frequency of Consolidated Health Status

	Health Indicators	Poor(Freq, %) (Freq, %)	Moderate (Freq, %)	Good (Freq, %)	Average Health Status (Mode)
1	CD4 Count	92 (60.5)	51 (33.6)	9 (5.9)	Poor
2	ART Line	4 (2.6)	18 (11.8)	130 (85.5)	Good
3	Body weight	39 (25.7)	54 (35.5)	59 (38.8)	Good
4	Incidence of STI	41 (27)	59 (38.8)	52 (34.2)	Moderate
5	Incidence of OI	43 (28.3)	90 (59.2)	19 (12.5)	Moderate
Consolidated Health Status		32 (21.1)	95 (62.5)	25 (16.4)	Moderate

It was herein observed that two out of every ten respondents (21.1 percent) had poor health condition while more than half of the respondent's consolidated health status seems to be moderate (62.5 percent).

The consolidated health condition of the respondents was found have high significance with extramarital sexual indulgences of the respondent using chi square test (p value=0.005 at df=2). Further significant correlations were found when cross tabulated with the following variables

Table 28 Factors influencing the consolidated health status

	Factors	Pearson's Sig.	Pearson's Value	Inference
1	Age of the respondent	0.002	-0.255	Increase in age implies decrease in Health
2	Personal income of the respondent	0.002	0.234	Increase in personal income implies increase in health
3	Family income of the respondent	0	0.313	Increase in Family income implies increase in Health
4	Total number of sexual partners outside marriage after ART	0.034	-0.172	Increase in sexual partners implies decrease in Health
5	Total number of sexual intercourses outside marriage after ART	0.024	-0.081	Increase in sexual intercourses implies decrease in Health

Factors like age, income and partners outside marriage have a direct impact on the health status of the MLHIV respondent. Thus proving true the formulated hypothesis

8.3. HEALTH PROFILE OF SPOUSE

Spousal HIV status: The spread of HIV among females is less of a physiological phenomenon but it is more of a behavioural and cultural phenomenon. In order to measure the risky sexual practices of MLHIV respondents, the HIV status of their spouses can also be considered an indicator (Anirudh, 2008). The HIV status of the respondent's spouses are as tabulated Table 29.

Table 29 HIV status of Respondent's Spouse

Spousal HIV status	Frequency	Valid Frequency	Valid Percent
HIV Negative	32	32	24.4
HIV Positive	99	99	75.6
NA since Not Tested	14	-	-
NA since unmarried	7	-	-
Total	**152**	**131**	**100.0**

It is important to note that 14 MLHIV respondents have not yet got their spouses tested for HIV in spite of they being on ART for at least 6 months. The ratio of HIV discordance amongst the respondents is thus observed to be one for every four couples. It is a matter of concern to note that three fourths of the MLHIV respondents (75.6 percent), who are on ART, have their spouses infected too. According to the Population Council of India report, spouses get HIV infected, since many do not have power to choose their sexual partner nor to choose the timing of sexual encounters nor to negotiate the use of male condoms. Moreover, neither do they have access to female condoms nor to another technology, which they can use to protect themselves. Many of them have little or no education on HIV and health and are relatively poor in accessing necessary prevention or care services. Many HIV infected women are also victims of gender-based violence or are forced to engage in transactional sex or are coerced into commercial sex work (Anirudh, 2008).

The consolidated health of the male respondent was found to have a significant positive correlation with the spousal HIV positive status, on Pearson's test with an asymptomatic value of 0.085. It is thus interesting to observe that respondents with better health conditions have reported that their spouses are also HIV positive.

Spousal CD4 count: With regards to the status of spousal CD4 count, it was observed that the spouses of only 85.6 percent respondents had tested for CD4.

Table 30: Spousal CD4 Status

CD4 status	Frequency	Valid Frequency	Valid Percent
CD4 count tested	85	85	85.6
CD4 count not tested	14	14	14.4
NA since Not Tested for HIV	14	-	
NA since HIV negative	32	-	
NA since unmarried	7	-	
Total	**152**	**99**	**100.0**

Amongst the spouses who were tested for CD_4, nearly half of the spouses (47 percent), were noted to have a poor CD_4 count of less than 350 (cells/mm^3), while 40 percent of the spouses had their CD_4 count in moderate range of 350 to 700 (cells/mm^3).

Spousal ART status: It was stated that of the 99 spouses, who were HIV positive, 43 respondents were on ART. As compared to men only a smaller percentage of woman know their HIV status, which may explain why they are less likely to seek and use ART and why they wait until much later stages of HIV infection to seek any government treatment (Marie Laga et al, 2001). Moreover, of these 43 spouses who are on ART, 40 spouses are on first line drugs while 3 spouses are on second line.

Incidence of OI among spouses: Amongst the spouses who were HIV infected, only 40 percent of had never suffered from of OIs. The OI incidence of the remaining 60 percent of the spouses is as tabulated below.

Table 31 Frequency of OI amongst spouses of MLHIV

Incidence of Spousal OI	Frequency	Percent
Very Often (infected 6 times or more)	9	9.1
Often (infected 4-5 times)	12	12.1
Sometimes (infected 2-3 times)	26	26.3
Rarely (infected only once infected)	12	12.1
Never Infected	40	40.4
Total	**99**	**100.0**

The consolidated health of the male respondent was found to have a significant association with the incidence of their spousal OI on chi-square test with a significance value of 0.009 and df=4. The cross tabulation between these variables illustrate that with increase in health conditions of the respondent there is a decrease in the incidence of OI amongst their spouses. It can thus be remarked that MLHIV respondents with poor health are more likely to transmit contagious infections to their spouses.

The types of OI that the spouses of the respondents suffered from are as enlisted below and the table shows that the most frequent OIs amongst the respondents spouses are TB, Herpes, Candidiasis and Diahorrea.

Table 32 Type of OI amongst spouses of MLHIV

	Frequency	Percent
TB	18	18.18
Herpes	12	12.12
Oral Candidiasis	11	11.11
Diarrhoea	9	9.09
Malaria	2	2.02
Pneumonia	2	2.02
Typhoid	1	1.01

(N=99)

Incidence of STI among spouses: The incidence of respondent's spouses suffering from STI was assessed and it was observed that more than half of the spouses (52.4 percent) spouses suffered from STI at least once. The frequency of STI incidence amongst the respondent's spouses has been collated Table 33.

Table 33

Incidence of Spousal STI	Frequency	Percent
Very Often (infected 6 times or more)	13	9.0
Often (infected 4-5 times)	16	11.0
Sometimes (infected 2-3 times)	23	15.9
Rarely (infected only once infected)	24	16.6
Never Infected	69	47.6
Total	**145**	**100.0**
NA since not married	7	—

The consolidated health interval of the MLHIV respondent was found to have a strong positive correlation with the incidence of their spousal STI, when using Pearson test, with a significance of 0.001, and value=0.275. The cross tabulation between these variables illustrate that with increase in health conditions of the respondent there is a decrease in the incidence of STI amongst their spouses. This finding indicates the likelihood of the respondents being the carriers of STI to their spouses.

Summary of PLHIV couples Health condition

Thus a comparative analysis is presented below summarizing both the respondent's and their spousal health profiles. Since this is a comparative analysis with the spouses, only married respondents (N= 145) have been filtered.

Table 34

Variable #	Health Condition Indicators	MLHIV's Health status	SpousalHealth status
1	**HIV status**		
	a. HIV Positive	145 (100%)	99 (75.6%)
	b. HIV Negative	*0 (0%)*	*32 (24.4%)*
	c. Not tested	0	14
2	**CD_4 Count Status**		
	a. Not Tested	8 (5.5%)	14 (14.1%)
	b. Less than 350	81 (55.9%)	40 (40.4%)
	c. 350 – 700	49 (33.8%)	34 (34.3%)
	d. Above 700	7 (4.8)	11 (11.1%)
	e. CD4 not applicable	*0*	*46*
3	**ART Status**		
	a. Not on ART	0 (0%)	56 (56.6%)
	b. First Line	123 (84.8%)	40 (40.4%)
	c. Second Line	18 (12.4%)	3 (3.0%)
	d. Discontinued ART	4 (2.8%)	0 (0%)
	e. ART not applicable	*0*	*46*
4	**Incidence of OIs**		
	a. Often	41 (28.3%)	21 (21.2%)
	b. Sometimes	85 (58.6%)	38 (38.4%)
	c. Never	19 (13.1%)	40 (40.4%)
	d. Not Applicable	*0*	*46*
5	**Incidence of STIs**		
	a. Often	38 (26.2%)	29 (20.0%)
	b. Sometimes	57 (39.3%)	47 (32.4%)
	c. Never	50 (34.5%)	6947.6%)

The spouses who have not been tested for HIV as yet, becomes a concern. The comparative chart shows how the spouses need to be counselled on increasing their CD4 count in order to prolong ART and also about measures to be taken to contain the incidence of OI and STI, which can further deteriorate their health status.

8.4 SEXUAL RELATIONS OF MLHIV OUTSIDE MARRIAGE

Effective research into long-term chronic illnesses requires longitudinal research efforts to study and compare the transitions within the life of the individual and not just across cases. This learning captured over time will provide an experience of managing chronic conditions and understanding attempts of behaviour change (Michael, 2004).

With this longitudinal paradigm, a comparative analysis is attempted within the cases in this study. Having an understanding of the health profiles the respondents from the above results, the MLHIV indulgence in Pre and Extra marital sexual activity has been studied in this segment, which includes number of sexual partners, frequency of sexual activity, number and type of sexual partners and the factors influencing sexual activity. Further, aspects like the respondents assessing the STI and HIV of sexual partners, level of sexual satisfaction with the partners, types and frequency of sexual acts, incidences of safe sex practices and disclosure were all explored.

8.4.1 Chronological events in the life of the respondent

This segment starts with capturing the milestones in the life of the MLHIV respondent at various age summits. This attempt was made to understand the chronological sequencing of events that happened in the respondent's life. The age wise distribution of the events in their life is represented in the table below.

Table 35

Events in the life of the MLHIV respondent	Valid Frequency (N)	Age in years					
		Mean	*Std. Deviation*	Median	Mode	Minimum	Maximum
Age since residing in Mumbai	152	8.86	*10.18*	4	0	0	40
Age of first sexual fantasy	152	17.72	*3.11*	17	18	14	42
Age of first sexual intercourse	152	20.75	*4.23*	20	20	14	42
Age of marriage	145	26.28	*5.05*	26	26	8	45
Age of HIV positive result	152	33.53	*6.06*	33	29	19	54
Age of receiving education on HIV	152	33.60	*6.18*	33	29	20	54
Age of ART initiation	152	34.76	*5.79*	34	31	22	54
Age when spouse was tested for HIV	131	35.17	*5.65*	35	35	24	52
Current age	152	38.09	*6.04*	37	40	23	56

A graphical representation of the chronological incidents happening in the lifetime of MLHIV respondents is represented below. The mean age has been considered for every variable.

Figure 21 Chronological Events in the life of MLHIV respondent

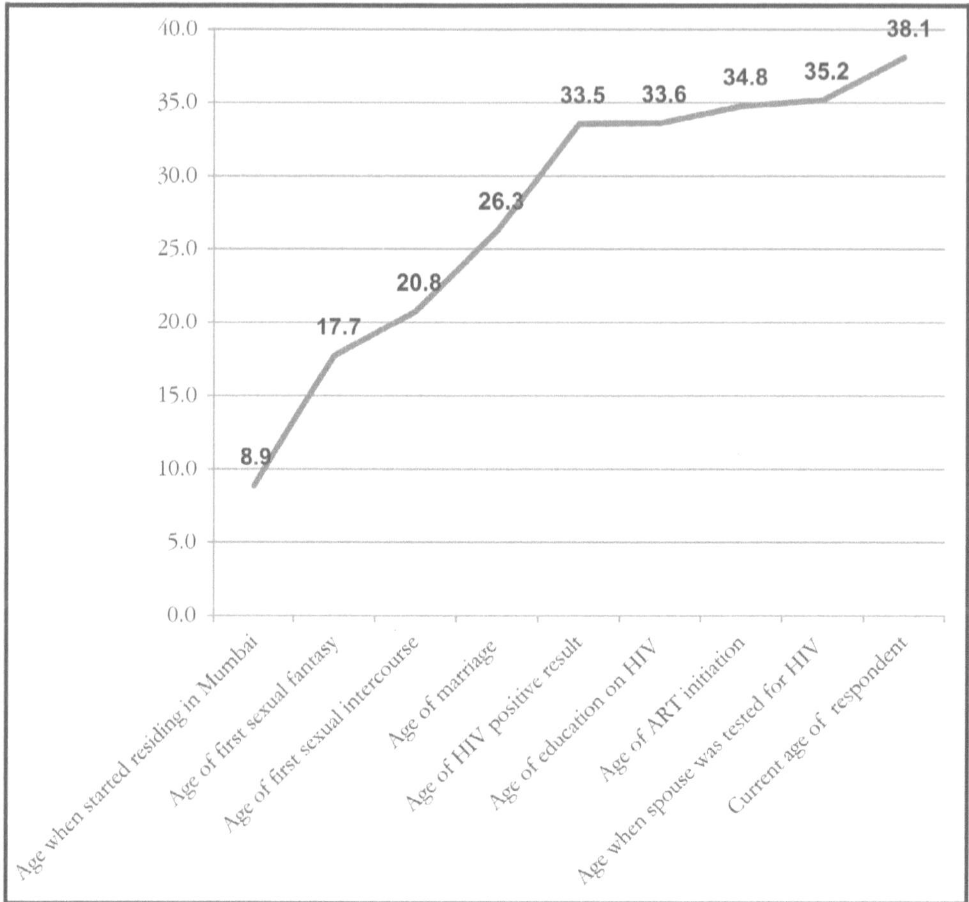

Age when started residing in Mumbai: The respondents were inquired about their duration of stay in Mumbai and it was found that about half of the respondents (48 percent) were born in Mumbai. Another 30.9 percent of the respondents have started residing in Mumbai at a very young age i.e. before the age of 18 years. Thus indicating that majority of respondents have spent their adolescence in Mumbai and the study findings should be understood in this context.

Age of Sexual Debut: The mean age of sexual debut, as recollected by the MLHIV respondent was found to be 20.7 years with a standard deviation of 4.2 years. The graph shows that the difference between the age of fantasy and sexual intercourse is just 3 years, implying that in case of the MLHIV respondents, actual sexual intercourse happened on an average of 3 years after they had fantasies about sex.

Age of Marriage: The mean age of marriage was observed to be 26.2 years with a standard deviation of 5 years. It is interesting to note that the age of marriage is 26 years, which is 6 years later than the age of their sexual debut. This span of time provides space for premarital sexual relations, especially in the context of the period of early adulthood, when sexual drives are at its peak. It needs to be further explored if this delay in the age of marriage is likely to be a prevailing condition for increased number of pre marital sexual relations.

Age of HIV test result: The respondents were enquired on when they had tested themselves for HIV and mean age of HIV testing was calculated to be 33.5 years with a standard deviation of 6 years. It is interesting to note that the detection of HIV amongst respondents happened 13 years after their sexual debut. This gap may indicate a lack of awareness about HIV and its routes of transmission. During the interview, a few of the respondents' additionally remarked that they had tested themselves only after they fell sick. The age range between the sexual debut and the HIV test is also an indicator pointing out that towards the long incubation time required for the virus to be symptomatically identified. Considering the potential risk of the 'male carrier' infecting the female in every unsafe sexual intercourse, this time span between the sexual debut and HIV detection is certainly a threat of HIV transmission to numerous sexual partners encountered during the period.

It is also noteworthy that the HIV test has happened 7 years after marriage, thus leaving a huge room for transmission of HIV to their spouses, in every act. The early years of marriage being highly sexually active, there is a chance of increased viral load transmission to the spouses. This is evident in the discussion above, where the three out of four spouses were identified to be HIV infected and most of them had a low CD4 and half amongst them had to start ART.

Age of HIV education: As seen in the graph above, most respondents have learnt about HIV and AIDS for the first time, only after the HIV test, when their mean age was 33.6 years (standard deviation of 6 years). This delay in the age of HIV awareness is in line with many KAP studies across the country and this miniscule awareness on HIV is also a factor influencing the respondent's indulgence in high risk sexual activities and also of their delay in accessing HIV testing facility. (UNAIDS, 2000)

Age of ART Initiation: It is observed that the respondents had to initiate ART within a year of HIV testing, at a mean age of 34.6 (with a standard deviation of 5.7 years). Thus indicating that a huge majority of respondents have initiated HIV testing only at the stage where their CD4 count fell very low and they had Opportunistic Infections.

On comparing within cases it was observed that most respondents started ART in the same year of the HIV test. Such a situation, leaves only a little time period for the counsellors to prepare the PLHIV for treatment and positive living. This is also a crisis situation for any PLHIV, since there is hardly any time for acceptance of HIV result and preparedness for treatment. An early diagnosis of HIV is essential to schedule appropriate follow up counselling sessions for the PLHIV, in order to prepare them and their support systems for ART. It needs to be explored if this insufficient time for preparedness before the onset of ART, is a reason for loss to follow-up / ART drop-out. On retrospection, it can be understood that in initial days of ART roll out, ART was started as soon as HIV was detected. The CD_4 count or viral load was not easily available or accessible as done now. This could be a possible reason why the respondents had to be initiated to ART immediately after the HIV test.

Age when spouse was tested for HIV: Of all respondents, whose spouses were tested for HIV, the mean age of the respondent when the spouse was tested for HIV was found to be 35 years, which is 2 years later to their own HIV detection! This long gap of spouse testing along with the probability of inadequate knowledge on safe sex practices puts the spouse at a high risk to acquire HIV/STI.

Spousal testing and spousal disclosure are variables, which are closely linked with each other with uncertainty in order of precedence (Cheewanan L. et al, 2007). In this context it seems that the respondents in this study too would have disclosed their HIV status around 2 years after their own test, thus leading to spousal testing.

Interestingly, the age of spousal HIV testing is also found to be 10 years after the marriage. Thus indicating that the infection has been transmitted vertically to their off springs too, most of which would have gone undetected.

The significance of this above chronological event chart is discussed further in Chapter 12 where the road map for the counsellor-counselee is laid out.

8.4.2 PREMARITAL SEXUAL RELATIONS OF MLHIV

The qualitative case studies with MLHIV reveal that sexual partners had been initiated before marriage, which has been further explored with the sample in this section. The respondents were inquired about their sexual relations before marriage and interestingly nine out of ten (89 percent) admitted to have had such pre-marital sexual relations. The respondents were further inquired on the number of partners with whom they had premarital sexual relations. Their responses have been summarized below:

Table 36 Pre Marital sexual partners

Number of Sexual Partners	Frequency	Percent
1 to 3 partners	60	44.44
4 to 10 partners	47	34.81
11 to 50 partners	24	17.78
Over 50 partners	4	2.96
Total	135	100.0
NA since did not have Pre Marital partners	17	—

As seen in this table more than half of the respondents (66.66 percent) had more than 3 sexual partners before marriage. Little has been explored about the number of premarital sexual partners of MLHIV in India and this finding holds a key to substantiate the understanding that most men, who have more than one partner, stand high chances to get infected with HIV.

The number of pre marital sexual partners of the respondents was cross tabulated with age, income, education and occupation. However significant relationships were found using chi square test only with occupation and spousal infection:

Table 37 Factors influencing pre-marital sexual relations

	Number of Pre-marital sexual partners of respondents	Chi SquareSignificance	df
1	Service occupation of the respondent	0.044	12
2	HIV positive status of spouse	0.002	9

The service occupation of the respondent as well as the spousal HIV status holds a strong association with the number of pre marital sexual partners. It is to be ascertained further if the service occupation offers greater access to more number of partners due to the time that these individuals have and also due to their peer contacts. This can be explored in future researches. Further, significant correlation was observed when cross-tabulated with the following variables

Table 38

#	Cross tabulation on No. of premarital partners	Pearson's value	Approx. Sig.	Inference
1	Educational achievement	0.061	0.162	An increase in number of pre-marital sexual partners was observed by more respondents, who were educationally better qualified in comparison
2	Consolidated health of respondent	0.059	0.498	An increase in number of pre-marital sexual partners was observed by more respondents, who had better consolidated health status
3	Frequency of protected sex	0.098	0.258	An increase in number of pre-marital sexual partners was observed by more respondents, who were less cautious about practising protected sex.

As seen in this table, number of pre-marital sexual partners of the respondents was found to be proportional to their educational background, health and less protected sexual behaviours.

8.4.2b Reasons for indulgence in Pre Marital Sex

Studies on male sexual behaviour point out the reasons for risky sexual behaviour to include "fun, curiosity, friendship and influence of alcohol". Machismo and patriarchal authority characterize male roles in many cultures and the negative aspects of machismo resulting in heavy drinking and sexual risk has been reported (Thomas et al, 2009).

The precursor qualitative interview conducted by the researcher reveals the reasons for indulgence in premarital sex to be driven by peer and alcohol influence, curiosity, relaxation need, easy availability of sexual partners or as a sign of intimacy. Whether these factors actually influenced pre marital sexual relations, was investigated with the respondents and the findings are as graphically demonstrated Figure 22.

The major factors which influence indulgence in pre marital sexual relations include:

1. Wanting to experiment by having sex (80.7 percent)
2. The need to relax and to enjoy (77 percent)
3. Peer influence (63.7 percent)
4. Easy availability and accessibility to sex (45.9 percent)
5. Influence of alcohol (44.4 percent)

Figure 22 Reasons for Pre Marital sexual indulgence

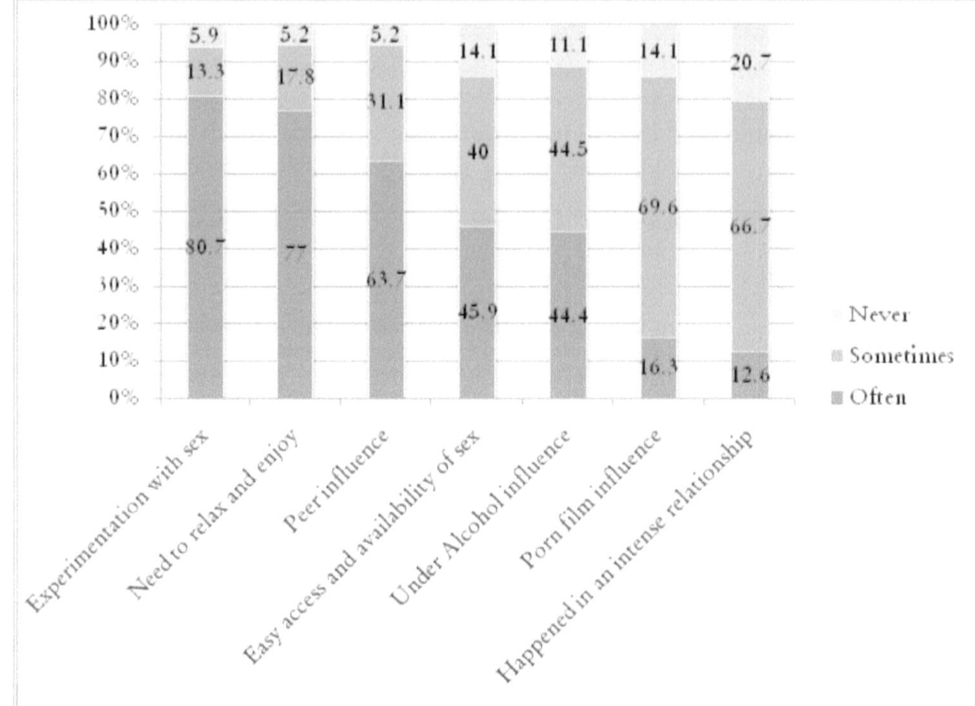

Thus the above reasons reveal that most of the times the sexual act is pre-meditative and was planned by the MLHIV respondents.

The above graph shows that one of the reasons for pre-marital sex was 'often' spurred out of intimacy with the partner (12.6 percent). It is debatable if premarital sex is encouraged as an acceptable behaviour to demonstrate love/ intimacy in a relationship. However, among the women, there is a feeling of helplessness and inability to refuse the premarital sexual relationship as the partner is usually their fiancé who promised them marriage or an employer who they were forced to oblige. The powerlessness of women to negotiate safe sexual practices has also been reported in other studies in sub Saharan Africa and Thailand (Thomas et al, 2009). This powerlessness amongst women to negotiate on safe sexual practices have also been explored in this Phase-3 of this study, from the FGD conducted with spouses.

8.4.2c Type of Pre Marital Partner

The pre-cursor qualitative interviews point out that the MLHIV's perception of risk is associated with the type of sexual partner. Sex workers operating from the brothels are considered to be core transmitters of HIV infection and if majority of the population engaging in pre-marital sex have easy access to brothels, they are at a greater vulnerability to HIV infection. Studies show that a high percentage of respondents who have had sex with a prostitute, visited them to for their first sexual experience. Also, younger men are more likely to visit prostitutes than older men. (Nguyen, M.T. et al, 2002)

The 135 respondents who had pre marital sex, were inquired about their type of pre marital sexual partner and it was found that over two third of the respondents (64.4 percent) had sexual relations with the brothel based partners, while just one out of every three respondents (31.1 percent) had sex with non brothel based partners. This finding indicates that the initiation of early sexual relations among the MLHIV respondents has been with sex workers (brothel based). Choosing brothel based partners for indulgence in premarital sex triangulates the information gathered in the above response on reasons for premarital sex, which include 'wanting to experiment', 'need to relax/ enjoy', 'peer and alcohol influence' easy availability and accessibility to sex.

The reasons to access brothel based partners as stated by the respondents also include

- Comparatively cheaper cost of the sex worker and the lodge
- Known sites of sex work are away from community of residence

Figure 23 Type of partner for pre-marital sex

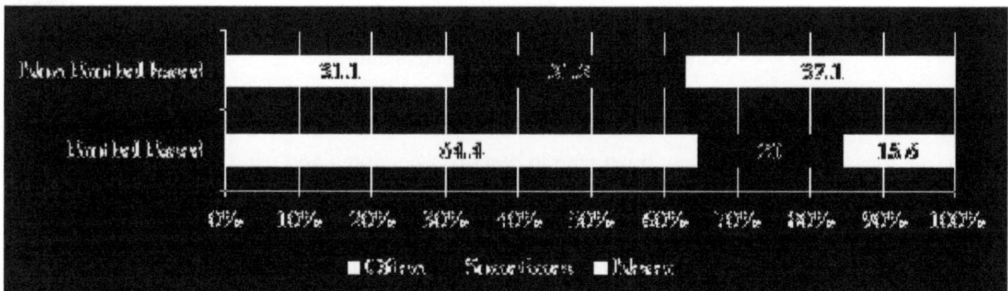

A descriptive analysis of MLHIV who have had sex with brothel based partners, revealed interesting facts about their sexual behaviour. Firstly the men in the median age group of 30 to 40 years mostly visited the brothel based partners, either 'often' (63.2 percent) or 'sometimes' (70.4 percent), compared to the men of younger or older age group. Secondly, more men (70.2 percent), who had resided in Mumbai for more than 20 years, have visited the brothel based partners, 'more frequently', than those men who started residing in Mumbai relatively later. Thirdly, MLHIV with lower levels of educational achievement, 'more often' visited brothel based partners (using Person's correlation as seen in above table). Fourthly, MLHIV with lower levels of personal income frequented brothel based partners *(Chisquare test with p=0.033 and df=6)*.

8.4.2 d Frequency of protected sex before marriage

Of all the respondents who admitted having indulged in pre – marital sex, only 7 percent of them stated that they used condoms 'every time' during the act. Every six out of ten respondents (57 percent) have never used condoms during their pre-marital sexual encounter. The respondents further stated that 'protected sex' was mostly practiced with brothel based partners and rarely with the non brothel based partners. The following reasons have been cited by few of them for not having protected sex every time:

Table 39

#	Areas	Reasons for not indulging in safe sex
1	Perceived that	- Sexual partners looked healthy and beautiful, so assumed that they had no disease
	partners were safe	- Had sex with Call Girls/ Non brothel based / non commercial partners and thought they were safer
		- Had regular partners for sex, considered them faithful
		- Sexual partner hailed from a good family background
		- Used condoms only when the sex worker insisted
		- Sexual partners would have used it if they had infections.
		- "Since I dint have any infections, I dint use condoms"
2	Issues with	- Could not use in intense relationship with partner
	condom use	- Used condoms with unknown partners only
		- Partner's objection on use of condom.
		- Partners never asked me to wear a condom
		- Condom was used only as a contraceptive tool
		- Condoms were not easily accessible
		- Condoms were not easily available, distribution of condoms was not as prominent as today
		- Did not have time to purchase condoms and used to rush into the act, whenever had an opportunity
		- Hesitation in buying and using condoms
		- Condom use diminishes sexual pleasure and did not enjoy using them
		- Condoms used to tear during the sexual act so stopped using condoms
3	Other reasons	- Under alcohol influence one forgot to wear condoms
		- "Had confidence in my health and thought I won't get infected"
		- "Some sexual acts were not planned and happened suddenly"
		- "HIV and STI infections were not a priority and focus was on enjoying the rub"
		- *javani ka josh* (spurt of youth hood)

It can thus be understood that protected sex in pre-marital sexual relations was not practiced either due to lack of awareness, issues with condom use or ignorance due to fatalistic approach.

8.4.3 EXTRA-MARITAL SEXUAL RELATIONS OF MLHIV

Extra marital sex in this study is understood as sex with a "non-spousal sexual partner after marriage". In the earlier segment the discussion revolved around non-spousal sexual partners before marriage.

When exploring about the respondents extramarital sexual relations, it was observed that more than half of the respondents (59.3 percent) have indulged in sexual relations with non-spousal sexual partner. These respondents were further inquired about the number of sexual partners they were associated with, and it was seen, as in the table below, that six out of every ten respondents, who had extramarital sexual relations (61.6 percent), had relations with 1 to 3 partners.

Table 40 No. of extra marital sexual partners

No. of extra marital sexual partners	Frequency	Valid Frequency	ValidPercent
1 to 3 partners	53	53	61.6
3 to 10 partners	29	29	33.7
More than 10 partners	4	4	4.7
NA since didn't have extra marital partners	66	-	
Total	152	86	100

8.4.3b Reasons for Extra Marital sex

The factors which influenced the respondents to indulge in extramarital sex were explored and the findings are graphically demonstrated figure 23. As per the pre-cursor qualitative interviews, the problems faced by MLHIV with their spouse were found to be reasons influencing their indulgence in extramarital sexual relations. In this context, to understand the factors influencing extramarital sex, the respondents were additionally checked on following variables associated with spouse like 'embarrassment to perform different acts at home', 'restrictions to sex at home', 'dissatisfaction with spouse', 'menstruation, menopause, pregnancy and HIV negative status of spouse'.

Thus the major factors which influenced extra marital relationships among the respondents included:

1. Need to relax and enjoy (83.7 percent)
2. Peer influence (55.8 percent)
3. Experimentation with sex (53.5 percent)
4. Under Alcohol influence (45.3 percent)
5. Wanted a change / variety in sexual relations (34.9 percent)
6. Embarrassment to perform varied sexual acts with spouse (25.6 percent)

The factors influencing extramarital sex 'often', has been arranged in the descending order of its frequency. It can be observed that the right hand side half of the chart have reasons specific to 'spouse' for indulgence into extramarital sex. It is interesting to note that factors such as dissatisfaction with spouse, spousal disinterest in sex, menstruation periods, HIV negative status of spouse, childbearing phase or even menopause of spouse were never major reasons influencing extramarital sex. Factors such as experimentation, peer influence, relaxation needs and long for a variety are common determinants of sex outside marriage (pre and extra). This finding helps to understand from the respondents' perspective that extramarital sexual indulgence may not necessarily indicate compatibility issues or sexual problems with spouse.

Figure 24 Factors influencing Extramarital sexual indulgence

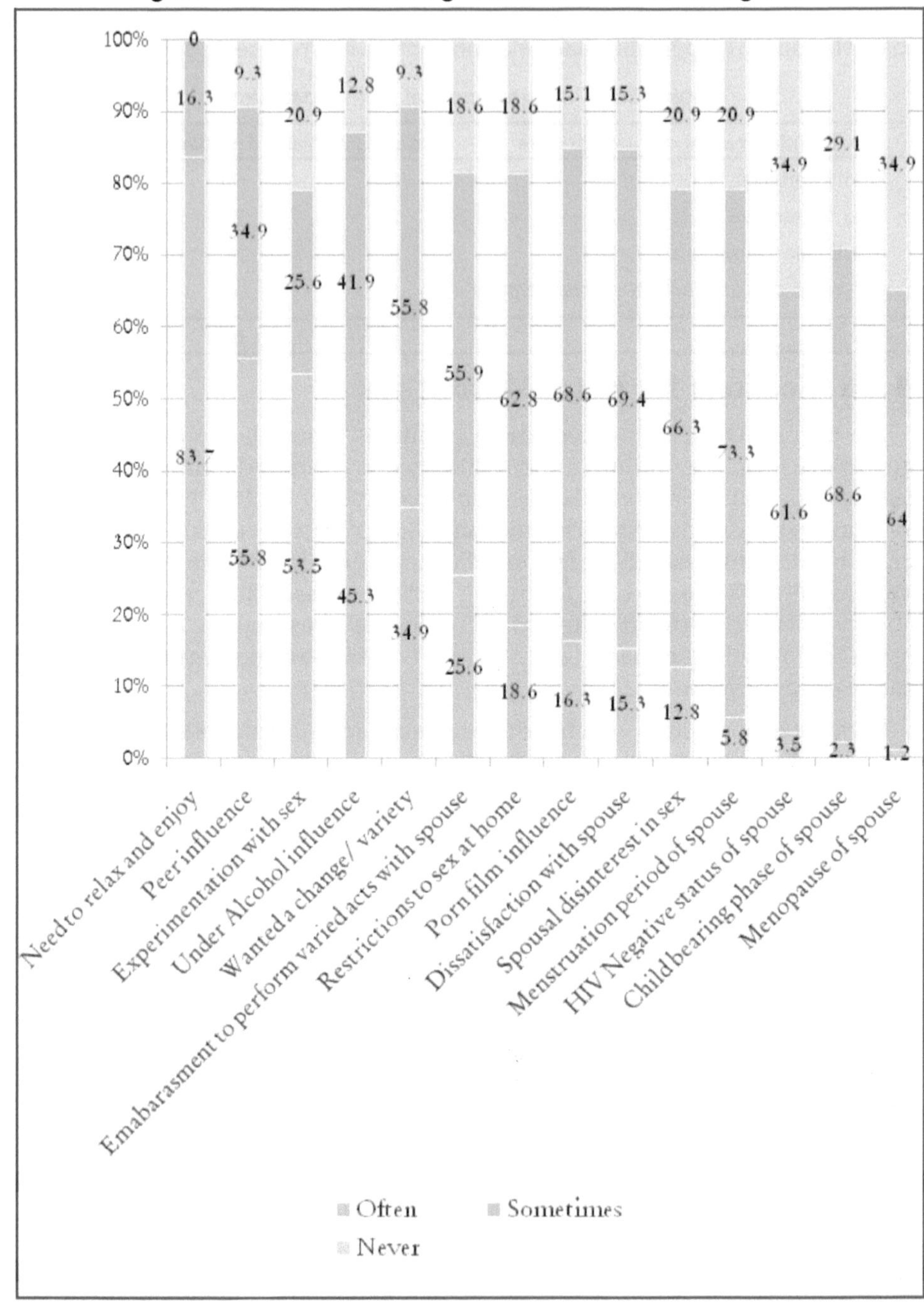

Additionally, the reasons mentioned by the respondents for their indulgence in extramarital sex include:

- Death of spouse (4 respondents)
- Spouse was in village (4 respondents)

- Had sex with men because afraid that brothel woman had HIV (1 respondent)
- After our child marriage, wife was kept at her home until the age of 21
- It was easier to have orgasm and sexual desire with women outside (1 respondent)
- The place of having sex is not disturbed by anyone else and we have complete freedom unlike home environment (1 respondent)
- Was involved in a live in relationship with a woman outside, with whom i had sex from the beginning and hence continued with her in her husband's absence
- The partner outside insisted that our sexual relations kept her happy in her husband's absence (1 respondent)

8.4.3c Type of extramarital Partner

As inquired in the pre-marital segment, the respondents were again inquired the type of their extramarital partner whether brothel based or non brothel based. The frequency of the respondents visit to these type of partners was also elicited on a scale of 'often – sometimes – never'. The findings are as demonstrated below:

Figure 25 Type of extramarital partners

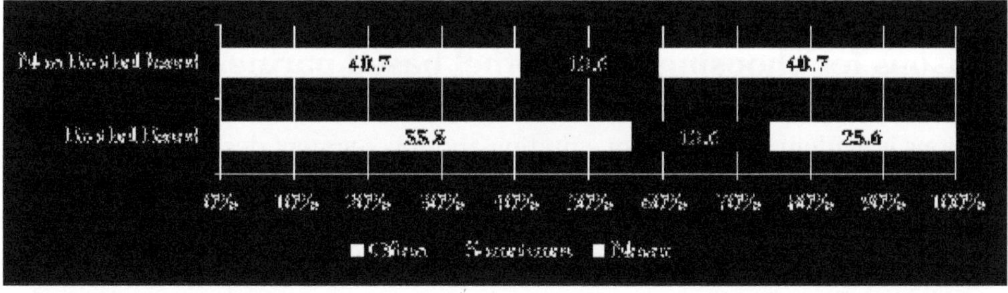

This graph shows that most of the respondents frequented with the brothel based partners again. However, in comparison to the type of pre-marital partners, it was observed that there is a drop in the frequency of visits to brothel based partners and a rise in frequenting non brothel based partners. This data points towards a trend where MLHIV respondents after marriage, prefer to associate with non-brothel based partners with whom long term relations are maintained.

The non brothel based partners of the respondents include:

1. Neighbourhood women whose husbands were not at home / widowed (non commercial) (19 respondents)
2. Call girls (6 respondents)
3. Bar girls (4 respondents)
4. Home based women who entertained sex for commercial benefits (snowballed through friends) (3 respondents)
5. Girlfriends (3 respondents)

6. Men attending gay parties (3 respondents)
7. Loyal Boyfriends (1 respondents)

Narratives of the respondent on the non brothel based partners, points out that they were in the age range of 25-45 years. It included married women residing in the neighbourhood, who were not sexually satisfied with husbands. In some cases, the respondent played the role of a guardian of these women and in return would offer them household support and be available for any needs. The respondent made regular visits to this partner without the knowledge of the spouse.

One respondent added that relationship building and physical proximity initiatives were often taken by some of these home based women. One married respondent shared that his partner was an office colleague, who was in agreement with his sexual advances and now they plan to marry each other. This respondent's wife deserted him when she got to know about this extramarital relationship.

Another respondent shared that when he used to deliver milk, one of his female customer (whose husband was absent at home), used to invite him into her house during the day. Her seduction instigated the respondent to have sex with her and thus the respondent's visits to her home regularized.

In case of one respondent, there was a bar close-by the place where he used to run his business and a woman used to come to his shop daily and seduce him. Thus his extra-marital relationship emerged and regularized.

Reasons for choosing non brothel based partners

The rise in the respondent's access to non brothel based partners for extramarital relations is evident from the above finding and this segment describes the reasons given by the respondents on why they chose non brothel based partners. The responses were:

- "Curiosity to know how non brothel based sex work happened"
- "There was easy access to non brothel based partners in the community and sex used to happen at their homes or in the fields. Some watched porn films together before the sexual activity."
- "Sexual relations were based on consensual interest in non brothel based partners leading to greater pleasure."
- "Other men offered behaviours like oral, anal and mutual masturbation"
- "The partner was a destitute women who desperately wanted money and had no objection in returning favour for sex"
- "Wife was too young and frightened to have sex since it was painful for her. His neighbour was loving and caring and allowed physical intimacy leading to sexual relations."
- "The partner was a woman in the community whom the respondent had advanced for sex, knowing that she was married housewife and her husband used to drink and not love her. The woman agreed to have sexual relations."

- "Used to spend more time with women at workplace, with whom quite some time was spent discussing each other's problems. This developed intimacy and we used to touch each other. The woman was in need of money, she exchanged with sex"
- "Call girls performed various types of acts and masturbated the respondent"
- "Although their charges are high, the service provided was rated good and their hospitality was appreciable"

8.4.3d Frequency of protected sex in extra marital sexual relations

The respondents were questioned on how frequently they indulged in protected sex within their extramarital relationships and about 16 percent of the respondents claimed to have indulged in protected sex 'Every time'. While more than half of the respondents (52 percent) admitted that they had 'Never' had protected sex and one third (32 percent) said that they used protection 'Sometimes'.

Summary of MLHIV respondent's Sexual Indulgence outside Marriage

This segment summarizes the sexual behaviour of the respondent outside marriage (ie. with premarital and/or extramarital partners), as discussed in length above.

Figure 26 Sex outside marriage among MLHIV and their age

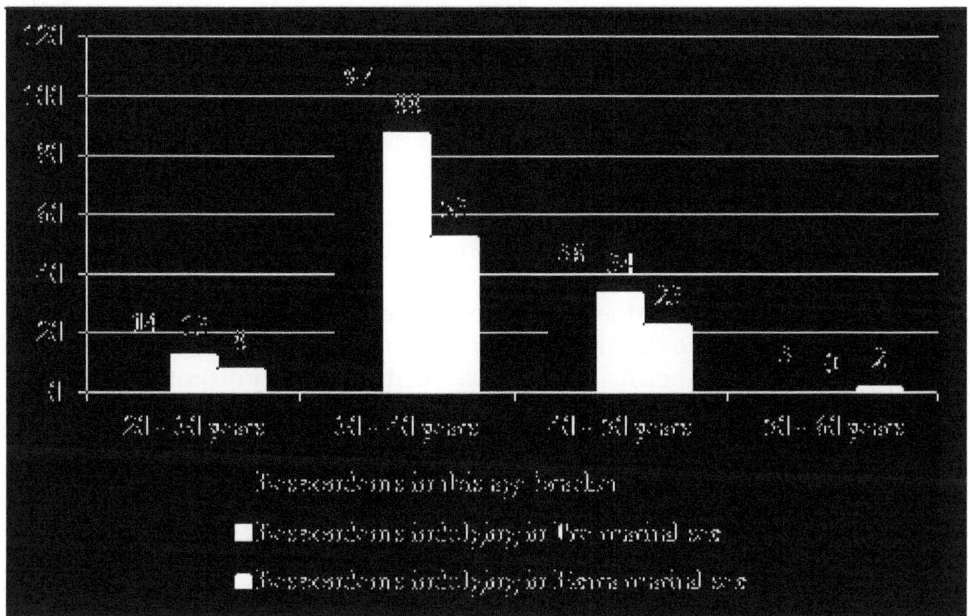

Pre Marital sex was practiced by many of the respondents, which was initiated at the age of 20 years and seems prominent right up to the age of 50 years (due to delay in marriage of some respondents). There seems to be a reduction in the number of respondents practicing extra-marital sexual indulgences, as compared to the pre-marital indulgences. From the above graph one can make out that sexual indulgence of men outside marriage does not cease even at the age of 50-60 years.

The table below gives an overview of the comparative findings between pre and extra marital sexual relations.

Table 41: Comparative Summary of sexual behaviours outside marriage

		Pre Marital	Extra Marital
Respondents having sex outside marriage (N)		135 (88.8 %)	86 (56.6 %)
1	**Number of sexual partners**		
	a. 1 – 3 partners	44.4 %	61.6 %
	b. 4 – 10 partners	34.8 %	33.7 %
	c. 11 – 50 partners	17.8 %	4.7 %
	d. Over 51 partners	3.0 %	0 %
2	**Respondents' who perform Penetrative** Sex "Often" in every intimate moment with partner	94.1 %	94.2 %
		Pre Marital	Extra Marital
3	**Source of sexual partners visited "Often"**	*N=135*	*N=86*
	a.Brothel Based	64.1 %	55.8 %
	b.Non Brothel based	31.1 %	40.7 %
4	**Frequency of Protected sex**		
	a.Often	14.1 %	18.6 %
	b.Sometimes	28.9 %	29.1 %
	c.Never	57.0%	52. 3 %

The above comparison shows that more number of partners are indulged with in pre-marital sex, which reduces significantly in the extra marital relations. Thus men seek more number of partners when having pre-marital sex. The type of sex most of the time is penetrative in nature. Seeking for non brothel based increases after marriage. There seems to be a marginal increase in the frequency of protected sex after marriage.

8.5. DIMENSIONS OF SEXUAL PRACTICES

The discussions in this segment will now look into aspects of sexual behaviour in general without categorization into premarital or extramarital.

8.5.1 Efforts taken to check for partner's STI status

The respondents were enquired on what efforts they took to assess the STI status of their non spousal sexual partners. Only about 12 respondents reported an attempt made to assess the partner's STI status and their style of assessment is as narrated below:

- "Looked if there are there any ulcers, rashes or boils in the area of urinals" (7 respondents)
- "Just observed if partner looks healthy by body weight" (2 respondents)
- "Had asked one partner about her STI status, but she got angry and in opposite reaction she asked me my status". The partner further said that she didn't call me to her and if the respondent was not interested in her, he should find someone else. After this the respondent never asked anyone (2 respondents)
- "Sometimes I could see ulcers on skin and that time we avoided sexual contact and partners" (1 respondent)

8.5.2 Frequency of partners STI assessment

The MLHIV were asked on how frequently they assessed their partners STI status. It was found that none of the respondent had ever "Always" asked their partner's STI status, while majority of the participants (91.5 percent) had "Never asked" for their partners status. The reasons for not assessing partners STI status have been listed below.

Fatalism

1. Since STI wasn't a common problem then (34 respondents)
2. "My priority was enjoying sex and I wasn't bothered about infections during the act" (10 respondents)
3. The respondent never thought that he would get infected (2 respondents)

Ignorance

4. Believed in their regular and known non-brothel based partner's health. "If they had STI no one else would have approached them" (20 respondents)
5. Not checked since had no knowledge about STI (24 respondents)
6. Was under influence of alcohol and was in a hurry to finish the act and leave (12 respondents)
7. The respondents used to have "hi-fi" partners never thought they would have such *'sadiyal'* (rotten) infections from them (5 respondents)
8. Could not assess since it was always dark inside the room (5 respondents)
9. Used condoms so never assessed (3 respondents)
10. Never assessed since did not have sex outside marriage (2 respondents)
11. The respondent never had any complains about STI themselves, so dint feel the need to check the regular partner (2 respondents)
12. One of my partners had infections in her genital areas but since she was regular I did not use condoms.

Partner Denial

1. It is difficult, embarrassing to ask women and they would not share the truth too (7 respondents)
2. Partner denied to have sexual relations with the respondent when he inquired about her STI status (2 respondents)
3. The partner (girlfriend) was a good family and claimed to have no other affairs.

8.5.3 Frequency of partner's HIV status assessment

The MLHIV respondents were then asked on how frequently they assessed their partners HIV infection status. Only 1 respondent had 'Always' asked his sexual partner's HIV status and majority of the participants (96.5 percent) had 'Never' asked for their partner's status.

The reasons for not assessing partners STI status have been listed below.

Fatalism

1. Never thought I would get infected, since partner was healthy, home/non brothel based and I thought she was faithful. (46 respondents)
2. Focus was on having sex and I didn't care about infection (3 respondents)
3. Did not feel that it was important to assess (2 respondents)

Ignorance

4. Did not have any information about HIV during that time (63 respondents)
5. Did not find the time to assess this (4 respondents)
6. We don't check such things of partner when we are in love. (3 respondents)
7. The rates of the sexual partner were very high so assumed that she will be healthy
8. No one assesses the HIV status of male partners

Fear of discord with partner

9. Embarrassing to ask the partner, for she may disallow sex or there will be break in relationship and trust. The true HIV status may not be shared too (13 respondents)
10. I myself was infected and I dint want them to know this. If I would have asked them, they would have asked me too (3 respondents)
11. I had made the choice of my partner and they didn't ask me to come to them. (3 respondents)
12. Tried once but the partner felt agitated and suspected me of being infected

Safe sex

13. Used condoms often so didn't have to ask (2 respondents)

8.5.4 Level of Sexual Satisfaction

In this segment the MLHIV respondents were inquired on their level of sexual satisfaction both within marriage and outside marriage. It is observed from the graph below that the respondent's level of sexual satisfaction within marriage is higher than that outside marriage. About one fourth of the respondents (25.5 percent) felt that the level of satisfaction outside marriage was not satisfactory at all, while only 6.2 percent of the respondents felt the same within marriage.

Figure 27 Comparison on Level of sexual satisfaction

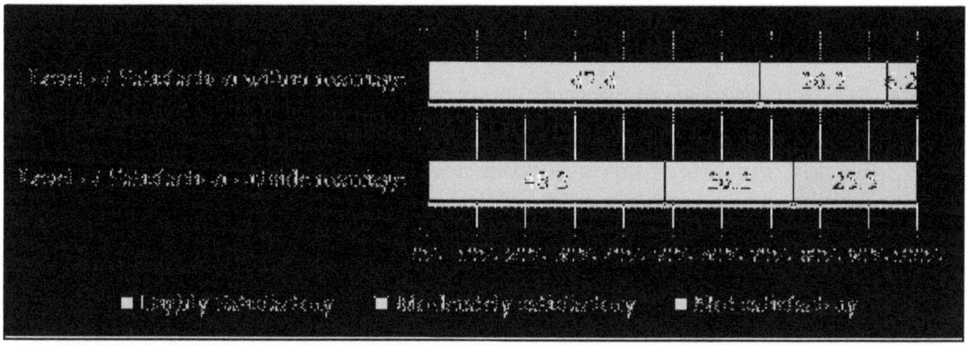

The respondents were further inquired on why some of them received greater satisfaction outside marriage as categorized below:

8.5.4a Reasons for greater level of satisfaction outside marriage

Reasons associated with spouse

- Regular conflicts at home had an adverse impact on sexual relations with spouse
- Spouse never took initiatives to perform sex
- Spousal disinterest in sex, "spouse doesn't have a good appetite for sex"
- Wife did not like oral and anal sex and couldn't have sex during menstruation

- I had to stay in different cities for purpose of work and had no access to wife and whenever I used to remember her, I felt like having sex outside.

Need for Variety

- "Greater interest and pleasure in having new sex partners, variety partners"
- "The partner outside marriage had better figure than wife"
- "I wasn't satisfied with my wife sexually and had greater interest to have sex with men"
- "Sexual partners outside performed various types of sexual acts and they had experience also. It is greater fun to do many things which can't be done with wife"

- "As commonly cited *'Ghar ki murgi daal barabar'*, my partner outside served my needs well and sex was fun with her unlike wife"
- "Sex outside happened only once in a while and with wife it was a regular event"
- "when the partner is new, the interest and pleasure is naturally double, I do get excited when girls outside have their hands over me and touch or hold me"

Social reasons

- Alcohol influence and paying for sex along with the time for intercourse being limited, helps deriving greater pleasure
- Restrictions to sex at home due to presence of parents n children
- Earlier the respondent roamed around together with spouse and had sex weekly, but after marriage when they had a child their responsibilities increased and couldn't enjoy. The respondents focus was then on earning and saving
- Wife being 11 years younger and showed immaturity, Neighbours wife was my partner then and she was satisfying

8.5.4b Reason for greater level of satisfaction within marriage

A few of the respondents, who had greater level of satisfaction with their spouses, have explained the reasons on why they claimed so.

- "I love my wife very much and she also loves me and hence sex with wife has greater pleasure" (love for spouse)
- "While having sex with wife I don't drink and am also not worried about restrictions of time, place, people watching etc., so the pleasure is greater" (not under the influence of alcohol)
- "There is no fear of people watching us and we can spend time and have as many encounters can have sex as much as we want without paying or worrying about time limits". (No fear of physical restrictions of time, space, money etc.)
- "Having sexual partners outside marriage on a frequent basis is a costly affair leading to dissatisfaction outside marriage"
- "The wife also enjoys the act simultaneously, unlike the sex worker, which gives satisfaction in the completion of the act" (mutual enjoyment and satisfaction)
- "Having sex outside was like fighting my own conscience each time, if I was doing something wrong and was feeling guilty. While with wife since this guilt was not there I was sexually satisfied after the act". (no guilt attached)
- "With my wife, I have a feeling of owning her and hence can perform whenever I am aroused. This gives satisfaction" (possession)

Thus the respondents enjoy greater sexual satisfaction with their spouses due to mutual love, non-influence of alcohol, no fear of physical restrictions of time, space, money, etc, no guilt of wrong doing attached and senses of possession of spouse.

8.5.5 Initiator of sexual activity within marriage

The married respondents were asked on who initiated the sexual advances within the marital relationship and more than half of the respondents (52 percent) stated that they by themselves have always initiated sexual relations. Less than half of the respondents (46 percent) felt that their spouses also took equal initiatives in sexual advances. A few respondents (2 percent) stated that their spouse always initiated sex.

This finding is crucial to understand why spouses are at risk to acquisition of the HIV infection and increased viral load, considering especially in the context of the above finding where only 5 percent of the male respondents claim to use condoms 'Often'.

8.5.6 Frequency of penetrative sexual act

Penetrative sex worldwide is understood in the paradigm of oral, vaginal and anal sex. HIV is more likely to be transmitted during anal sex than during vaginal sex, because the anus is not naturally lubricated, and small tears and lesions, that allow HIV to pass from one partner to another, can easily occur. This is especially true for the receptive partner, because sperm and other body fluids will remain in the anus after the inceptive partner has withdrawn (Map Report, 2005). While oral sex may not be entirely without risk, unprotected oral sex is much safer than unprotected anal sex. However, it is important to bear in mind that there is still a chance of HIV being transmitted from an infected person to an uninfected person during unprotected oral sex.

In the context of this understanding of risky penetrative behaviours, the MLHIV respondents were inquired about the types of penetrative sexual act that they were involved in, across their sexual careers and their response is demonstrated below.

Figure 28 Type of penetrative sex and Frequency of indulgence

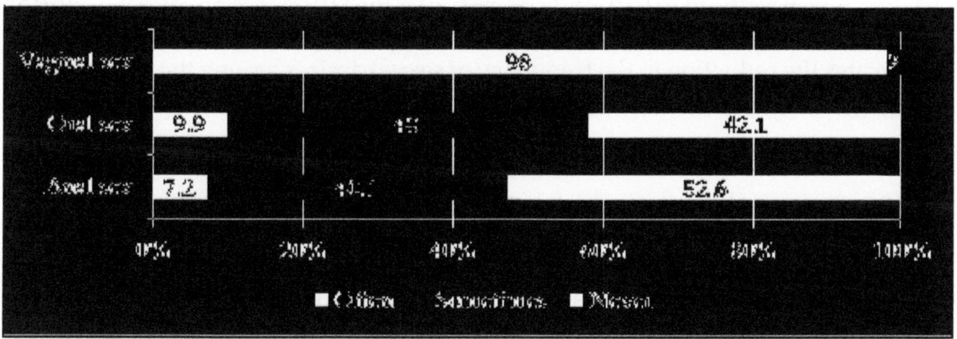

As seen in the graph above, almost all respondents (98 percent) performed vaginal sex during every sexual act, while only one in ten respondents performed oral and anal sex often during the sexual act. About half of the respondents as seen in green colour (52.6 and 42.1 percent respectively) in the graph had never ever tried oral and anal sex. According to most counsellors' perception (Phase-1), only around 3 percent of their MLHIV were believed to have anal sex, 2 percent have oral sex and 90 percent indulge in vaginal sex. However, the actual number of MLHIV indulging in penetrative behaviours, in the selected sample seems to be higher than what was perceived by the counsellors.

On cross tabulation, it was observed that 78 percent and 71 percent of the men who had oral and anal sex respectively did not have any male partners. Thus the frequency of anal sex and oral sex as depicted is to be contextualised with women. More men performed oral and anal sex with brothel based partners.

8.5.7 Frequency of Sexual Desires across phases of HIV

The MLHIV were inquired about the incidence of sexual desires in their lives across the phases of HIV infection. The phases of HIV infection have been compartmentalized as 'Before the HIV test', 'After the HIV test', 'After onset of ART'.

Figure 29: Frequency of sexual desire across stages of infection

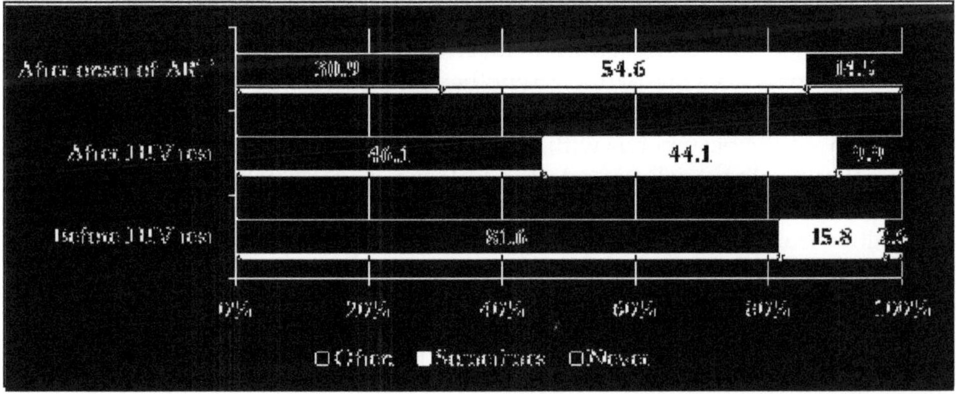

Majority of the respondents (81.6 percent) had sexual desires 'Often' before the HIV test, which reduced to half (46.1 percent) after the HIV test. And after the onset of ART the sexual desires further reduced to 30.9 percent. The graph below clearly demarcates the reduction in the frequency of sexual desires among the respondents, as they progressed in their phases of HIV infection.

8.5.8 Frequency of non penetrative sex across phases of HIV

On inquiring about the incidence of non penetrative sexual relations with their sexual partners, it was interesting to note that even the frequency of non penetrative sex reduced with growing 'phases of HIV infection'. This shows the lack of awareness amongst the MLHIV respondents about the fact that non penetrative sex is a safe sex tool to prevent HIV infection. This aspect of education need be stressed in counsellor's training so that in turn the MLHIV can be educated too.

Figure 30: Frequency of Non Penetrative Sex across stages of infection

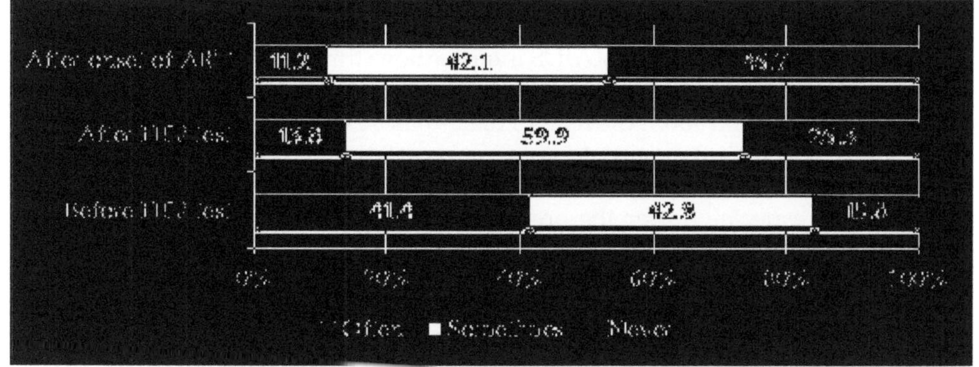

The above figure shows that the number of persons who indulged in non penetrative sexual practices are half of those who had sexual desires. Thus all those who desire may not be aware of non penetrative practices. There is scope for this education.

8.5.9 Frequency of using condoms across phases of HIV

It is noted that the use of condoms "Often", increased 5 times after the detection of HIV (ie. from 5.3 to 31.3 percent). And after the onset of ART six out of every ten respondents reported the use of condoms 'Often'. However, it is a matter of concern that more than half of the respondents 'Never' used condoms before the HIV test and about two out of every ten respondents (19.1 percent) continue not to use condoms after ART.

Figure 31: Frequency of condom use across stages of infection

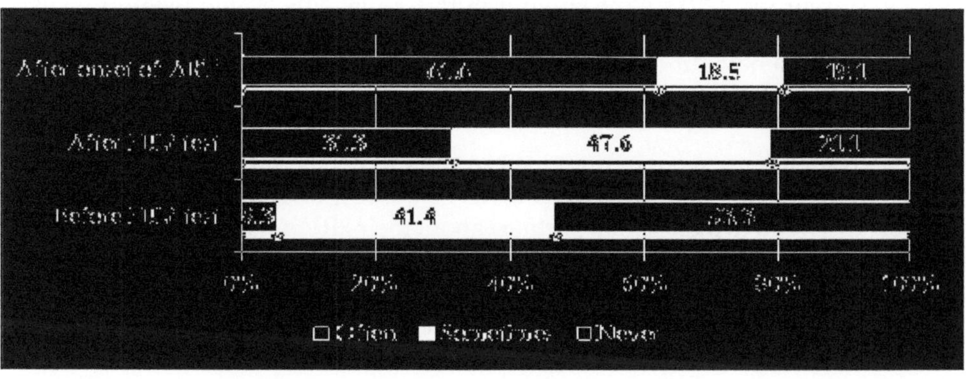

Consistency of condom use 'Often' as reported by 61.6 percent of the subjects after the onset of ART is certainly suboptimal but better than expected from earlier studies of male adolescents and HIV sero-positive adults. A 1990 national survey found that only 39 percent of sexually active young men (12 to 17 years of age) used condoms consistently. Another study of sexually active male and female high school students found that 32 percent reported always using condoms during sex (Gary Remafedi, 1997).

Almost everywhere it has been measured, condom use in commercial sex between males and females is consistently higher than condom use in commercial sex between males, even though male-male sex carries a far higher risk of HIV transmission. This is probably in part because HIV/AIDS interventions throughout Asia have focused attention on the issue of unprotected heterosexual sex. This has left many people inadequately informed about the risks of male-male sexual behaviours (Map Report, 2005). However, it is interesting to note in this study that respondents have often used condoms with their male sexual partners in the increasing phases of HIV infection and especially after the onset of ART with a moderate significance of association on Chisquare with a p value of 0.029 and df=6.

It is widely known that the STIs increase the likelihood of HIV transmission from one person to another during sexual encounters. STIs constitute a neglected epidemic even among males, in whom infections are more likely to be symptomatic. This is particularly so among women, in whom asymptomatic infections are common. But infections that are transmitted in anal sex are not just overlooked, they are almost completely invisible. So much so, that there is very few data available about this serious problem. The information that does exist is not encouraging (Map Report, 2005). It is interesting to note that in this study that the respondents who had STI did not use condoms consistently before the HIV test. However after the onset of ART, the frequency of condom use by respondents having STI was higher. This association was found moderately significant using chisquare with p value=0.052 and df=4.

About 60 percent of the counsellors (Phase-1) were of the opinion that their MLHIV clients would be indulging in protected sex. This is similar to what was reported by the MLHIV 'after ART' and thus triangulated. In the instances above, of increased condom use after ART both in case of homosexual partners or having an STI, points towards initiation of significant behaviour change attempts post treatment. Although from the above association it appears that safe sexual health practices have been attempted by the MLHIV, there is still room to build a crucial strategy to generalise this behaviour change and make it more consistent.

8.5.10 Frequency of disclosure across phases of HIV infection

The respondents were inquired about the frequency of HIV status disclosure and it was found that about three fourths of the respondents (75.5 percent) had "Never" disclosed to their sexual partners about their HIV infection. Two third of the respondents (66.9 percent) continued not to disclose their HIV status to their sexual partners even after the onset of ART *(pink shaded bars)*. However it is noteworthy that the frequency of disclosure "Often" is doubled 'after the onset of ART' from what it was 'after the HIV test'. The probable reasons for this are explored in the next chapter.

8.5.11a Number of sexual partners outside marriage

The number of lifetime sexual partners and knowledge about HIV/AIDS are significantly and positively associated with the use of condoms to prevent HIV infections (Nguyen, M.T. et al, 2002). To understand this, the total number of sexual partners outside marriage of the respondent, during their phases of HIV infection is explored in this segment.

It was found that before the HIV test, except for 7.2 percent respondents *(refer blue bar)*, all others had more than 1 partner before HIV test and interestingly 22.4 percent reported to have more than 10 partners. However after the HIV test result, it was seen that four out of ten respondents (40.8 percent) decided not to have any partners outside marriage. Further after the onset of ART, it was seen that it increased to six out of ten respondents (63.2 percent) abstained from partners outside marriage.

Figure 32 Frequency of Disclosure across stages of infection

Figure 33 Number of Sexual Partners outside marriage across stages of infection

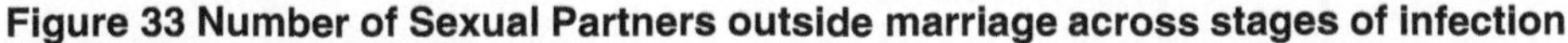

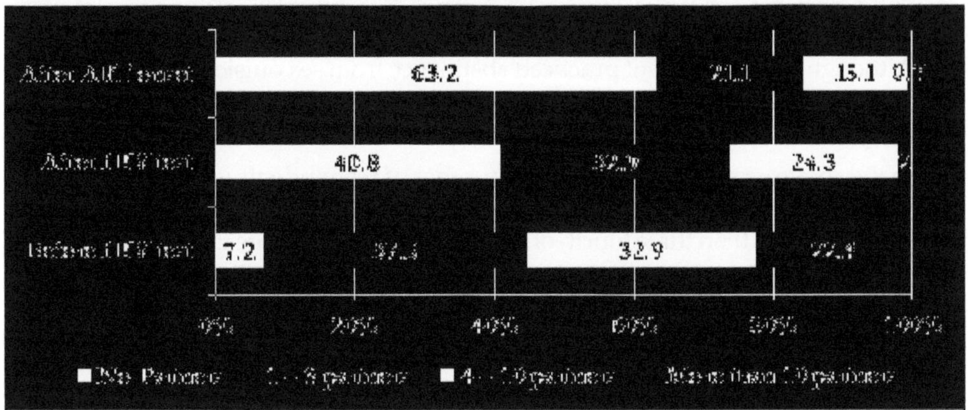

It is evident from the graph below that the multiple sexual partners outside marriage have drastically reduced after the onset of ART, proving true the set hypothesis. An average respondent before the HIV test had about 5 partners (median value), which reduced to about 2.53 partners, after HIV test and further reduced to 1.28 partners after the onset of ART.

8.5.11b Frequency of sexual indulgences outside marriage

With the understanding on the total number of partners outside marriage it was also important to know the frequency of sexual acts with them so as to understand the risk of acquisition and transmission of HIV. Thus the total number of sexual intercourses with partners outside marriage was elicited in the different 'phases of HIV infection'.

It was found that an average respondent had about 40 sexual intercourses (median value) outside marriage before the HIV test. This reduced to about 10 intercourses (median value) after being detected HIV positive and to 0 intercourses (median value) after the onset of ART.

Figure 34 Number of sexual indulgences outside marriage across stages of infection

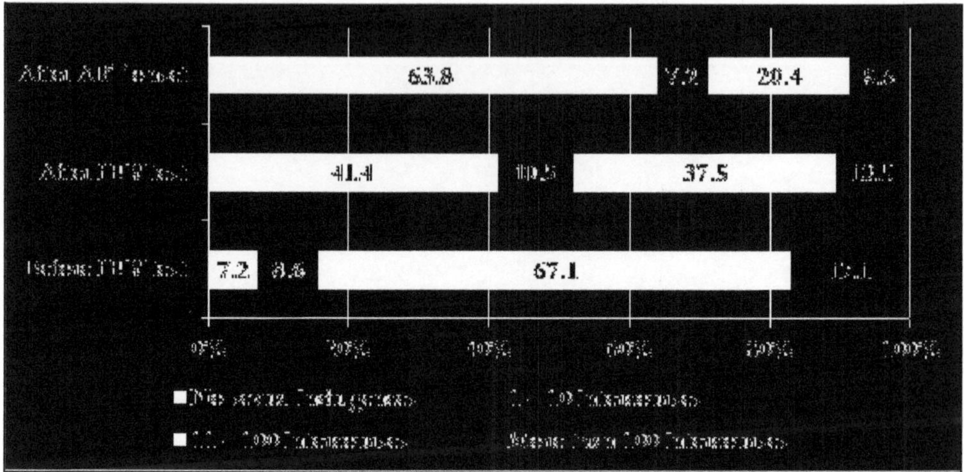

Although only 7.2 percent practiced abstinence from sex outside marriage, before the HIV test, it was observed that abstinence increased six fold (41.4 percent) after the HIV positive test and further to 63.8 percent after the onset of ART.

In the above graph, if we look at the number of respondents who had more than 10 sexual intercourses outside marriage *(colour coded green and purple)*, it is noteworthy that although more than three fourth of the respondents had more than 10 intercourses outside marriage, before the HIV test, it reduced to nearly half of the respondents after the HIV test and further reduced to nearly one fourth after the onset of ART. This indicates that the 'HIV test result' and the 'onset of ART' have both changed the risk indulgences of MLHIV.

8.5.11c Frequency of sexual indulgences with spouse

The respondents were probed on the frequency of sexual relations *(on an average)* with their spouses in a month, before HIV test and that after ART onset. In the graph below it is clear that eight out of ten respondents (82.8 percent) had 'Upto 4 sexual acts' with their spouse every month before the HIV test. This frequency of 'Upto 4 sexual acts' a month reduced to 63.4 percent after the onset of ART.

Interestingly, after ART, about three out of ten respondents (26.9 percent) abstained from sexual relations with spouse, which was not seen as a practice by any of the respondents before HIV test. The reasons for no sexual indulgence with spouse after ART also include death of spouse, divorce by spouse or because spouse stays at native place. The chapter on 'Behavior change' will further explore the influencing factors.

Figure 35 Number of sexual indulgences with spouse across stages of infection

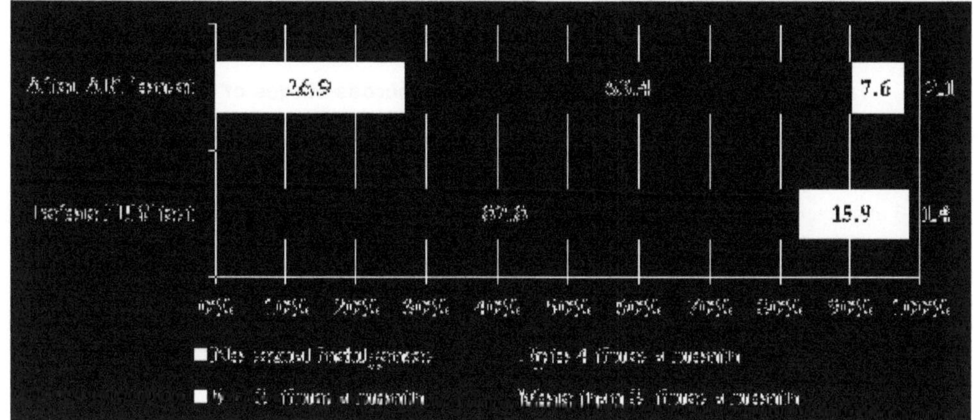

The counsellors interviews (Pase-1) show that spouses would be indulging in sex, in spite of HIV infection since the most spouses lack negotiation skills or because some are coerced into sex or seek procreation. According to one third counsellors, the spouses may continue to indulge in sexual relations since their sexual desires have to be met. This data shall be further triangulated in Phase-3.

8.5.12 Frequency of sexual indulgences with other men (MSM)

In many industrialized countries, a majority of people classify themselves relatively easily into one of three behavioural categories: homosexual, heterosexual or bisexual. But in Asia, people's sexual behaviours, occasional sex with male or transgender sex workers, for example, may not match their overt social identities (such as heterosexual family men). A high proportion of males reporting same-sex behaviour also have reported having heterosexual sex (Map Report, 2005).

In this study, out of the 152 respondents, about 22 respondents (14.6 percent) claimed to have had sex with men too and that they were behaviourally bisexual. None of the respondents accepted to be identified as a 'gay' and only one confessed that he had sex with a 'transgender'. The stigma often attached on 'male to male sexual behaviour' can encourage MSM to be secretive about this aspect of their lives. In most Asian countries, there is an unfavourable social and political climate for discussing issues related to MSM, and it is even more unfavourable for organizing communities to respond to the HIV/AIDS epidemic. As a result, MSM populations can remain hidden in many Asian settings, making it difficult for service providers to reach them. MSM may be more accessible to their peers, which means that the MSM community has a vital role to play in promoting HIV prevention measures within their community (Klitzman et al, 2004).

While "gay" social identity and norms are beginning to emerge in some Asian cities, a high proportion of men who have sex with other men do not consider themselves "homosexual," and also have sex with women. This plethora of identities and behaviours, illustrate the difficulty of even finding an appropriate term for the risk of anal sex between biological males in Asia. For the sake of brevity, this report will refer to people who engage in male to male sex as MSM (Map Report, 2005).

These 22 respondents who admitted MSM behaviours were inquired about their sexual relationships during the phases of HIV infection and the responses are classified:

Table 42 Frequency of homosexual acts across stages of infection

MSM Frequency of sexual act	Before HIV test	After HIV detection	After ART onset
No Male Partners	130 (85.5%)	143 (94.1%)	147 (96.7%)
1 to 3 anal intercourses	9 (5.9%)	4 (2.6%)	1 (0.7%)
4 to 10 anal intercourses	6 (3.9%)	0 (0%)	1 (0.7%)
More than 11 anal intercourses	7 (4.6%)	5 (3.3%)	3 (2%)
Total	**152 (100%)**	**152 (100%)**	**152 (100%)**

The table above points out that 'Before the HIV test', there were 22 respondents (ie. 9+6+7 respondents) (14.6 percent), who indulged in sex with men, which reduced to 9 respondents (5.9 percent) after the HIV test and further reduced to 5 respondents (3.4 percent) after the onset of ART. Thus to some extent there is reduction in bisexual behaviour among respondents after the HIV infection. However, those 5 respondents continuing to have unprotected sex with their male partners is a matter of concern.

It should be noted that the prevalence figures of above data are unlikely to represent HIV infection in the whole population of MSM. Still, this should act as a wake-up call to focus attention in identifying men from general community who depict homosexual behaviour but refuse to identify themselves as 'gay'.

In comparison with the counsellor's perception (Phase-2), it was observed that over half of the counsellors felt 1 to 5 percent of their MLHIV indulge in MSM behaviour. This finding is corroborated in this phase.

Summary of sexual indulgences in Phases of HIV Infection

The above findings explored in the context of phases of HIV infection have been summarized in the following table:

Table 43 Summary of sexual behaviours across stages of HIV infection

		Before HIV test	After HIV test	After ART onset
1	Experiencing sexual desires	81.6 %	46.1 %	30.9 %
2	Non Penetrative sexual practices	41.4 %	13.8 %	11.2 %
3	Incidence of condom use 'often'	5. 3 %	31.3 %	61.6 %
4	HIV status disclosure to sexual partners	NA	10.2 %	24.3 %
5	Frequency of sexual partners outside marriage (Average Median)	5 partners	2 partners	0 partners
6	Frequency of sexual intercourses outside marriage (Average Median)	40 intercourses per month	20 intercourses per month	0 intercourses per month
7	Frequency of sexual intercourse with spouse	1 – 4 times per month	*Not recorded*	1 – 4 times per month

8.6. ATTITUDES OF MLHIV TOWARDS MALE SEXUALITY

This research tried to explore whether the men's beliefs about manhood were the strongest predictors of risk-taking behaviour. These beliefs include the idea that "real" men have uncontrollable sexual needs, multiple partners who are often younger, drink alcohol, and use violence or intimidation to get what they want. Expectations that men should be more knowledgeable and experienced than women about sexual matters may also prevent them from seeking information about sexual health problems. Studies also demonstrate the link between these attitudes and behaviours, and women's increased vulnerability to HIV. A 2004 survey of 1500 South African women found those with violent or controlling male partners were at a higher risk of HIV infection (Bujra, 2000).

Traditional gender roles also increase the risk of a man being infected by and passing on HIV. Driven partly by stereotypes equating an increased number of sexual partners with increased sexual prowess, UNAIDS says that men - regardless of culture - tend to have more sexual partners than women. Although men might be aware of the dangers posed by HIV, ingrained notions of masculinity will often lead them to put themselves - and their partners - at risk. For example, the idea that "real" men have only "skin on skin" (unprotected sex) thrives in many African countries. Stereotypes also put men and their partners at greater risk: some men believe only promiscuous women carry condoms. Men might also be pressured by their peers to use alcohol or drugs, which often results in lower condom use and riskier, more careless behaviour. In one South African survey, young men were twice as likely as women to report having sex under the influence of alcohol (Hallman, 2004). A series of such questions have been developed by the researcher to understand the attitudes of MLHIV towards sexuality as below.

MLHIV Respondents Consolidated Attitude score

It was important to understand the attitudes of the MLHIV respondents towards their understanding on sexuality. Hence the need to derive a consolidated heath score of the respondent was felt, so as to ease the analysis of respondent's attitude with the other variables on sexual behaviour and disclosure.

A 14 point scale for MLHIV attitude was developed by the researcher, such that its responses are framed in the ascending order of the respondent's sexist attitude. The attitude of the respondents towards each item was scored in ascending order from Low to High sexist attitude as per this scale,

1 = Strongly Disagree, 2 = Disagree, 3 = Agree, 4 = Strongly Agree.

Thus indicating that respondents who strongly disagree with the statement is of low sexist attitude and the respondent who strongly agrees with the statement reflects his extreme sexist attitude. This scale was calculated to be highly internally reliable with a value of 0.758 for the 14 items taken together. The frequencies of responses have been tabulated Table 44.

Table 44

	MLHIV's Attitude towards Sexuality	Valid Percentage			
	1 = Strongly Disagree, 2 = Disagree, 3 = Agree, 4 = Strongly Agree	**SD1**	**D2**	**A3**	**SA4**
1	Male sexuality is always superior to female sexuality	3.3	17.8	53.3	25.7
2	Male sexual urges are stronger than the sexual urges in females	3.3	21.1	46.1	29.6
3	Infidel sexual expressions are not to be considered immoral	2.6	55.3	37.5	4.6
4	Male sexual behaviour has a greater degree of societal sanction	4.6	40.8	49.3	5.3
5	Male sexual behaviour need not be controlled as such, like female sexual behaviour	5.3	25.0	63.2	6.6
6	Men to men sexual expressions are acceptable as pleasure activities	25.7	46.7	17.8	9.9
7	Having multiple sexual partners, for a man is socially important	12.5	60.5	20.4	6.6
8	Sex with a virgin partner gives greater pleasure and satisfaction	1.3	19.7	36.8	42.1
9	Age doesn't diminish sexual desires in men, unlike women	6.6	27.0	52	14.5
10	Use of Condom diminishes the sexual pleasure in men	3.9	21.1	37.5	37.5
11	Men lose their mental and emotional stability 2.0 if their sexual needs and fantasies are not satisfied	24.3	38.8	34.9	
12	Elder male peers influence the sexual activity	3.9	18.4	71.7	5.9
13	Men should always take initiatives to perform sex	1.3	51.3	29.6	17.8
14	The wives unruly behaviour leads the man to practices illicit sexual behaviours	3.9	18.4	71.7	5.9

This Attitude scale has been designed such that the increasing order of agreement indicates a highly sexist attitude. As observed in this table, all respondents except one are seen to have a sexist attitude varying from moderately sexist to highly sexist attitude.

Attitude on Sexuality Cumulative Index: Theoretical classification

This being a 14 point Likert scale and all respondents having responded to all items in this tool, the minimum score the respondent can achieve is (14x1point) = 14 points and the maximum score being (14x4points) = 56 points. Based on the range of 14–56 points the set of values in the range is 43 points. Thus to classify the respondent's attitude, the range of 43 points have been divided into 3 theoretical class intervals of 14 points each, as designated below:

14 points : No sexist attitude

15 – 28 points : Low level of sexist attitude

29 – 42 points : Moderate level of sexist attitude

43 – 56 points : High level of sexist attitude

Based on this calculation the frequency for 152 respondents has been tabulated below

Table 45

Attitude on Sexuality: Cumulative Index	Frequency	Percent
No sexist attitude (14 points)	0	0
Low level of sexist attitude (15-28)	1	0.7
Moderate Level of Sexist attitude (29-42)	113	74.3
High level of Sexist Attitude (43-56)	38	25.0
Total	**152**	**100.0**

The table shows that almost all of the respondents had a sexist attitude, with three fourth of the respondents (74.3 percent) having a moderate level sexist attitude while one fourth of the respondents (25 percent) having a high level sexist attitude.

The **Attitude on Sexuality Cumulative Index** as seen in the table above was cross tabulated with various other dependent variables and associations with the following variables were found significant:

Table 46

#	Cross tabulation of MLHIV Attitude with	Pearson's value	Approx. Significance	Inference
1	Duration of stay in Mumbai	-0.003	0.976	Increase in the years of stay in Mumbai indicates a lower sexist attitude.
2	Personal income of respondent	0.061	0.457	As the respondents income increases, their sexist attitude seems to increase
3	Consolidated Health of respondent	0.066	0.422	Respondents with better health conditions seem to have a sexist attitude
4	Indulgence in pre-marital sex	-0.053	0.513	Respondents who have indulged in pre-marital sex show sexist attitudes
5	Indulgence in extra-marital sex	-0.039	0.639	Respondents who have indulged in e xtramarital sex show sexist attitudes

These results highlight that the sexist attitudes of the respondent seem to have associations with the greater income class of the respondents, higher order of occupation, greater number of sexual partners outside marriage and especially the ones having greater number of non brothel based partners.

It is the attitude, which influences any human behaviour and the fact that the respondents demonstrate a sexist attitude speaks volumes about their coercive and risky sexual indulgences. Although this interview does not capture the coercive behaviours of men in sexual indulgences, it captures the risky sexual indulgences as evident in the findings above. The association of masculinity to sexual behaviour is evident on a whole. The attitude scale results show the respondent's ideas of masculinity are still strong although they seem to have adopted safe behaviours and reduced risky practices. This understanding is further researched in the next 2 chapters which will speak of disclosure and behaviour change.

8.7 Major Findings

This chapter of Phase 2 dealt with the profile and sexual behaviours of 152 interviewed MLHIV and the major observations have been summarised below:

Major Findings: MLHIV Profile

- Most MLHIV were in the age bracket of 30 – 50 years and residing in Mumbai since 29 years. More than half of them had completed their primary education.
- Only one third of them were employed in service and the others were on daily wages (28 percent), business (20 percent) or unemployed (9 percent).
- Mean age of respondent's marriage was 26 years with 16 percent of them marrying before the age of 21 years. Re-marriage was observed in 7 percent of the MLHIV. Nearly 79 percent of the MLHIV currently lived with their spouses. All those who married at an early age were observed to have an STI.
- One tenth of the respondents did not have a personal income, while the mean personal income of more than half of the respondents was Rs.5,000. The mean family income (mostly supplemented through spouses) of most respondents was nearly Rs.10,000.
- The consolidated health of an average respondent was found to be 'Moderate' and poor health conditions held significance with greater age, lesser personal and family income, greater number of sexual partners and frequency of penetration.
- One fourth of the MLHIV's spouses were HIV concordant and they were observed to have a poor CD4 count, with half of them being on ART.
- The MLHIV respondents started residing in Mumbai at the median age of 8 years, their sexual fantasies erupted at the median age of 17, penetrative sexual debut happened at 20 years. However they got married at 26 and were found HIV infected at 33 (median age), after which, they were immediately enrolled on ART at 34 (median age). The spouses were tested after all this, when the MLHIV were 35 years old (median).

Major Findings: MLHIV Sexual Behaviours

- HIV detection in MLHIV happened at the age of 34 and ART was soon initiated at the age of 35 and spouses were also tested around the same age.
- 90 percent MLHIV admitted to pre-marital sexual relations and most of them had more than 3 partners. Respondents who had greater educational achievements and with a better health status indulged in pre-marital relations. Majority of the respondents did not use condoms consistently with their pre-marital partners. The major reasons for such indulgence include

experimentation, relaxation, peer influence and easy access. Most of the respondents had more relations with brothel based partners than with non brothel based partners.

- 60 percent of the MLHIV continued with extra marital sexual relations with most of them having 1-3 partners. The major reasons for such indulgence include relaxation, peer influence, experimentation, alcohol influence, wanting a change and issues with spouse. The respondents seemed to increase their access to non brothel based partners for extra-marital relations. Only 16 percent of the respondents were consistent in the use of condoms.
- Majority of the respondents never assessed the HIV or STI status of their sexual partners before penetration.
- More than half of the men claim to be the 'always' the initiator of sexual act
- The respondents confessed to a comparatively a greater level of sexual satisfaction within marriage than that outside, for reasons of greater comfort, more time, space and frequency for the act, no fear or guilt and better response from spouse.
- Nearly a tenth of the respondents 'often' indulged in oral and anal sex and most of them did so with their female counterparts.
- The onset of ART comparatively reduced the sexual desires, number of sexual partners outside marriage, frequency of non-penetrative acts, frequency of sexual indulgences and MSM behaviours, in comparison to the behaviours before the HIV detection. On the other hand the onset of ART positively enhanced the use of condoms and frequency of disclosure.
- The attitudes of MLHIV about sexuality were observed to be either moderately or highly sexist. The sexist attitudes seemed to reduce with longer duration of stay in Mumbai. These sexist attitudes were inflated by higher personal income, better health status or with indulgence in pre/ extra – marital sex.

Conclusion

This chapter of Phase-2 certainly brought to light a dip in risky sexual behaviours of MLHIV in comparison to that before the HIV detection. The risks faced by the spouses and feminisation of the epidemic are evident from the respondent's behaviour. Although some respondents have made attempts to change some of their high risk practices, there are areas of sub-optimal behaviour change, which should be a cause of concern for intervening organisations. These major areas where intervention is needed shall be triangulated with the findings of the other Phases in the last chapter. In line with the sexual practices, the next chapter shall to explore level of risk indulgences through the disclosure attempts made by the MLHIV.

Chapter 9

PHASE - 2 FINDINGS ON MLHIV DISCLOSURE

INTRODUCTION

Disclosure of one's HIV status to another significant person in life of PLHA can be one of the factors affecting Behaviour Change in them. Disclosure in a socially secured environment will help to reduce the stigma, discrimination and denial that still surround HIV/AIDS. People may suspect the clients HIV status, particularly if they show symptoms of AIDS. Fear and stigma is caused by ignorance and lack of complete information on the issue (NACO, 2006). The chapter on theoretical framework of disclosure points out strong associations between Disclosure and Behaviour Change.

This chapter is in continuation of the Phase-2 MLHIV interview, wherein the study objective is to trace the process and consequences of disclosure, to study the factors influencing disclosure and the barriers faced by the MLHIV respondents in disclosure. It includes the opinions of the respondents if their spouse or sexual partners had the right to know their HIV status, whether actual disclosure has been done. In cases of non-disclosure, the reasons are explored, the measures attempted for prevention of HIV transmission and help required for the same are some areas which have been explored. In cases of spousal disclosure, the reasons for disclosure, the consequent feelings after disclosure, the time required, words used, the spousal reactions and the impact of disclosure on sexual relations have been studied. Lastly, the processes of disclosure amidst other sexual partners as well as respondent's suggestions have been solicited towards encouraging partner disclosure.

9.1. SPOUSAL DISCLOSURE

9.1.a Right of the spouse to know the respondent's HIV status

The respondents were asked if they were of the opinion that their spouse reserves the right to know their HIV status. It was seen that 90.1 percent of the respondents were in favour of their spousal right to know the respondents HIV status.

9.1.b Legal Compulsion on Spousal Disclosure

The respondents were probed as to whether spousal disclosure should be made compulsory by law and it was found that four out of every five respondents (80.9 percent) were in favour of the need for such a legal binding. These respondents, who were in favour of legalization for disclosure, were further inquired on why they thought that spousal disclosure should be made compulsory by law. Out of them, 104 of the MLHIV gave reasons as follows:

Table 47 MLHIV's views on legalisation of spousal disclosure

#	Reasons	Frequency
1	Since spouse is primary caretaker and will be there till the end - *Spouse provides daily support in coping and treatment* - *She will be there for the children until the end*	58
2	Legalisation will help introduce safe practices and prevent the spread of infections - *Life of the spouse is precious and needs to be protected from infection* - *To prevent the spread of epidemic to innocent victims* - *To prevent a second generation of infection* - *Legalization will also help positive people to marry a concordant partner*	34
3	If not disclosed there will be discord in relationship - *One day or the other spouse will come to know of the husband's status, so it is better to disclose than they finding it out if such information is disclosed timely the relationship between the couple is not hampered*	6
4	Early diagnosis and treatment of other family members - *Helps prepare for spouse's failing health*	6
5	No reasons mentioned	18

Table 48

	Harm in legalization of spousal disclosure	Frequency
1	Stigma & Discrimination - *Legalization of spousal disclosure will automatically lead to public HIV status disclosure* - *None other than the wife will show acceptance to the positive status* - *The self esteem of PLHIV will be reduced. Although now the infection has normalized yet general community still don't come close to PLHIV*	10

Contd...

2	Breach of individuals right to privacy - *The choice of HIV status disclosure should be left to the individual and no legal compulsions should be made, people can be encouraged to do so"* - *"disclosure should be self initiated and not forced,* - *Instead of legalization condom use should be insisted, this will prevent the spread of the infection* - *The sexual partner should share truthfully about their infection. But the spouse need not be disclosed of HIV status since she has no option but to accept it.*	11
3	Discord in relationships - *Legalization will adversely affect marital relations*	4
4	Loop-holes in legalisation - *In spite of legalization, no one will speak the truth*	3
5	No reasons mentioned	2

9.1.c Disclosure to spouse

Men's reluctance to test their spousal HIV status can have devastating effects on their spouse. Lack of male involvement has been identified as a major impediment to the success of prevention of mother-to-child transmission (PMTCT) programmes. Studies show that pregnant women are less likely to agree to an HIV test, if they fear their partner's reactions. For those women who do accept the positive result, their participation in PMTCT programmes or their freedom to make appropriate feeding choices may be limited without disclosure to partners (Siti et al, 2007).

In this context, the respondents were inquired if their spouses were aware of their HIV status. This question was not applicable to the 7 respondents who were unmarried. Of the remaining married respondents (N=145), about nine out of ten respondents (92 percent) claimed to have honestly disclosed to their spouses of their HIV status. It has to be noted that the 92 percent of the respondents, who now claim to have disclosed their HIV status, have all done so mostly after the onset of ART *(as seen in the earlier chapter in the section age of spousal disclosure)*. This is a dangerous delay, since the viral load and the poor health conditions are at its peak and may lead to treatment failure.

There were 12 respondents (8.3 percent) whose HIV status continues to remain unknown to their spouses, in spite of their onset of ART. The reasons behind non disclosure were explored and are tabulated as below:

Table 49

#	Reasons for Non Disclosure (Multiple Response)	Frequency(Respondents)
1	Is preparing oneself to disclose the status later	6
2	Fear of being disallowed sex	5
3	Fears that the spouse will get upset after disclosure	4
4	Fear about loss of spousal support to the extent of marital discord	3
5	Fear of accusations of infidelity	1

(N=12)

9.2. NON DISCLOSURE

a. Help required in the process of disclosure

These 8.3 percent male respondents, who did not disclose their HIV status with their spouses, were asked what help they would require to disclose their status with their spouses and their responses were:

1. "I need a good counselling session for my partner and education on safe sexual practices and life after HIV." (5 respondents)
2. "I need help, to mentally prepare myself, in sharing the HIV positive status and related information with spouse." (3 respondents)
3. "I don't think there is a need to disclose to my spouse and hence no help required." (1 respondent)
4. "I don't want to disclose to my spouse now and if someday I have to, I will bring her to the counsellor." (1 respondent)

In order to counteract and assuage these fears, familial interaction, friend involvement, and generic social support are strongly encouraged (Johnson et al., 2001). Involvement is cited as the key towards an easier and more "successful" medical continuity (Ryan et al., 2007).

b. Respondent's plan towards spousal disclose

Considering the delay in disclosure, the respondents were in addition inquired on when they plan to disclose their status to their spouses and their responses are as below:

Table 50

	Intended plan for disclosure	Frequency
1	"Not decided now and will disclose whenever comfortable"	6 respondents
2	"Plan to disclose before sexual intercourse with spouse"	2 respondents
3	"Shall disclose during sickness"	2 respondents
4	"Shall disclose during pregnancy/ child birth"	1 respondent

The plan for disclosure as shared by the respondents (except one who had no plan) seem to be crucial incidents in their lives and the event of disclosure at these points of time may lead to negative reactions from spouse and impact reversely on their relationships, as seen in the discussions below.

a. Efforts made to prevent HIV transmission in the absence of disclosure

Of the 8.3 percent respondents, whose HIV status were not known to the spouses, the following efforts were claimed to be made by the respondent in prevention of HIV transmission to their spouses:

Table 51

	Efforts made in prevention of HIV transmission	Frequency
1	Uses condoms with spouse	4 respondents
2	Avoids sexual relations, especially during infection in the genitals	2 respondents
3	Has sex with partner very rarely since spouse resides in village	2 respondents
4	Spouse expired and hence not applicable	2 respondents
5	No attempts of prevention have been made so far	1 respondents
6	Spouse is also infected and hence no efforts are made towards HIV prevention	1 respondent

The efforts made by the respondents seem to follow the risk reduction model of behaviour change as explained in chapter 3, wherein the respondents continue to have sexual indulgences with reduced risky indulgences. The respondents yet need to be educated to transform their behaviours towards approaching the Harm Reduction Model.

9.3. DISCLOSURE: Process and Outcome of Disclosure

Voluntary disclosure refers to when a client shares information about their HIV status with other people. The counsellors training module highlights on 2 types of disclosure namely partial (where only a few people are chosen by the client for status disclosure) or full (client discloses status to everyone) disclosure. (NACO, 2006)

Most of the respondents (92 percent), who claimed that their spouses knew about their HIV status, were inquired more about the process and outcome of disclosure, as documented below:

a. Feelings after Disclosure

HIV status Disclosure is associated with ventilation as seen in chapter 3 and it is found that such ventilation can have both positive and negative feelings attached to the subject. The immediate feelings of the respondents after the act of disclosure with spouse were explored and their responses have been categorized into positive and negative feelings. This question was not applicable to 26 respondents, of which 7 respondents were unmarried, 12 respondents had not disclosed the status to spouse and another 7 respondents, whose health care provider directly disclosed the HIV status to their spouse.

The remaining 126 respondents hereby recollected their immediate feelings after disclosure and it was mentioned that more than half of the respondents (52 percent) felt negative after their disclosure. Less than one fourth of the respondents (24 percent) claimed to have felt positive after their disclosure. The remaining (24 percent) shared mixed feelings. Both the positive and negative feelings stated by them have been collated as seen in the two consecutive tables below:

Table 52 Positive Feeling after HIV status Disclosure

Feelings	Frequency	Percent
Sense of relief, relaxed, de-stressed and peaceful	33	55.9
Pleased, since it did not affect spousal relationship	16	27.1
Content with spousal acceptance, care and support	10	16.9
Total	59	100.0

Table 53 Negative Feelings after HIV status Disclosure

Feelings	Frequency	Percent
Felt ashamed to face spouse, fearing her reaction	37	40.2
Guilt of illicit behaviour persisted even after disclosure	21	22.8
Lonely, Depressed and Hopelessness	20	21.7
Anxious about health and future of family	14	15.2
Total	92	100.0

Thus as evident from the above tables, more respondents have associated negative feelings with disclosure (73 percent) in comparison to those who have associated positive feelings (46.8 percent). In spite of these negative feelings a large number of them agree for legalisation of spousal disclosure!

The negative feelings housed within oneself, as shared by the respondents seem to be short-lived and based on the respondent's coping skills it would have been outlived sooner or later. Thus it can be perceived that the process of ventilation vis-a-vis disclosure has a positively loaded 'Impact on Self feelings', although it may have interim hick-ups initially. It will now be interesting to observe the other dimensions of the impact of disclosure.

On cross tabulating the respondent's feelings after disclosure with other variables, the following significant relationships were observed when using a Chi-square test.

Table 54 Factors influencing feelings after disclosure

#	Factors	p value	df	Inference
1	Duration of stay in	6 Mumbai	0.044	Longer the duration of the respondent's stay in Mumbai, higher the chances of positive feeling associated with disclosure
2	Currently living with spouse	0.001	2	Those respondents who currently lived with spouse show greater negative feelings associated with disclosure. Most of those respondents not living with spouse have positive or mixed feelings after disclosure
3	Frequency of STI of respondent	0.004	4	Increased frequency of STI incidence leads to greater chances of acquiring Negative feelings after disclosure
4	Indulgence in Extra marital sex	0.031	2	More respondents who indulged in extra-marital sex had negative or mixed feelings after disclosure
5	Initiator of sexual activity within marriage	0.036	1	More respondents whose spouses initiated sexual activity claimed to have had positive or mixed impact of disclosure.
6	Time taken by respondent for disclosure	0.000	6	Greater the time taken by the respondent for disclosure, higher the positive the feeling associated with disclosure

#		Spearman's r value		Inference
		Asym. Sig.		
1	Age of respondent	0.534	-0.057	More older MLHIV have faced Negative reaction from spouses
2	Period of time required for disclosure	0.389	0.095	Most respondents who had a positive feeling associated with disclosure had taken more than a week's time to prepare themselves for disclosure

b. Reasons influencing HIV status Disclosure

The respondents were inquired on what were the reasons which encouraged them to disclose their HIV status to their spouses and their responses are as follows:

Table 55 Reasons for spousal disclosure

	Reasons :	Frequency	Percent
1	Sense of responsibility towards partner or concern for partner's health	95	75.4
2	Need for spousal support to cope with treatment	91	72.2
3	To prepare spouse for failing health /severe illness	89	70.6
4	Disclosed under doctor's/ counsellor's insistence	45	35.7
5	To alleviate the distress associated with non-disclosure	42	33.3
6	To facilitate HIV-preventive behaviour	14	11.1
7	To help wife get tested and prevent the child from infection	4	3.2
8	Since spouse tested HIV positive, it was obvious that she was infected through me and hence disclosed	4	3.2
9	Organizations like CHIRAG motivated me to disclose the status to spouse	3	2.4
10	Spouse insisted on sex often and I could not deny always without any reason	1	0.8

The factors influencing spousal disclosure thus seem to include concern for spousal health, need for spousal support, to alleviate distress of non disclosure, to facilitate preventive behaviours, early spousal testing. These factors being self initiated by the respondent is an empowering attempt. Additionally it is seen that the insistence and influence NGOs, counsellors, doctors and spousal test results have also played an important role in encouraging disclosure. It has to be understood that due to the influence of these stakeholders, the respondents have taken initiatives to disclose.

c. Disclosure was initiated by

Studies show that disclosure initiatives made in presence of the HCP is beneficial in order to control the immediate reactions of the spouse very skilfully (Hays et al., 1992). However, only 6.8 percent of the respondents undertook this strategy, while more than half of the respondents initiated spousal disclosure by themselves in solitude (56.4 percent), indicating that disclosure is treated as a very private affair.

Sadly, in one third of the cases either the HCP revealed the respondent's status to the spouse (27.8 percent) or the spouse herself discovered the respondent's HIV status (9 percent). Both these cases seem to be potential dangerous for the spouse to react negatively. The MLHIV responses on status disclosure initiatives to their spouse are as under.

Table 56 Initiator of Disclosure

Initiator	Frequency	Percent	Valid Percent
Self initiated	75	49.3	56.4
Health Care Provider (HCP) revealed	38	24.3	27.8
Spouse discovered my status	12	7.9	9.0
Self in presence of HCP	8	5.9	6.8
Total	133	87.5	100.0
NA since unmarried or not disclosed	19	12.5	-
	152	100.0	-

On cross tabulating with the respondent's negative feelings after disclosure it was observed that when disclosure was self initiated, in most cases the respondents had a fear and anxiety about spousal reaction, ashamed to face her, or felt lonely/ depressed/ hopeless. Most respondents also continued to feel guilty about their illicit behaviour.

However, in cases where the HCP revealed the status to the spouse, the respondent was at the receiving end of spousal blame, abuses and fights. This phenomenon was observed to be highly significant when using Pearsons test with a significance value of 0.009. Disclosure attempts initiated by 'Self, in presence of the HCP' did not seem to have any negative reactions attached to it. Thus the spousal reactions and implications after disclosure are dependent on the type of individual who initiated it. Thus it can be considered that the HCP should not directly disclose the status to the spouses and should encourage the MLHIV to disclose in their presence. The HCP can then supplement the education on HIV and handle their anxieties in this regard.

The counselling training module highlights the role of a counsellor to help the client identify possible impacts of the decision to disclose. A counsellor needs to assist the client in exploring who to tell, how and when to tell. In this way, the client can remain in control of what to say and how to say it and also be prepared for the range of possible out comes before disclosing their status (NACO, 2006). This is an area where the counsellors need to help their MLHIV clients as they prepare to disclose.

a. Situation of disclosure

As seen in chapter 3, the 'when' and 'where' are the factors which influence the implications of disclosure. Accordingly the 83 respondents, who initiated disclosure either by themselves or with the help of their HCW, were inquired of the situation in which they disclosed their HIV status. As seen in the doughnut below, there were only 7 percent respondents, who took time out to discuss about their status. This indicates that the communication pertaining to disclosure of the respondent's HIV status rarely happened in a healthy/ enabling environment. Descriptive analysis show that many of these respondents (59 percent), who have disclosed in stressful situations underwent an immediate negative reaction of the spouse as discussed above.

Figure 36 Situations of Disclosure

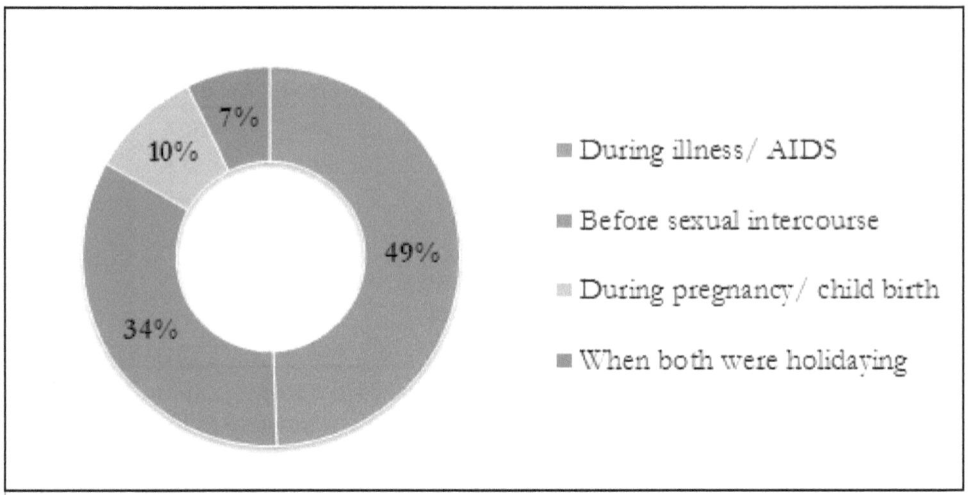

Instances of disclosure initiated by the others

Of the 50 respondents whose status disclosure was not self initiated were inquired of the instance in which spousal disclosure occurred and their responses have been recorded in the doughnut below.

Figure 37 Situation in which Disclosure was not initiated by self

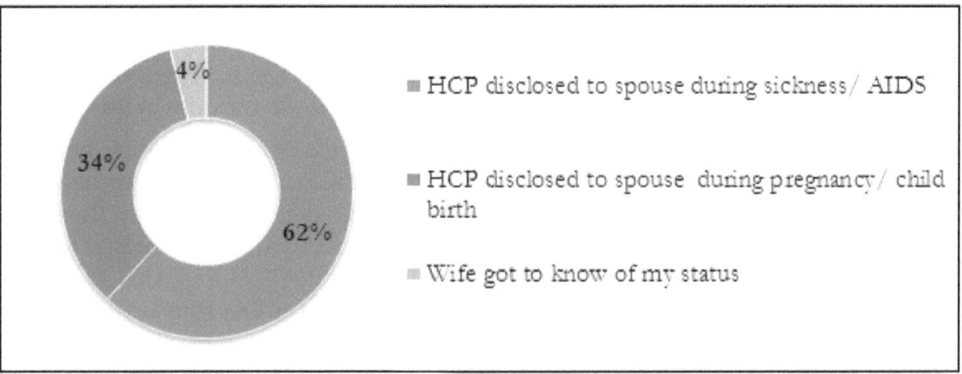

As seen above, disclosure by HCW in situation of illness/ AIDS, predominates the disclosure during child birth indicating that the spouse come to know of their husbands HIV status only at a later stage of their infection. This is not just a concern for the spouses to meet appropriate care and treatment needs for their husbands but also it becomes pretty late for them to initiate health seeking facilities for their own self. In other words sickness and pregnancies are precipitating factors which put certain compulsion on the individual PLHIV to go for disclosure. A voluntary disclosure can thus be based on an enabling situation, which makes the process of disclosure easier for the MLHIV. However, a delay in the occurrence of such enabling situations can lead to delay in disclosure causing greater harm. The MLHIV clients therefore need to be empowered on how disclosure can be initiated without waiting for enabling situations.

a. Time spent on spousal disclosure

It is essential that an individual spends considerable amount of time with the partner (if required in phases) to explaining about one's status. The reactions of the spouses is obvious and time has to be given to respond to this too (Serovich, 2005). An attempt was made in this study to understand the time taken by the respondents in disclosing their status with their spouses and it was interesting to observe that the process of disclosure took less than 5 minutes for about half of the respondents (49 percent).

Figure 38 Time spent for disclosure process

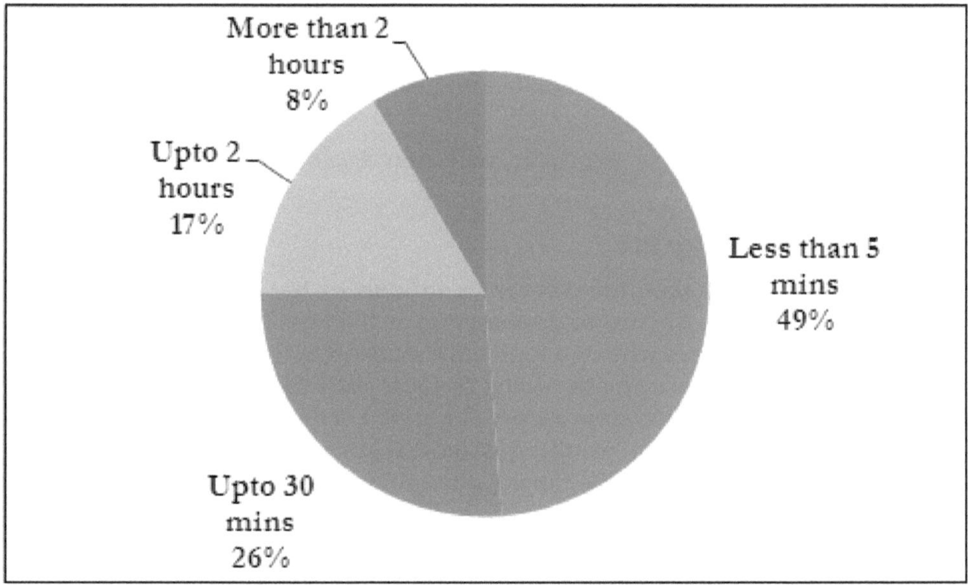

On cross-tabulating the time spent in disclosure with the negative feelings of the respondents after disclosure, it was observed that none of the respondents who had spent more than 2 hours in disclosure harboured any negative feeling as the outcome of disclosure. Moreover as seen in the table below, the greater the time spent in disclosure, the lesser the negative reactions faced. A significant positive correlation has been observed between these 2 variables with on Pearsons test with a significance value of 0.47

Table 57 Cross-tabulation on time spent on disclosure and negative feelings

	Negative feelings harboured after disclosure			
Time spent in disclosure	Lonely, Depressed and Hopelessness	Fear and anxiety about spousal reaction, ashamed to face	Anxious about health and future of family	Saddened by guilt of illicit behaviour, cried a lot
Less than 5 mins	13	14	6	5
	81.30%	53.80%	50.00%	55.60%
Upto 30 mins	3	10	6	2
	18.80%	38.50%	50.00%	22.20%
Upto 2 hours	0	2	0	2
	0	7.70%	0	22.20%
Total	16	26	12	9
	100%	100%	100%	100%

Similarly on cross-tabulating the time spent in disclosure with the positive feelings after disclosure, it was observed to be moderately significant using a Chi-square test with a value of 0.074 with df=6, indicating that greater amount of time spent in disclosure is proportional to the positive feelings. Greater time spent in disclosure also had moderate significant association with the following variables related to reasons of disclosure

1. To prepare spouse for failing health/ sickness (Chi-square value = 0.009, df=3)
2. To alleviate distress associated with non disclosure (Chi-square value = 0.034, df=3)

a. Period of Disclosure

The time period taken for disclosure influences the impact of disclosure negatively, with shock, distrust and separation as the possible outcome (Siti et al, 2007). The 84 respondents who had initiated disclosure were inquired on the time required in preparing themselves in doing so. Over one tenth of the respondents (13 percent) mentioned that their spouses were informed of the respondent's HIV status on the same day of the HIV test result, while more than one third (34 percent) claimed to have disclosed after a month's time. Although no significant associations were found on the negative impact of such early disclosure, it raises concern on the type of preparation undertaken towards such disclosure.

Figure 39 Period of Time taken in preparation for disclosure

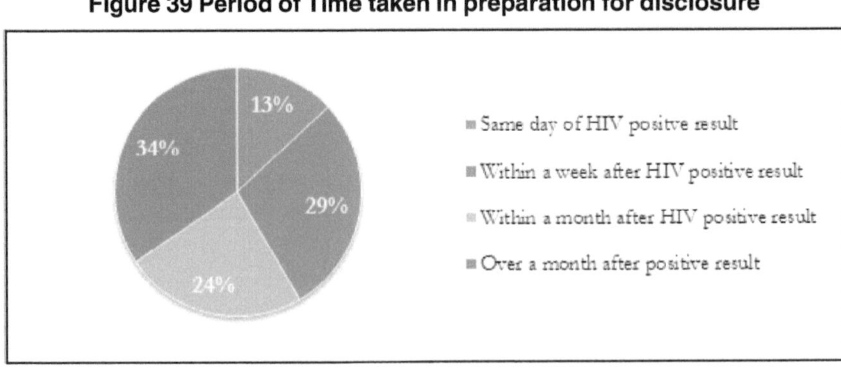

The time taken in disclosure was cross tabulated with Incidences of condom use after HIV infection and the significant association was observed with a chi-square test significance value of 0.067 at df=6. This indicates that the condom use have increased after disclosure in the studied sample even though it shows a very weak significant association. This association can be further tested in future with higher number of samples. This finding somewhat proves true the study hypothesis "Longer the duration of living with HIV, greater the comfort level of HIV status disclosure to spouse"

a. Words used for disclosure to spouse

These respondents who initiated disclosure with spouse were asked on the words used in disclosure so as to better understand the attempt made towards disclosure.

Table 58

#	Table 58Words used for Disclosure	Frequency	Valid Percent
1	Stating Confidently: *I have HIV but there is nothing to worry. Thereafter motivated family for testing*	53	48.2
2	HCP helped explain infection and result to spouse	17	15.5
3	Stating with Self Guilt : *Confessed to spouse about past behaviour, pleaded forgiveness, promised behaviour change*	14	12.7
4	Stating to elicit sympathy: *I have HIV and won't live long.*	8	7.3
5	Eliciting Mutual support: *Now that both are positive we need to support each other and live for our children*	8	7.3
6	Confessing timidly: *When spouse asked me, I calmly accepted to be infected*	6	5.5
7	Blaming the spouse for the infection: *I don't know how I got HIV infected*	4	3.6
	Total	**110**	**100.0**

Additionally, the respondents as mentioned in the above table used the below mentioned statements like in disclosing their status to their spouses:

a. Blaming the spouse for the infection

- *"I don't know how I got infected. I did no wrong activity else you and our children would have been infected too."*

b. Confessing with Self Guilt

- *"Don't leave me, I made a mistake, forgive me"*
- *"I have tested positive for HIV, you also need to test. I may be infected because of you since I never had sex with a female outside marriage and hence I see no other reason of being infected".*
- *"I took her out to a garden, told her that I'm afraid to share the problems of my life with her and that I was guilty about my past behaviour, which led me to infection. I told her that I was being cheated by my sexual partner with whom I had sex once. She didn't tell me about her infection"*

c. Stating to elicit sympathy

- *"After wife was tested positive, I disclosed that I am also HIV+ve, and I told her "we both need to live for our elder daughter who is negative"*
- *"Gave examples of a few other illnesses and how it took peoples' lives, later after seeing spousal reaction, I mentioned that I have HIV and that I will have to be on medicines life-long."*
- *"I had severe TB and was hospitalized, shared with my wife that I have TB and HIV infections, within my body which is making me sick"*
- *"I'm wanting to have poison and end my life"*
- *"what had to happen has happened, you don't worry, if I take the drugs on time everything would be alright"*

d. Stating Confidently

- *"I have AIDS and I'm HIV positive" (she then responded negatively and I was handling her emotions, we discussed HIV and its impacts related knowledge that I had)*
- *I informed the spouse that I underwent a blood test and the result showed HIV infection*
- *I made her understand that this infection is spread through blood*
- *"I'm falling sick often due to HIV infection"*
- *I phoned her and told her that I'm suffering from TB, health is going weak, falling ill often and doctors say that I have AIDS too*
- *"My blood is infected, I said I dint know how" and asked her to test her blood, after test doctor shared the result with both of us and instructed not to have sex*

9.3.2 Spousal response to MLHIV's status disclosure

The MLHIV respondents were asked on how their spouses reacted on the disclosure; the following reactions were recollected by the respondents:

Table 59: Spousal response to MLHIV's status disclosure

#	Response of spouse	Frequency	Valid Percent
1	Spouse was shocked, anxious about OI, self treatment and concerned over the death of family members	37	30.1
2	Spouse cried, cursed and dint talk for some days	21	17.1
3	Periodic anger, irritated behaviour of spouse and blamed the husband (respondent) for spoiling her life	20	16.3
4	Disclosure was accepted without any reaction since spouse dint understand HIV	17	13.8
5	Spouse deserted husband or divorced	15	12.2
6	Verbal and physically abusive behaviour of spouse	13	10.6
	Total	**123**	**100.0**

9.3.3 Impact of Disclosure on sexual life

The MLHIV respondents were questioned on the impact of disclosure on their sexual lives. Interestingly, 105 respondents (69.1 percent) shared negative impact of disclosure while 84 respondents (55.3 percent) shared the positive side of disclosure. This indicates that there are more chances of a MLHIV respondent facing a negative impact of disclosure. This negative impact can be because of the improper situation chosen or inadequate time taken in disclosure as explained above.

The impact of disclosure, as stated by the participants, has been classified into negative and positive as explained in the tables below:

Table 60 Negative impact of Disclosure

Nature of impact	Frequency	Valid Percent
Sexual Abstinence, spouse shows disinterest in sex	48	45.7
Have to performs non penetrative sex, safe practices	28	26.7
Reduced sexual relations with spouse	19	18.1
Spouse insists on condom use	7	6.7
Ashamed to have sex with spouse	3	2.9
Total	**105**	**100.0**

Table 61 Positive impact of disclosure

Nature of impact	Frequency	Valid Percent
Sexual intimacy was gradually accepted by spouse	55	67.9
Joint decision on safer practices to prevent re-infection	10	12.3
Couple approached counselling on sexual relations	6	7.4
Reduction in guilt feeling about past infidelity	8	9.9
Took necessary precautions in child bearing	2	2.5
Total	**81**	**100.0**

Those who shared of a positive impact of disclosure spoke of one's own feelings as well as better relationship with the spouse.

9.3.4 Further assistance required in process of disclosure

The respondents were inquired if they needed any assistance in disclosure and except for 5 respondents, the others did not seem interested in external support for disclosure. Those who said they needed assistance elaborated it as under:

- *"Need help in bringing back my spouse from village and making her understand to spend rest of the life happily together and provide me care and support during illness."*
- *"Need counselling on HIV and in keeping the marriage intact."*
- *"help required to make the spouse understand that HIV is not a serious infection"*
- *"Family counselling required for my spouse to make her understand implications of HIV better and cope with our situation."*
- *"Need more information on how to protect oneself from the infection."*

9.4. NON SPOUSAL DISCLOSURE

a. Right of the non spousal sexual partners to know of your status

The MLHIV respondents were asked if they thought that it is the right of their sexual partners to know of their HIV status. Over half of the respondents (57 percent), have agreed that it is the right of the non spousal sexual partner (sexual partners outside marriage) to know their HIV status. It is a matter of concern that 43 percent respondents do not agree about the right of the sexual partner to know about their infection. This may lead to unsafe sexual practice and the spread of the infection. The respondents have stated the following reasons that explain their stand:

Table 62

	HIV status disclosure to non spousal sexual partners	Frequency	Valid Percent
+	Disclosure will help prevent our partners from getting infected from us	64	54.2
-	It's the commercial sexual partners responsibility to take self care with every client they cater to	14	11.9
-	On disclosure, partners will refuse to have sex straight away	11	9.3
-	Disclosure is the individual's choice of sharing and this decision cannot be seen as our partners right	10	8.5
-	"Even the sexual partners will never disclose their status truthfully, so why should we"	7	5.9
+	"Partners outside marriage also have a right to lead a healthy life and hence need to be disclosed"	6	5.1
+	Disclosure will enable the use of condoms and practice safe sex during the act with sexual partner.	6	5.1
	Total	**118**	**100.0**

c. Frequency of disclosure to non spousal sexual partners

The MLHIV respondents were inquired on the frequency of their HIV status disclosure to their non spousal sexual partners. It was found that only 3 percent of the MLHIV disclosed their status to their partners 'Every time', while another 3 percent disclosed 'Sometimes'. This finding proves true the hypothesis "HIV status Disclosure to other sexual partners would be minimal"

The remaining majority of the respondents 94 percent of the respondents have 'Never' disclosed their status to their non-spousal sexual partners and this is certainly a concern in the spread of the infection. Their reasons for not disclosing to the sexual partners ones HIV status have been as stated by the respondents as below (multiple response):

1. "Did not know of my HIV status" (60 respondents)
2. "Afraid that partner won't permit sex" (60 respondents)
3. "Since I pay for sex I dint need to disclose" (46 respondents)

4. "Partners would anyways be infected due to their high risk behaviours" (31 resp)
5. "Did not need to disclose, since I performed protected sex" (15 respondents)
6. "I knew that sexual partner was also infected" (5 respondents)

d. Disclosure to long term partners

As seen in the literature review, some studies have pointed out that non spousal disclosure is positively associated with sexual partners, who serve a long term relationship with the male (Jourard, 2005). Accordingly, the respondents were inquired if they had disclosed their status to those sexual partners with whom they were associated for a long period of time. In response, 28 percent of the respondents stated that they did not have a partner, with whom they were regular for a long period of time.

In contrary to the above study results, only 6 percent of the MLHIV respondents in this study had disclosed to their long term partners. It is interesting to note that these respondents, who had shared their HIV status with their sexual partners outside marriage, stated that it did not have a negative impact on their relationship and they started using condoms in their relationship. An attempt was made to study more about the behaviours of these respondents, who had a long term (non spousal) sexual partner, and had disclosed to their HIV status to their partners. Cross-tabulation results of within case analysis show that All of these respondents were married and

- 4 of them (out of 9) were not living with their spouses
- 8 of them (out of 9) had also shared with their spouses about their status
- 8 out of 9 were also using condoms, although none used it before the HIV test
- 7 of them (out of 9) frequented a non-brothel based partner with whom they had disclosed their status.

Thus indicating that disclosure with long term non spousal sexual partner may also be predictive of spousal disclosure, increased use of condoms and that the sexual partner is of a non-brothel based origin.

9.4.2 Suggestions to encourage disclosure to sexual partners

Based on one's life experiences, the MLHIV respondents were requested to suggest how a PLHIV should proceed with disclosure and their suggestions include:

a. *Strategize the steps of initiating disclosure*

- "Don't worry too much, take help of ORW at the hospital and they will guide you by making home visits and speaking to spouse" (3 respondents)
- PLHIV couples who have already disclosed their status to spouse should share at the hospital on how they got better care and support of the spouse. (2 respondents)
- When counselling on HIV prevention the counsellor should encourage clients to disclose to their sexual partners

- Spouses can be brought to ART Centre, and their fears regarding HIV be removed first by individual counselling and later disclosed.
- PLHIV peer counsellors sharing their self experiences is very encouraging
- Conduct awareness programs on disclosure amongst couples at ART Centre
- People other than close family members should not be involved in disclosure.
- The decision of whom and when to disclose should be left to the individual
- People working in this field should bring an end to the spread of this epidemic first, through medicines and then disclosure will not be a problem

b. Show clients benefits of disclosure

- Early disclosure brings peace within oneself and builds better relations.
- Disclosing will help save many people's lives from acquisition of HIV
- Disclosure leads to reduction in high risk activity
- Disclosure is beneficial to one's own treatment since you have to take drugs daily and come to hospital monthly, before the spouse suspects it is important to tell them so as to receive assistance in treatment. (2 respondents)
- Disclosure is important for early diagnosis and treatment of spouse (2 respondents)
- Early disclosure helps have safe sex and will help your wife remain healthy and keeps her from being infected (3 respondents).

c. Motivating messages that one can give PLHIV

- "Every possible step should be taken to prevent spread of HIV to partners, it is our responsibility as infected individuals"
- "Sharing your status will help prevent the spread of the epidemic"
- "Negative persons can continue to remain negative with HIV status disclosure. Help the negative persons protect their lives"
- "It is our responsibility not to spread the infection for a healthy society"
- "Its better that the MLHIV withdraws and terminates the sexual relationship"
- "Your wife should not come to know from someone else about your HIV status else it will cause marital discord"
- "How long will u keep this away from your wife? She may say no to condom one day and would thus get infected."
- "Even if you don't tell anyone else about your HIV status you should tell your wife, as this is what makes them responsible husband"
- One has to take courage to initiate disclosure, reality cannot be hidden for long, *dar ke mat bolo hakk se baat karo* (don't disclose with fear, speak with might)

- Information sharing is important and hiding it will only aggravate the discomfort and pain, it is our responsibility to share in order to protect health of partner
- PLHIV should be happy and told that disclosure will keep partners happy too

9.5 Major Findings: MLHIV Disclosure

- 90 percent of the respondents felt that their spouses have the right to be disclosed and 81 percent agreed that there should be a legal compulsion to spousal disclosure stating that such disclosure was important since the spouse is primary caretaker, also to prevent the spread of infection to spouses, to prevent discord in relationship and enable care, support and treatment processes.
- 92 percent of the MLHIV claimed that their spouses knew of the MLHIV status. While the others are preparing themselves for disclosure and most of them are taking efforts towards prevention of HIV transmission.
- Nearly half of the respondents had negative feelings immediately after disclosure (shame, fear, guilt, lonely, anxiety, depression and hopelessness), while only one-fourth expressed positive feelings (relief, relaxed, peaceful, pleasant and accepted). Positive feelings showed strong associations with longer duration of stay in Mumbai, currently residing with spouse, those who spent more than a week in preparation for disclosure, those who spent greater time spent on disclosure and in those MLHIV where the spouses initiated sexual intercourse. Negative feelings showed associations with older age of MLHIV, presence of STI and indulgence in extramarital relations
- The reasons for MLHIV disclosing their status comprised of: sense of responsibility towards partners health, need for spousal support to cope with treatment, to prepare spouse for failing health, doctors insistence and to alleviate distress associated with non-disclosure.
- Disclosure was initiated by MLHIV only in half the cases and otherwise the spouse got to know of MLHIV status either through HCP or self discovery. Direct disclosure by HCP seemed to have a negative impact on the couple's relationship.
- Self Disclosure was mostly made during illness of MLHIV or before sexual intercourse / holidaying or during pregnancy.
- Nearly half of the respondents spent less than 5 minutes in disclosure. Greater amount of time spent in disclosure showed positive co-relations with positive feelings associated with disclosure.
- More than half of the MLHIV took at least a week's time to prepare themselves for disclosure and these cases also showed increased condom use.
- The immediate spousal response included shock, anxiety about her health, fear of death, reduced communication, periodic anger and weeping. Tenth of

the MLHIV reported spousal behaviours like verbal / physical abuse and separation.

- The negative impact of disclosure from the spouse included sexual abstinence, disinterest in sex, non penetrative practices, insistence on condom use (reported by 70 percent MLHIV). Over half of the respondents reported positive spousal reaction like acceptance, greater intimacy, taking joint decisions on safer practices, initiatives to attend couple counselling sessions and careful child bearing.
- Over half of the respondents agreed on the need for disclosure to non spousal partners and the need for legalising the same as a measure for HIV prevention. However 94 percent MLHIV reported to have 'Never' disclosed their status to non spousal partners and those MLHIV who had disclosed, did so only with those partners with whom they were associated since long.

Conclusion

This chapter pointed out contrasting features within spousal and non spousal disclosure explaining the period, process and consequences of disclosure. The next chapter would probe into understanding behaviour change amongst MLHIV.

Chapter 10

PHASE - 2 BEHAVIOUR CHANGE

Introduction

The efforts to change the unsafe sexual behaviour are an important factor to reverse the HIV epidemic path in India. The Existing literature generally points to limited changes in sexual behaviour in India, but fail to take into account possible differences across individuals (Rowman, 2008). Behaviour Change is the third segment in the MLHIV Interview for Phase-2 of this study, with an objective to understand the impact of HIV and ART on sexual behaviour and to also ascertain the factors influencing behaviour change.

This segment has to be understood in sync with Chapter 9 (Findings on Sexual Behaviour) since quite a deal of behaviour change initiatives of the MLHIV across the phases of HIV infection have already been discussed therein. The findings there proved beyond doubt the null hypotheses namely "Frequency of Sexual indulgences have comparatively decreased after the onset of ART" and "Condom use with sexual partners have increased after ART."

This chapter will specifically address the respondent's understanding of safe sex, the hurdles in its practice and the support required for sustenance of safe practices. The use of condoms and reactions of sexual partners towards condom use is also discussed. The use of substances and its impact on the sexual behaviours of the respondent is witnessed. The impact of ART on the behaviours and other factors that influence behaviour change is discussed herein.

10.1a MLHIV Understanding of safe sex

Safe sex is the key component of behaviour change to reverse the epidemic (Parker, 1995). The counsellor's interviews revealed quite a lot of information being transferred to the client on safe sex, which is being triangulated here. The MLHIV clients being the agents of behaviour change, were inquired of their perceptions of safe sex will highlight their understanding on safe sex and it will be interesting to assess later if it reflect their practice.

As seen in the table below, most respondents (94.7 percent) associate safe sex with the use of condoms.

Table 63 MLHIV's Understanding of safe sex

	Safe Sex is	Frequency	Percent
1	Correct and consistent use of condoms	144	94.7
2	Reduce/ Avoid Multiple partners	23	15.1
3	Kissing and cuddling	13	8.6
4	Complete Abstinence from sex	7	4.6
5	Being faithful to one sexual partner	7	4.6
6	Masturbation	3	2.0
7	Not having wild sex, which will have bruises	3	2.0
8	STI assessment of partner	2	1.3

The counsellor's interview in chapter 8 points out that most counsellors approach towards safe sex counselling was focussed on abstinence and risk reduction as tools in prevention of sexual transmission. The MLHIV respondents focus on condom use can therefore be understood in the context of the education received from the counsellors. The need of the hour is further education on harm reduction models of safe sex to both the counsellors and the MLHIV, so that sexual lives of PLHIV can be rejuvenated in a truly safe manner. Moreover, it has to be understood by the counsellors that maintenance of safe sexual behaviours over time depends on interventions that are continuous and repetitive in nature (NACO, 2006).

10.1b Hurdles faced in practicing safe sex

The respondents were inquired on the hurdles they face in practicing safe sex. As seen above, since most respondents associated safe sex with condom use, they have mentioned here about their difficulties in using condoms. The difficulties in using condoms have been explained in detail in the section below. Besides the hurdles faced in the use of condoms, the following hurdles in practicing safe sex were mentioned by some individuals:

- "Easy access to sexual partners and alcohol addiction is not conducive for safe sex practices" (2 respondents)
- "Inadequate knowledge on HIV and lack information on masturbation"
- "Fear of being caught while masturbating"
- "Cannot indulge in 'body rubbing' since partner has skin infections"

- "Since we are old now, safe sex is not important to us as a couple, the frequency of sex has reduced due to age and I don't want to start using condoms with my wife."
- "Do not feel the need of safe sex with spouse since both wants to die together"

These comments point out that there are certain issues and hurdles in practising 'safe sex' and it would be important for the counsellors to probe these behaviours tactfully during the process of counselling their clients.

10.1c Support required in practicing safe sex

In consideration of the hurdles in practicing safe sex, the respondents were asked on what kind of support was required to help them practice safe sex and induce behaviour change. Most respondents affirmed that they did not need any support in the practice of safe sex since they knew about it but chose not to practice. However, few respondents solicit support from intervening agencies to address their issues as below:

- More information on safe practices
- Different techniques of having safe sex and yet feeling satisfied, "How to have fun in sex without the fear of infection"
- Resisting temptations of having sexual contacts with partners
- "How to use condoms and not miss pleasure", "How to have safe sex without using condoms", "Make easy access to condoms, eg: placing condom boxes in the brothels"
- "Should we have sex when there are cuts/ scars on the body of partner"
- "How to convince spouse for sex when she knows of my HIV status"
- "How to prolong the sexual act", "How to handle reduction in sexual desires"

The researcher in his capacity tried to address some of these queries of the respondent at the end of the interviews and encouraged them to discuss these issues with the NGOs or counsellors in the ICTCs.

10.2 Impact of ART on sexual life

The literature review points out a mixed response on impact of ART on sexual lives of PLHIV, as some studies claim a decreased interest in sex and sexual desires, while others state greater indulgences (Bunnell, 2004). However, Chapter 9 of this study points that there has been significant reduction in sexual indulgences outside marriage after the onset of ART and that the sexual indulgences within marriage remains almost the same, across the phases of HIV infection. There may be various factors influencing the behaviour change in sexual indulgences of the respondent. In this segment, the respondents were specifically questioned if it was the 'Onset of ART' that had any impact on their sexual lives. It was interesting to note that 61.2 percent of responded in affirmation. The respondents were asked to further explain on how their initiation on ART had an impact on their sexual lives.

Table 64 Impact of ART onset on sexual life

	Impact of ART	Frequency	Valid Percent
1	Reduction in multiple sexual indulgences	102	67.1
2	Had to curb sexual excitements	96	63.2
3	Initiated protected sexual practices	62	40.8
4	Dislike for sex	43	28.3
5	Decrease in sexual satisfaction	41	27.0
6	Early ejaculation after ART	39	25.7
7	Unable to maintain penile erection	30	19.7
8	Observing complete abstinence	28	18.4
9	Feeling of impotence/ sexual dysfunction	21	13.8

(N=152)

Thus the process of 'treatment initiation' by itself seems to be influential in the respondent consciously choosing to reduce their multiple partners, curbing their sexual excitements and initiating protected practices. The highlighted sections of the table, which include 'dislike for sex', 'decrease in sexual satisfaction', 'early ejaculation', 'inability to maintain penile erection' and 'feeling of impotence' are also similar to the complaints of MLHIV brought to light by researchers from the medical fraternity (Sgombich et al 2001), which have been proved true in a meta-analytic review of studies conducted between 1996 and 2003 (Nicole, 2006). These are significant psychological aspects which have to be considered, while devising training curriculums on counseling for MLHIV on sexual health.

10.3 Reaction of spouses to condom use

Chapter 9 reveals that 61.6 percent of the MLHIV use condoms 'Often' after the onset of ART. In this context, the respondents were inquired about the reaction of the spouse when the respondent uses condoms. Some respondents (18.1 percent) claimed to have never used condoms with their spouses as seen in the pie below. While the spousal responses of MLHIV who used condoms have been depicted below:

Figure 40 Reaction of spouses to condom use

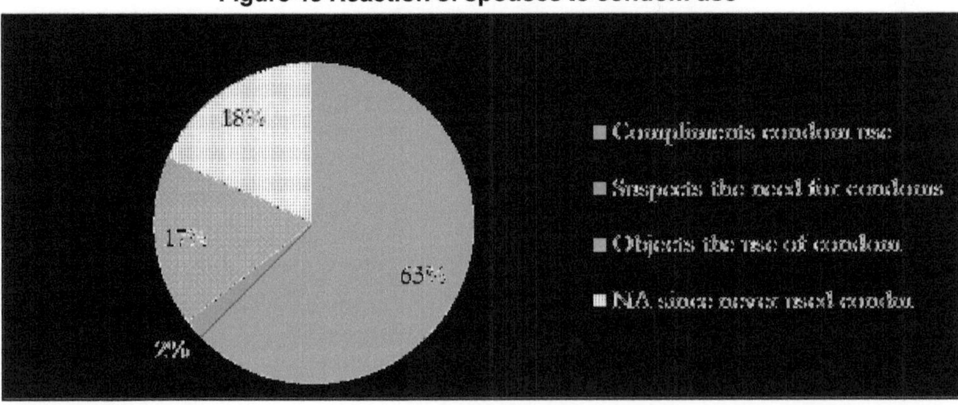

It is interesting to note that 17.1 percent of the spouses were objecting condom use, although no further probing was done here to find out the reason for the spousal objection. However, this can be understood from the counsellor's interview, which explores the reasons for the spouses indulging in unprotected sexual relations in spite of their knowledge of their husband's HIV status. The results show 37.6 percent of the counsellors feel that spouses want their sexual desires to be met too and 29.4 feel that the spouses may object protected sex in lieu of their need for procreation. This can be triangulated further in the FGD with spouses of MLHIV in the next chapter (Phase-3).

Difficulties faced in consistently using condoms

Nearly half of the counsellors (Chapter 8) believe that consistent condom use is practiced by less than 80 percent of their MLHIV clients and this data is triangulated with the findings of MLHIV interviews (Chapter 9), which also reveal that 40 percent of the MLHIV stating that condoms are not used consistently, even after onset of ART. This is an area of concern and hence to address this issue, the MLHIV respondents were inquired of the difficulties they face, due to which condoms are not used consistently. The concerns of MLHIV have been listed categorically as below:

Table 65 Difficulties faced in consistently using condoms

#	Areas of concern	Specific Issues/ Concerns
1	Issues at Individual level	- Can't trust free condoms distributed by the government, since not sufficiently lubricated - How do I start using condom when I have not shared with wife my HIV status - Feel hesitant to immediately introduce condoms in a marital relationship - Although condoms are carried for using during intercourse, it is always left out during the act since both get busy with foreplay and sex happens quickly. - Afraid about condom slipping off into the vagina and its consequences. (2 respondents) - Incomplete knowledge on the correct way of using - It is difficult to maintain erection with condom on, - Afraid about condoms tearing during the act, - Wearing condoms makes you conscious of slowing the speed of intercourse - due to weakness of penis can't use condom, condom comes out frequently
2	Issues at Partner level	- Have never used condoms with regular partners so far and hence it is difficult to use it hereafter since they will understand that there is something wrong in us (3 respondents) - Regular and faithful partners objects the use of condoms as they claim to have no infections (2 respondents) - Sexual partner objects the use of condoms - Spouse says that we will die together and isn't bothered about infections any more - Condom use leads to skin irritation in partner - Partner questions the need of condoms in marital relations she feels that now both are infected what more can happen
3	Social issues	- Feels embarrassing to buy condoms frequently for the shopkeeper will come to know of our sexual behaviours. - Feel embarrassed to pick up condoms from the ART centre-Peer pressure on not to use condoms

Contd...

Table 65 Contd...

4	Structural issues	- Why to use condoms with wife - Non brothel partners object the use of condom while brothel based partner's compliments the use. - Condoms are costly to buy and its quality is poor too (2 respondents) - condoms are not available at the right time and at the right places
5	Issues with condoms	- Condoms are considered as a barrier in god's gift of sex - The pleasure in having sex is reduced with the use of condoms (2 respondents) - condom diminishes pleasure since the skin contact is lost - Condoms are difficult to use - Condom causes itching on the skin, at tip of penis - Have to use double condoms for extra protection from tearing - The focus is on holding the condom during the act and hence not comfortable - Condom slips off and doesn't fit me - It is difficult to remember to wear a condom in the middle of foreplay - condom use creates discomfort during sex

It is expected that some behaviours will change as an individual's life changes, eg. condom use may no longer be necessary when an uninfected person enters a monogamous relationship with another person who is HIV-negative (NACO, 2006). However, there is a dimension of one's own belief system strongly playing a role of influence in the actions taken up. It affects a person both psychologically as well as socially. As seen in the above table, the sexual acts of MLHIV individuals are influenced by elements which are both personal as well as social. There is the efficiency of skills involved at the personal level for the correct use of condom. The sexual act is also a cognitive act for which the mind has to be trained. The issues faced by MLHIV in consistent condom use as stated above needs to be focussed in counsellor's trainings. However, one should also be aware that use of condom is also not an absolute protection from the infections. This is where the education on safe sexual practices will prove beneficial to MLHIV clients.

10.4 Consumption of Substances before the sexual act

Substance use amongst PLHIV shows strong positive association with unprotected sex, anal sex, multiple partners, and non disclosure (Manif, 2002; Lurie, 2004). The respondents were inquired of the consumption of any substances to enable the sexual act and it was found that alcohol was the only substance consumed before the sexual act. The frequency of the use of alcohol before the sexual act both before ART and after ART were elicited and have been compared as depicted figure 40.

The graph above shows that majority of the respondents (63.8 + 23 = 86.8 percent) of the respondents had consumed alcohol before the sexual act. However after the onset of ART, it has reduced to (13.2+53.9=67.1 percent), which is still an issue that needs to be addressed. It is also to be acknowledged that the consumption of alcohol "Often" before sexual act, which was found to be practiced by 63.8 percent respondents has reduced to one fifth (13.2 percent) after the onset of ART. This significant reduction in the consumption of alcohol post ART, was found highly significant on Chi-square test with a p=0.000 and df=4. This establishes the initiatives taken by the respondents towards behaviour change and it seems that the ART education on non alcohol use has had a major impact.

Figure 41 Extent of Alcohol Intake before and after ART

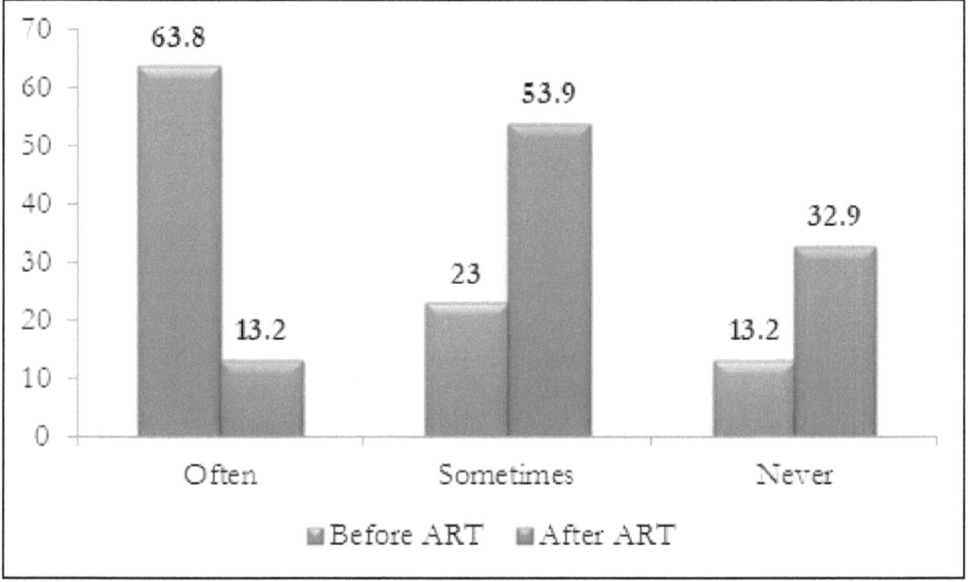

There is also a moderate significant association between the respondents age and their 'alcohol consumption after ART' when using chi square test with p=0.016 and df=6. This indicates that respondents used alcohol only 'Sometimes' in the age range of 20-30 years which increased to 'Often use alcohol' between 30-50 years and in the ages thereafter the alcohol use comes down to 'never'. Similarly, strong significant associations were found when cross tabulating 'alcohol consumption after ART with the respondent's:

1. Educational achievement (chi-square p=0.005 at df=8)
2. Current personal income (chi-square p=0.007 at df=6)
3. Current health status (measured on a scale of poor, moderate, good) showing a p value of 0.001 at df=4.

10.4.b Need for consumption of alcohol before sexual activity

The researcher did not come across studies, which have explored the need to consume alcohol before the sexual activity amidst PLHIV and hence to supplement the above data holistically, this area was probed. It was thereby reported by three fourths of the respondents that alcohol consumption was helpful in prolonging the sexual performance and in providing courage to take risks. Over half of the respondents (51.3 percent) felt that alcohol reduces the inhibitions in having sex outside marriage.

Table 66

	Alcohol consumption was helpful in	Frequency	Percent
1	Increased and prolonged sexual performance	117	77.0
2	Providing courage to take risks	114	75.0
3	Reduced inhibitions on having sex outside marriage	78	51.3
4	Reduced inhibitions in performing non-traditional sexual acts	46	30.3

(N=152)

The respondents in the above discussion on impact of ART mentioned on how the onset of ART has affected the sexual performance. The above table reflect that alcohol is mostly consumed in increasing sexual performance. However, since there has been a dip in the frequency of alcohol use it remains to be studied on how the MLHIV deal with issues of their decreased sexual performance.

In order to further understand the sexual practices after alcohol consumption, the researcher probed with the respondents on the type of partners with sexual contacts were established after alcohol was consumed. Herein, three fourth of the respondents (75.7 percent) mentioned that alcohol was consumed before indulging in sexual activity with commercial sexual partners, while 36.8 percent did so with non commercial sexual partners. Nearly one fourth of the respondent (23.7 percent) consumed alcohol before having sex with their spouse as seen in the table below.

Table 67

	Alcohol is often consumed before having sex with	Frequency	Percent
1	Commercial sexual partner	115	75.7
2	Non commercial sexual partner	56	36.8
3	Spouse	36	23.7
4	Never consumed alcohol before sex	28	18.4
5	Male partners	16	10.5

(N=152)

As seen in Phase-2 Chapter 9, there were 22 respondents, who indulged in MSM behaviour out of which 16 (73 percent) have claimed here to have consumed alcohol before having the sexual activity. This finding highlights the reason behind the high incidence of unprotected anal sex among MSM. One respondent also shared additionally that under the influence of alcohol he also had sex with his pet dog.

10.5 Behaviours changed post ART

The respondents were checked on which of the below mentioned behaviours they have induced change, after the onset of ART. The behaviours, on which the respondents have changed, have been ranked as per the frequency responses.

Although there is a reduction in alcohol intake and high risk activities, there is a long way to go to abstain from these. It is pleasing to see two thirds of the respondents abstaining from sex outside marriage.

Table 68

	Behaviours changed after ART	Frequency	Percent
1	Reduced Alcohol intake	114	85.1
2	Reduced High risk sexual activities	102	71.8
3	Abstinence of sex outside marriage	97	68.8
4	Consistent condom use	85	64.4
5	Spends greater time with family	94	62.0
6	Greater Social/ community involvement	62	40.8
7	Greater focus on Non penetrative sex	60	39.5
8	Have become more Spiritual	56	36.8
9	Active participation in peer networks	35	23.0
10	Complete Abstinence from sex	25	16.4

(N=152)

The findings on condom use from both chapter 8 and 9 have been triangulated in the above table to state that only 64 percent use condoms consistently. Consistent condom use education, has received highest priority in all counselling sessions yet it has not transpired into changing behaviours of over one third of the respondents.

Besides these, a couple of respondents additionally mentioned that post ART the focus is on children's future and family is the priority and not sex. The last five areas in the table namely spending time with family, involvement in community and peer networks, religious involvement are indulgences which can help sustain the behaviour change attempts as explained in the social ecological health promotion model (chapter 4). Emphasis on these, along with the education on non penetrative sex will result in better coping capacities for MLHIV to deal with their sexual health.

10.6 Factors influencing behaviour change

Considering the behaviours that have changed as per the discussion above, it is also important to understand the factors that have influenced these changes so as to help intervening agencies plan their intervention strategies appropriately. Laying adequate focus on the factors that influence behaviour change will only help sustain these attempts. Thus the factors which influenced behaviour change in the life of the respondent are:

Table 69

	Factors influencing behaviour change	Frequency	Valid Percent
1	Counselling at ART Centre	139	91.4
2	NGO Outreach work or Community interventions programs	107	70.4
3	Counselling at Testing Centre	83	54.6
4	Peer Education/ Support Group meetings	77	50.7
5	Self determination to stay healthy for family and children	71	46.7
6	Reading IEC materials	56	36.8

Contd...

Table 69 Contd...

7	Attending Religious services	25	16.4
8	Fear of HIV re-infection	25	16.4
9	Occurrence of STI or Opportunistic infections	20	13.2
10	Guilt about illicit past	19	12.5

Most respondents (91.4 percent) have attributed behaviour changes in their lives to the 'counselling' received at the ART Centre and the NGO outreach intervention (70.4 percent). About half of the respondents felt that the counselling at Testing centre and the peer group meetings were also the stepping stones to their behaviour change initiatives. This is certainly an appreciation of the services provided by governmental and non governmental agencies in the field of HIV counselling.

Nearly half of the respondents (46.7 percent) also acknowledged the fact that the behaviour change in their lives is mainly because they wish to remain healthy for the sake of their family and children.

It is interesting to note the emergence of factors like involvement in religious activities, reading of IEC materials and consciousness of re-infection of HIV/STI along with the guilt associated about past behaviours, being instrumental in maintaining behaviour change amongst MLHIV. It will be useful for the counsellors to focus on these aspects too to help sustain behaviour change attempts made by MLHIV. The rates of high-risk behaviour and new infections will increase if such interventions are withdrawn. Therefore, continued risk reduction depends on continued behaviour change programmes, and continued encouragement and support from counsellors are encouraging in maintaining behaviour change amongst PLHIV (NACO, 2006).

10.6 b Persons found comfortable to discuss sexual problems

The MLHIV respondents were asked to rank persons in order of which they would feel comfortable to discuss their sexual problems with and the results

Table 70 Sexual queries would be addressed with

#		Frequency	Percentage
1	Male Counsellors	150	98.7
2	Doctor	136	89.5
3	MLHIV Peer	73	48.0
4	Female Counsellors	18	11.8
5	Sexologist	1	0.1

(N=152)

As seen in the table above the MLHIV respondents seem to hold traditional beliefs on speaking comfortably on issues related to sex with Male counsellors, doctors or MLHIV peers. It is interesting to note that MLHIV are not comfortable speaking to female counsellors about their sexual concerns and this is also found true in Phase-1 Chapter 8, where most female counsellors, especially those who were less than a year experienced, reported that no MLHIV had ever asked them questions related to sex.

Since counsellors are a great asset to the HIV program and the counsellor has to interact with people of both the same as well as other sexes. In such circumstances, it is important that counsellors be trained to proactively speak about issues concerning sex and sexuality to their PLHIV clients. Only such an initiative from the counsellors will help break the ice on gender taboos that continue to exist in the society.

10.7 Self Assessment of Behaviour Change satisfaction

The MLHIV interview of Phase-2 ended with a self perception by the respondents, of how they valued the behaviour change attempts that they induced in their lives. It was interesting to note that over one tenth of the respondents (13 percent) rated their behaviour change strategies used as "excellent", while most of them (71 percent) were "just satisfied" with it.

Figure 42 Self Assessment of Behaviour Change attempts

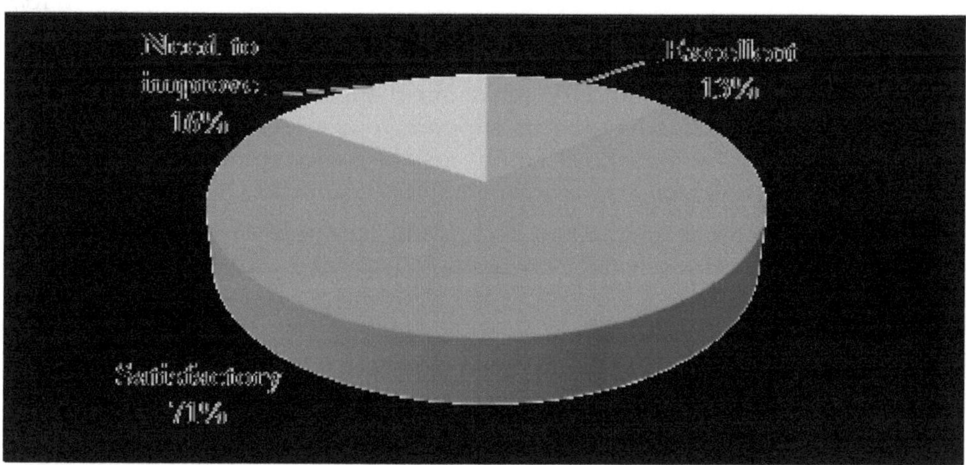

10.8 Major Findings: MLHIV Behaviour Change

- Safe sex practice was mostly understood by MLHIV as correct condom use and only a few felt that it included reduction in multiple partners or kissing.
- Sixth of the respondents claimed that the onset of ART had an impact on their sexual behaviours. The onset of ART has led to reduction in multiple sexual indulgences, curbing sexual excitements, protected sexual practices, dislike for sex, decrease in sexual satisfaction, early ejaculation after ART, loss of penile errection, abstinence and sexual dysfunction.
- Two tenths of the MLHIV's sexual partners seemed to suspect and object condom use respectively, while that of the others complimented condom use.
- Difficulties faced in consistent condom use were mostly individual based (like fear of introducing condoms in the relation, forgetting to carry condoms for intercourse, discomfort to self and partner, monogamous partner, etc.) or were because of issues with condoms (like reduced pleasure, difficulty in using, fear of slippage/ tear/ breaking, etc.)

- After the onset of ART, the intake of alcohol before sexual activity although has considerably reduced, nearly half continue to use alcohol even after ART. Reduction in alcohol use after ART was found significantly associated with educational background, personal income and health status of the respondent.
- Alcohol was mostly consumed before having sex with non spousal partners
- MLHIV mentioned that alcohol use enabled prolonged sexual performance, provided courage to take risks, reduced inhibitions in having sex outside marriage, and reduced inhibitions in performing non traditional sexual acts.
- MLHIV's Behaviour changes inferred after the onset of ART were: reduced alcohol intake, reduction in high risk activities, abstinence of sex outside marriage, consistent condom use, spending greater time with family, greater involvement in activities of the community, focus on non penetrative sex, spiritual inclination, active participation in peer network, complete abstinence from sex.
- Factors influencing MLHIV behaviour change were counselling at ART/ ICTC, NGO outreach programs, support group meetings, self determination to stay healthy for sake of family, insight gained through IEC materials, attending religious services, fear of re-infection/ STI/ OI, guilt about past.
- MLHIV rate male counsellors, doctors and male peers as persons whom they feel can be approached for discussions on sex and sexuality related issues.

Conclusion

This chapter brings to light the differences between the behaviour change related knowledge of the MLHIV and the barriers in practice. The onset of ART and the fear of resistance, re-infection/ super infection have naturally influenced behaviour changes in MLHIV. Some initiatives have been taken by MLHIV to bring about behaviour change and further emphasis needs to be laid during counselling on various layers of safe sex practices. The agents of behaviour change in the life of MLHIV (counsellors, doctors and peers) should be tapped as channels for further education. Most MLHIV are only satisfied about their behaviour change initiatives and can be moulded further.

The findings from Phase-2 interviews with MLHIV end here and the next chapter presents the findings of FGD with spouses of MLHIV on the study topic.

Chapter 11

PHASE - 3
SPOUSAL PERCEPTION ON MLHIV BEHAVIOURS

Introduction

This study has a strong focus on the male sexual behaviour, in trying to understand how it has implication on the health status of men, their spouse and their disclosure of the HIV status to the spouse. Gathering the counsellor's views on sexual behaviours and disclosure amongst MLHIV, in Phase-1 of this studying and then in Phase-2 directly interviewing the MLHIV, did project quite some information pertaining to the spouses of MLHIV. It was therefore important to validate these findings and also in order to triangulate the data; the views of spouses of the already interviewed MLHIV (Phase-2), on the researched topic were considered significant. The objective of data collection with spouses was to study the spousal perception of their male counterparts towards disclosure and behaviour change initiatives in general. Focus Group Discussion (FGD) was held best an instrument for data collection in view of the sensitivity of the issue being discussed and also since the need was to only produce the generic experiences of these spouses with their male counterparts.

FGD is a research methodology in which a small group of participants gather to discuss a specified topic or an issue to generate data. The main characteristic of a focus group is the interaction between the moderator and the group, as well as the interaction between group members (Wong, 2008). The objective of this FGD was to give the researcher an understanding of the spousal perspective on the MLHIV behaviours.

Study design

Some of the spouses of MLHIV were associated with the SHGs of the project CHIRAG, where data collection was carried out. The SHG meeting was a platform chosen purposefully for the convenience of both the sample (easy access for spouses) as well as project CHIRAG to get hold of the sample in a secure environment. It was also considered that women may not prefer talking openly in an unknown group, on the subject of MLHIV sexual behaviours, in our cultural context. Since the project CHIRAG's SHG of women have been formed a year back, sufficient rapport has been established within the women, which would ease their inhibitions to respond to the group discussion. In order to maintain anonymity and confidentiality of the MLHIV sample, the women were informed that data has been collected from several MLHIV in Mumbai and no reference related to any individuals was made to the data being gathered from their husbands. Thus with the given constraints of both time and resources of the researcher, only 2 FGDs were conducted with the spouses of interviewed MLHIV, conducted in the period May - June 2010, in which 10 and 11 spouses consented to participate respectively. A female moderator was appointed to facilitate the group discussion, in anticipation of the comfort level of the gender of participants.

The Moderator started the discussion with a brief introduction of the study, its purpose and explaining the objective of this FGD. The participants mentioned that they were informed in brief about the study by the project CHIRAG, who had mobilized them for this and provided consent to participate in this discussion. The participants consent form, prepared in Hindi, was circulated to the members and was read aloud for the group. The participants confirmed their interest of participation by signing the consent form.

Findings from the FGD

This chapter covers the profile of participants, their knowledge about the HIV status of self and spouse, their reactions to being HIV infected and the impact of HIV on relationships. It also speaks of the condom use of MLHIV, their alcoholic behaviours, STI infection and finally ends with understanding their level of sexual satisfaction.

11.1 Health Profile of Participants

There were 21 spouses in all, who participated in the 2 FGDs and their health profile is summarised as tab le 71.

Table 71 Health Profile of Spouses

Health Status	Number of spouses
HIV status	All women participating in the FGD were HIV positive
ART status	17 spouses out of the 21 women were on ART
CD_4 status	The CD_4 count was tested by all the spouses, through the encouragement of the project CHIRAG. Over one third of the spouses on ART reported that their CD_4 count was less than 200, when they started ART. The spouses claimed that their CD_4 count as well as their weight increased subsequent to ART. The latest CD_4 count of these women (as tested within the last 6 months) ranged from 249 to 1238 except for one whose count was 115.
Opportunistic Infections	Nearly half of the spouses shared that they suffered from OIs at least once
STI	Nearly one fourth of the spouses shared that they suffered from STI
Observed health	Most of the spouses (19/21) seemed to be physically healthy on direct observation by the researcher
Husband's HIV status	All their husbands were HIV infected and were on ART (they have been interviewed in Phase-2)
Children infected	One third of the spouses stated that their children were infected too

Coincidentally, all spouses were HIV infected and thus bringing homogeneity to the sample. The findings can thus be understood in the context of HIV concordant couples.

11.2 HIV status Disclosure by MLHIV

The discussion started by exploring the knowledge of the spouses about their husbands HIV status. All spouses stated that they knew that their husband was HIV infected. One of the spouse added that men are mostly infected first and HIV is later transmitted to their wives. The spouses were further probed on how did their male counterparts come to know of their HIV status and when did they disclose it to the spouse. The responses are as tabulated below:

Table 72 HIV status Disclosure to spouses by MLHIV

Situation	Explanation
Non Disclosure by MLHIV	- "Some men don't share their status with their wives for they fear rejection and fights at home. They fear that their parents will not accept them and ask them to leave the house."
	- "Women often share about their status to their spouses but men never share their HIV status thinking how others will react"
	- "If a man wants to share his status, he would do so only if the wife has patience and only if she is understanding because he may fear that the wife would have arguments at home and desert him. Hence men generally don't share"
Men are not aware of illness	"Some men take treatment from private hospitals not knowing what they are being treated for, since the doctor does not share with them about their HIV infection. Thus men are not to be blamed, since they themselves aren't aware of the truth behind what they are suffering from."

Contd...

Table 72 Contd...

During sickness of MLHIV	- "Men often do not know their HIV status unless they fall sick/ diseased and are taken to the hospital. Here they get to know their status and they then share with their wives"
	- "In the hospital, most of the time doctors inform us about the HIV status of our spouse"
Before marriage	"I came to know about my husband's HIV status two days prior to our marriage. He came to my place and told me that he was infected with HIV.""
	When we were dating before marriage, my husband explained to me about his leg's operation and then he told me that he was HIV positive"
When holidaying	"My husband shared with me after our marriage when we were holidaying that he had HIV"

When a couple of spouses shared of their helplessness, when they were disclosed immediately before marriage, another spouse from the group added "I feel that all men should be tested before marriage. In fact, people should now stop asking for *Kundalis* and start looking at HIV status compulsorily". This comment on making HIV testing compulsory before marriage is certainly encouraging and depicts the critical consciousness that these women have achieved. The spouses agreed upon their right to know the HIV status of their men and when one spouse mentioned that HIV test should be made mandatory before marriage, everyone supported the idea. She further explained that this will help infected people marry other infected partners and thus not spread the infection to innocent girls. When probed about the benefits about such an event, it was mentioned that both of the couple can take good care of each other and support each other and thus it reduces the additional burden of an HIV negative woman to take care of their husbands.

As seen above the MLHIV seem to have maintained confidentiality of their high risk behaviours. Some of them have not shared their HIV positive status with their spouses and waited for their spouses to find it out on their own when they fell ill and got themselves tested. This was done for the fear of rejection and fear of desertion. In one case the husband did not know what he was being treated for and was under false perception of the disease.

As seen in the table, the common situations in which MLHIV disclose their status include, during the period of their illness, before marriage or during holidaying. This is in line with the findings from both the counsellor's perspective and MLHIV disclosure pattern. The spouses also claim that some men are unaware of their HIV status and that the spouses were tested positive for HIV, earlier to their men.

What comes out clearly from the above sharing of the women is the vast gap in their status and that of their husbands where they can never doubt or question the sexual fidelity of their spouses in the marriage.

11.3 Spousal Knowledge about their HIV infection

Between 70 and 90 percent of all HIV infections in women are acquired through heterosexual intercourse, and women are twice as likely as their male partners to acquire HIV during sex, due in part to their biological factors that make them more susceptible (Lisa, 2010). In the context of limited disclosure by the husband about his HIV status, the spouses were inquired on 'how' and 'when' they got to know their status. The spouse claimed that they were detected HIV infected in the following circumstances.

Table 73 Spousal Knowledge about their HIV status

Situation	Explanation
Spouse found out	- "When husband fell sick I asked him what happened and he said that he had Jaundice. I got to know that he had HIV when I saw his reports. After this I was tested and found infected too"
Self tested during illness	- "When I used to fall ill often, I was advised for blood tests and found positive"
Self tested during illness of child	- "Child used to fall sick often and when hospitalized, she was tested positive and subsequently the couple was tested positive"
	- "When my younger child was a year old, he used to fall ill frequently. He was consequently tested positive and then we both tested ourselves and found positive. Then the elder daughter was tested positive too. Thus all in our family are infected."
Through HCP during pregnancy	- "During the third trimester of pregnancy, when underwent routine testing" (8 spouses confirmed a similar situation)
Through HCP during HIV	- "When my husband was sick and admitted, doctor informed me about his Illness of MLHIV status and then I tested myself for HIV"
	- "When my husband was admitted the doctors asked who the next responsible person in the family was and thus shared the result with me."
	- "My husband got infected one year back when he was sick and hospitalized and during this time doctor advised me and our children to be tested too.
Disclosure by MLHIV	- "My husband had tested himself and he had shared his HIV positive status within a few days. He confessed to me that he had 2 partners before marriage. He also said that if he had known of his HIV status before marriage, he wouldn't have married me and spoilt my life. He was very regretful about infecting me and child. He now takes good care of us now"
	- "My husband showed his report to me and said that he was HIV positive. I didn't understand what that means. When I had gone to test I came to know of my status and about HIV infection as well."(7 spouses confirmed similar situation)

As seen in the table above, a few spouses got to know of their HIV status, either during the illness of self or child. In nearly half of the cases, the status was disclosed by the HCW either during their pregnancy or when the husband was admitted for OI. Thus in many cases the woman or child was tested HIV positive first and only when they disclosed it to their husbands, did the MLHIV get them tested. These findings on the situations of disclosure can be corroborated with what the counsellors and MLHIV had stated about HIV status disclosure to spouse.

One third of the spouses claimed that their husband directly disclosed their HIV status to them and encouraged the spouse to test too. The case where the husband was tested first, the disclosure was voluntarily initiated in a few days in a confession mode, he encouraged the wife to get tested and when the wife and child were found positive, he was regretful and seem to have invested extra care in the relationship to live in mutual concord after that. Sickness and inability to care for one self have been the major causes for the husbands to make the disclosure.

11.4 Spousal Reactions on knowledge of their HIV infection

With the understanding from above discussion on how and when the spouses got to know of their infection, they were further probed on "what were their reactions on the knowledge of their HIV infection". The spousal reactions were classified as 'Negative', 'Naïve' and 'Positive' as reported in the table below:

Table 74 Spousal Reactions on knowledge of their HIV status

Reactions	Explanation
Negative	- "Felt bad that I had to bear the brunt of the infection due to my husband. I stopped going to office, skipped my meals and also had reduced food intake in the initial days" (self harm)
	- "My husband was hospitalized and I came to know that he had HIV. I also was tested for HIV then. I told my parents that I am going to eat poison and give poison to my children and die instead of living with this *'ganddi bimari'* (shameful disease). My family members prevented me from doing anything like this and convinced me that I will be fine." (inducing self harm)
	- "Coming to know of the infection was painful, since there is a fear on how the in-laws would treat you and that they would hold you responsible for bringing the infection home." (perceived discrimination)
	- "I was afraid when I heard of this infection. I was asked to abort the child so that the child wouldn't have to live with HIV. However since it was 6 months doctors did not permit abortion. The child is now two and half years and he is infected too." (discrimination by family)
	- "Doctor shared that my husband's HIV status when he was admitted. I was told not to tell him then, since his health condition was critical and advised me to share this when he is alright and back home. When he was brought home and was well, I told him that he was infected with HIV. He got angry and questioned me on how he got infected. I was speechless after hearing his reaction and did not talk to him further." (being blamed)
Naïve	- "Whenever I get angry I blame my husband for making me sick, But later I pacify myself saying that this is my destiny and a result of my actions in the past life, that I am punished in this life."
	- "My husband came to me 2 days before the marriage to share about his infection. But I had already distributed cards and organized everything. He asked me not to share with anyone. But I told him that it was not possible and I shared his status with my family. So that tomorrow I would not be blamed for having infected him. I thought that I should not get married at first and cried a lot. It was too late to cancel the wedding and I was afraid if I would find another bridegroom, if I cancelled this wedding. If I dint get married, my life would be spoilt and even if I get married, my life is spoilt. I thought to myself that I had to die some day in any case and that this is how I'm destined to die. So I accepted the marriage. I knew that this is not a contagious infection since my *chacha* also had this infection. I remembered him that time and how he died. (helplessness)
	- "I dint know what HIV was during that time. Got more information after starting ART and joining the project"

Contd...

Table 74 Contd...

	- "After HIV, we have sex with condoms and only when we wanted to have children did we not use condoms. That too I did not want to have children after knowing about this infection, since I did want to knowingly spoil their lives with HIV. But my husband used to insist regularly that he wanted children and for few times we had sex without condoms. When I missed 2 of my menstrual cycle, I was told that I m pregnant. I asked the nurse to abort the child since I dint want my child to be infected. However people there made me understand that I can give birth to a healthy child also. I decided to refrain from breast feeding and did top feed, whatever the cost be so as to protect the child. My children are both negative luckily." (helplessness) *(Although this spouse shows informed consciousness about HIV, but in the context of her reaction to the husband, her reactions are considered naive.)*

The oppressive nature of patriarchal system is evident from the above responses, wherein the decision of having sex is always taken by the husband. Another manifestation of this was observed where the man shared his status at the last minute before marriage, by when the damage done was irreparable. It is also evident that the HIV status and the related stigma on a woman have far greater implications on her social relationships as compared to men.

The discussion reveal that immediate spousal reactions after disclosure include, the feeling of being deceived by their husbands, reduced interest in work, lack of appetite, reduced communication with the husband, fear of being blamed for bringing home the infection, fear of in-laws holding them responsible. Except in one case all the women have faced humiliation, rejection, were blamed, made a scapegoat, kept ignorant and remained fatalistic. In cases where the wife was tested positive before their husbands was discriminated by both, the husbands as well as the in-laws, who blamed the woman for bringing home the infection. In one case the husband till his death was not willing to accept that he was infected first and claims his wife to be unfaithful.

From the table, it can be inferred that there were no positive reactions from the spouse, when they came to know of their HIV status. Most of the spouses seem to have reacted negatively, while some chose to be naïve. The reactions of the spouses highlight their helplessness, self harm attempts, actual discriminations, fear of being discriminated and anger against their husbands. Luckily, the suicidal tendency of one spouse was prevented and managed due to her family support.

The counsellor's interviews also corroborate the above finding depicting that the most spouses insist on safe sex, while some give up to fatalism. Moreover, the MLHIV interviews in disclosure also highlight that majority of their spouses reacted negatively or had mixed feelings. However, half of the MLHIV respondents had reported that their spouses reacted positively to disclosure, which contradicts the response of the spouses chosen for the FGD.

It is to be noted that the role of the HCW in giving correct information and guidance changed the lives of some spouses. It is also pleasing to note that the hospital system went a step further on helping a deserted spouse find a new life companion and instilled hope in her about the future too.

11.5.a Impact of HIV on spousal relationship

Moving on from understanding the spousal reactions to the knowledge of their HIV status, the Moderator proceeded to explore the impact this status knowledge of self and the husband, on their mutual relationships.

Table 75: Impact of HIV on spousal relationship

Impact	Explanation
Abandonment by in laws	- "My in-laws did not take me home or allow me to interact with other members of the house"
	- When I told my in-laws about my husband's HIV infection and how he transmitted it to me, he left me and ran away from home. He was absconding for months and I was pregnant. Doctor told me that I will live long and that my children will also be fine. That's when I felt relieved and then I met another positive person in the hospital who was willing to marry me and accept my child. Thus I remarried."
Violence by MLHIV	- "When I was first tested positive in the family, my husband never listened to what I had to say, he used to hit and beat me."
Reduced communication	- "There was reduced communication at home"
	- "When I heard about this infection I was afraid and thought I would die now. The distance in marital relationship has widened after knowing our status and I used to get irritated each time I heard my husband's name. My husband used to ask me to massage his hands and legs since it was paining. I refused to take care of him and he continues to fall sick"
Care and support	- "My husband was serious and his family did not take care of him. My mother accepted him to our home and cared for him. We both share a normal relationship as earlier."
	- "When my husband knew that I too was infected we loved each other more intensely and care for each other more than ever. We frequently go out together and spend time with each other and with our child.

It is seen from the table that the impact of HIV on spousal relations are mainly in the negative realm ie. Abandonment, Domestic Violence, Reduced communication. It is important to note that a few spouses have willingly accepted the result and offers care and support to MLHIV. Thus the accommodative nature of women in consoling and supporting their spouses is evident from this discussion.

A spouse added, "I was shocked to know of husband's infection, when he was admitted and when I shared with him he did not react and was silent. After a couple of hours his eyes were full and he was worried about what will happen to me and our children after his death". This concern about the future of the family and children seems to be integrating stability and mutual support within martial relationships.

11.5.b Impact of HIV on sexual relationship

Now that the spouses spoke about relationships in general, the moderator narrowed the attention of the group to speak, in particular, about the impact of HIV disclosure on sexual relationships within the couple.

Table 76 Impact of HIV on sexual relationship

Impact	Explanation
Sexual abstinence	- "My husband forces me for sex and threatens me that he will go outside and have sex if I don't permit. I told him to go outside and that he was anyways going to die whether he goes outside or not. He has infected me and now he wants sex from me, how can I accept this?
	- "I never kept sexual relationship with my husband ever since I knew of my status. We deserted after the test. He used to stay with his family and I moved to my family. I refrained from sex after my HIV test result"
	- "Since he was continuously sick for 4 years, we never kept sexual relations during this period."
	- "I felt like slapping my husband each time he approached for sex. I feel very irritated when he speaks about sex. I do not entertain him for sex as I am angry still"
	- "We never had any relation as he was continuously ill."
Reduced sexual	- "There is now a reduction in the frequency of sexual intercourse"
relations	- "He used to forcefully has sex with me but not very often"
Non penetrative	- "My husband told me that we should not keep sexual relations as my viral load will increase and we may acquire other infections as well. We had become intimate in sharing our daily chores and loved each other even more after the HIV positive test result."
	- "We have sex but its non penetrative..*(upar upar se hi sambandh rakhte hain)*, we only hug and kiss each other and not have that actual sex. My husband ejaculates outside my body, keeping me safe. *(mera admi bahar ja ke dhatu chod deta he...)*"
	- "I have no intercourse with husband since the knowledge of my status. On bed we hold each other, hug and kiss. That's all we do"
Condom use	- "We used condoms very rarely earlier but after the knowledge of the status, we started using condoms."
	- "Husband did not like using condoms initially but we understood the need for controlling the viral load."
	- "We have sex with condoms now and our sexual lives are not affected with HIV. We have sex 2-3 times a month."
Unsafe sexual	- "After the infection husbands still wanted to have sex and he takes initiatives practices for this" (Giving in to sex)
	- "When I was tested for HIV during pregnancy I came home running to share with my husband of my infection. At that time he told me that he is infected too. After that day his love and care for me has increased than ever before. I find that HIV has increased our relationship with each other and I'm happy now. I have sex with husband to keep him happy. I am not bothered about HIV anymore"

It was interesting to witness the spouses voice out loud, their anger and breach of trust, when the Moderator, facilitated discussion on this issue. The anger of most spouses against they being HIV infected was evident from the confronting reactions like initiating sexual abstinence and reduced sexual relations. One spouse seemed to be so angry about acquiring the infection that she did not permit her husband any sexual relations with her, even when he blackmailed her of going out to have sex.

Impact of disclosure on sexual relations include in some cases spousal refusal to have sex, while in other cases sex was refrained from as long as the MLHIV suffered from OIs or STIs. Two women shared that their husbands abstained from sex after the knowledge of their HIV status and focused more on the needs of the spouse and family members. Some spouses shared how they avoid penetrative sexual relationships and indulge in non penetrative sex or were cautious enough to encourage condom use practices. Only a couple of them shared unsafe sexual indulgences still, wherein one seemed unable to negotiate and in the other, who felt that her husband's love towards her increased after the knowledge of her HIV status, there seems to be naïve consciousness.

As this discussion was being summed up, a spouse who was vocal throughout the discussion added, "We women have *himmat* (strength) to live and we at one time used to fear 'death' and 'disease'. We are the ones, who now give strength to our spouses. In my case, my spouse wouldn't have been alive had it not been for my backing and consoling"

The interviews with MLHIV in Phase 2 also reveal that their frequency of sexual indulgences with spouses have come down to less than 4 times a month after the onset of ART, thus triangulating this finding.

11.6 Condom use

The concordant spouses were then probed on the condom use and only few spouses reported that they used condoms during their sexual relations post the knowledge of their HIV status. This is in line with the finding of Phase-2 where only 60 percent of MLHIV reported condom use. However, most spouses agreed that they are empowered enough to tell their husbands to use condoms during the intercourse and were sure that their husbands would co-operate in the same.

One spouse shared that it was her doctor, who advised the couple to abstain after detection of HIV. She was not content with this solution and she acknowledged the project CHIRAG's staff, who gave her the information that with condoms they can continue to have sex and there were no problems in doing so. She further stated that educated people like doctors should not give wrong messages which may hamper the lives of a couple.

Consistent condom use is the most effective way to reduce the likelihood of HIV being transmitted during sex. However, spouses are still frequently unable to obtain condoms, or negotiate its use, and are reluctant to use them in marital relationships. Making condoms easily accessible to spouses and teaching negotiation skills need to have primary attention (Marie et al, 2001)

11.7 Sexual practices under Alcohol influence

The researcher wanted to probe of sexual indulgences of the couple under the influence of alcohol and wanted to be cautious of receiving a socially desirable response. Hence, the spouses were indirectly inquired of their response to a hypothetical situation of their husbands coming home under the influence of alcohol and insisting on having sex. Most spouses agreed that they would avoid keeping sexual relations when the husband is drunk. A couple of spouses stated that this would never happen and that their husbands have never had sex under the influence of alcohol.

The spouses were asked to think of a situation where they would be approached by an HIV negative woman, whose husband is HIV positive and under the influence of alcohol forcing her to sex with him. The spouses were asked to respond to this situation. Herein, one pointed out that abstinence would be advised to the HIV negative woman. A couple of them suggested that they would advise them to use condoms. One spouse voiced that she would advise the woman to give a police case if her husband would refuse to use condoms, as it is her right to be protected from HIV. Another said, "Such a woman should make her husband understand that she is in no mood to have sex and that having sex under the influence of alcohol is not acceptable to her. The husband should be convinced on having sex on another day when he isn't drunk"

One spouse shared of how use of alcohol has a negative impact on health as she said, "I think my husband, due to his frequent alcoholic intake, continues to remain sick often. Further, when he is drunk, he never takes medications properly hence he is not getting well at all". This indicates high consciousness amongst the spouses, on the ill-effects of having sexual relationships, under the influence of alcohol.

One spouse, who was passive during the discussion, shared of her experience with an alcoholic husband as she said, "After my husband was tested positive, he tested the 3 year old child who was not infected. Then one day when my husband was drunk, he took out his blood in a syringe and added alcohol to it and he pricked me with it. I dint know of his HIV infection then and thought that he is behaving foolish under the influence of alcohol. Later when he had 'Nagin' (Herepes Zoster), he showed me his HIV report. We took him to the hospital for treatment and there I asked the nurse that I wanted to be tested for HIV. She showed me where to test and there I found myself positive too". Such experiences of women living out clearly that they suffered not only by the HIV infection of their husbands but also suffered social rejection and were ostracized.

Other studies from India found that violence was a barrier in discussing fidelity and refusing sex, and that economic dependence and social pressures limit women's response to violence from their partners. The characterization of women as being unable to change situations or of complying with male demands results in women being dependant on their male partners and prevents them from asserting themselves in sexual relationships (Thomas et al, 2009)

11.8 Suggestions for sex among concordant couples

All of them being concordant spouses, their opinion was solicited on how they would maintain sexual relations hereafter. In response, most spouses shared that they would promote condom use as it was considered safe and would protect them from an increase in viral load. Some women stated that the knowledge of the HIV infection should not interrupt their sexual lives and that the couples should continue to have sex as earlier.

The concordant spouses were asked if they would consider indulging in the practice of kissing and cuddling without any penetration, the group though felt ashamed, nodded their heads in agreement. A couple of spouses boldly stated that they are already practising this thanks to the education of the project CHIRAG staff.

11.9 STI assessment and treatment

Higher levels of asymptomatic and untreated STI, such as gonococcal or chlamydial infections among young women compared with young men further add to the increased susceptibility to HIV (Marie et al, 2001). All the women nodded positively when asked if they knew what Sexually Transmitted Infections were. When asked about sexual encounters during an STI, one spouse stated that men do not have sex during their STI, since it is very painful for them to have sex when they have any STI. Another spouse added her experience with STI saying, "When my husband refused to have sex with me I asked him what the problem was and why he doesn't have sex these days. He shared that he can't urinate and had pain and had boils there. I was tensed about this and took him to a doctor who shared that this was an STI. We dint have sex this time until he was fine". A third spouse joined in to share her experience saying "My man too had boils and I had sex with him during this time. I thought that this boil was due to heat 'garmi' , but later he knew that it was and STI and dint have sex". All other woman did not seem interested to talk about it.

11.10 Level of sexual satisfaction for the spouse

The spouses were asked if they were satisfied with their sexual lives, wherein 4 spouses wittingly questioned back "How can we be satisfied now that there is no sex". Another stated, "From the time I have heard that I have HIV I have lost interest in sex. *'dil ud gaya hai sex se'*". While most of the spouses responded in agreement when one declared that "We never wanted to have sex after knowing our HIV status".

11.11 Social relationships after HIV

A few women in the end also added on how their social relationships have changed after HIV. A spouse shared that "Some people in my workplace tease me and ask me out *'bahar chalta hain kya'*. I tell them *'HIV hai mujhe, ab bol chalta hai kya'* (I have HIV, now tell me if u still want to have sex). On hearing this they run away and never come back or even talk to me. They keep a distance now from me. Well that's good. I am openly disclosing my status and I have no fear now to speak about it."

Another stated a positive outcome stating that "When I go to the ART centre to take medicines I am friendly with other men and I have lost my interest in sex now. I see these men as my brothers and talk to them. Some of them have shared with me about how they got infected. Some have gone out or had sex with their girlfriends only once and they got infected. I feel sorry for them."

11.12 Major Findings: Spousal perception of MLHIV behaviours

The women involved for FGD were spouses of the MLHIV who were interviewed in Phase 2. Their perceptions are as highlighted below:

Major Findings: Profile of MLHIV spouses

- All spouses were HIV concordant and most of them were on ART, with an average CD_4 count. Most spouses were observed to be healthy.
- Half of them had suffered from OI at least once and one fourth from STI
- One third of these concordant couples children were HIV infected too.

Major Findings: Perception of MLHIV spouses on Disclosure

- The Spouses gets to know of MLHIV status when they are admitted for some illness, or through HCP, or immediately before their marriage date or when holidaying. In some cases MLHIV were not themselves aware of their illness as the spouse had tested first. Some spouses felt that their MLHIV did not disclose their status for fear of spousal reaction.
- The spouses get to know of their HIV status mostly during their illness, illness of the child, during pregnancy, through HCP during illness of MLHIV and only in a few instances through direct disclosure by the MLHIV.
- Spouses shared that their reaction to HIV infection was mostly negative (inducing self harm, feeling deceived by husband, reduced interest in work, perceived discrimination and being blamed for bringing home the infection). Some spouses also reacted naively to the news of HIV feeling that it was a punishment for sins of past life, or feeling of helplessness. Ignorance about HIV infection and oppressive nature of patriarchal system, also appears to bring about naive reactions.
- Spouses face humiliation, rejection, being blamed and are made a scapegoat as a result of being tested first for HIV. Further abandonment by in laws, physical violence by male counterparts, reduced communication with MLHIV were some of the common impact faced by the spouses. A couple of spouses contradicted saying that they only received greater love, care and support post HIV detection.
- As a result of knowledge of HIV status the spouses claimed to abstain from sexual relations with MLHIV (especially during STI/OI) or have reduced contacts, non penetrative practices were performed and they insisted the MLHIV to use condoms. A couple of spouses stated that they continued to give in to MLHIV's unsafe practices due to their fatalistic approach.

Major Findings: Perception of MLHIV spouses on Behaviour Change

- The spouses claim to have lost their sexual satisfaction post HIV detection.
- The use of condom was practiced consistently only by a few spouses although all knew of the relevance of condom use as a preventive strategy.
- Although the spouses did not claim that their husbands had sex under the influence of alcohol, they mentioned that they would say 'no' to sex in such situations. One spouse complained of how her alcoholic husband attacked her child physically.

- All spouses claimed to know what STI was and some stated that their husbands never had sexual relations during STI since it was painful.
- The spouses have engaged in bolder social relationships after the HIV infection with the help of support from the organisation.

Conclusion

In conclusion, all spouses unanimously agreed that they have accepted the infection from the husband and that they had forgiven their husbands in this regard and declared that they kept no grudges against the husband. However, one added to say that "On the contrary, if the husband would have been discordant, they would have never accepted or forgiven us". Some spouses acknowledged their family members and the project CHIRAG, who have accepted them with their infections and that they are receiving adequate support to access treatment services.

One spouse summed up the discussion with a very reflective insight on which the researcher wishes to end this note. She mentioned, "A man's need for extramarital partners is particularly urgent, when a man has lost control over his household and is humiliated/ rejected by his wife for sex. Here the man's ego has been hurt, and he needs peace on his mind and desires to be comforted. One way to meet these needs is to go to the bar – to socialise with friends – where 'money-hungry women' are waiting for a catch. Wives do not have the time, energy or money to provide the comfort and pleasure like such women." This was an eye-opener for the researcher to understand two new variables 'the ego of the man' and the dynamics in the 'pleasure provided by women outside marriage', which encourages extramarital relationships.

Chapter 12

MAJOR FINDINGS AND RECOMMENDATIONS

This research was conducted in three phases based on the type of population targeted for primary data. The findings of the study with Counsellors, MLHIV and their spouses have been highlighted in the earlier chapters. This chapter aims to thematically collate and triangulate the major findings across the 3 phases under the categories of Respondents Profile, Sexual behaviour, Disclosure and Behaviour Change. It also provides appropriate recommendations to counsellors, training institutes, intervening organisations and SACS, in the light of these findings. A thematic "Counsellor-Counsellee" roadmap is also worked out to enhance the crucial role of the counsellors in combating the spread of the epidemic and in upholding the welfare of PLHIV.

12.1. FINDINGS FROM RESPONDENTS PROFILE

In better understanding the findings of the study an overview of the respondent's profiles across the 3 phases have been summarized herein.

12.1.a Profile Counsellors from ART & ICTC (Phase 1)

The counsellor's knowledge and perceptions were gathered using a questionnaire, when they came for their refresher training in counselling at CSWNN Institute. The aim of this interview was to assess the content of knowledge and skill level of counsellors when dealing with issues pertaining to sexuality. When saturation was obtained with 85 counsellors, the sample size was freezed. Hence as explained in Chapter 7, this sample may not be representative of the population. The emphasis of these findings is to identify the knowledge and skills of counsellors in the area of sexuality counselling and to understand their response to the concerns of MLHIV. These issues are triangulated with the findings from other groups of respondents in the study. Most of the respondent counsellors were employed with ART centres of MSACS.

Around two third of the interviewed counsellors were males. Of these, 15 percent of the respondents were fresh graduates and were new in the field of counselling with less than 25 years of age. Only 7 percent of the counsellors had retained with the ACS for five years or more. Greater number of female counsellors continued in this job. Over half of the counsellors were in the age bracket 26 – 30 years, with a mean age of 29 years. More men seem to be employed in this profession than women and at more or less the same age. Only one fifth of the counsellors were from the Psychology discipline.

12.1.b Profile of MLHIV on ART (Phase 2)

Through purposive sampling method, 152 MLHIV respondents were selected. Most MLHIV interviewed in this study fell in the age bracket of 30 to 50 years, with a mean age of 38 years. They have been residing in Mumbai since 20 to 40 years, with an average 29 years of stay. Only one third of the MLHIV had completed secondary education while nearly half of them were educated less than the primary level. More than half of the MLHIV were either into service or business, while others were daily wage labourers (28 percent) or did home based work (8 percent) and about 9 percent of the MLHIV were unemployed during the time of the interview. The MLHIV's educational achievement was directly proportional to their occupation.

Apart from one tenth respondents, who did not have a personal income, the mean income of the others was found to be around Rs.5000/- . In most cases (89 percent), the respondent's total family income was less than Rs.10,000/-. It was calculated that the respondent's personal income was supplemented by additional family income in only 29 percent cases, while all other respondents were the only source of income in their family.

The mean age of marriage amongst the MLHIV was calculated to be 26 years, even as 16 percent have married before the legal age of marriage ie.21 years. All those who married at an early age were observed to have suffered from at least one episode of STI. Moreover, 8 percent of the respondents had re-married, since their first spouse had either died of AIDS or had separated. Remarriage was initiated by the ORWs of the NGO they were associated with. Over three fourths of the respondent resided with their spouses in Mumbai, while the spouses of others were either expired or had separated/ divorced on the knowledge of their male counterparts HIV infection. One fourth of the respondents had either one, two and three children respectively, while 14 percent of the respondents did not have a child yet.

About half of the MLHIV had a CD_4 count of less than 350 (cells/mm^3) at the time of the interview. Most respondents looked 'healthy' with their body weight ranging from 50-70 kg. Nearly 86 percent MLHIV were on first line ART and more than half of them complained of the incidence of STI and OI, at least 2 or more times prior to data collection. None suffered from OI at the time of the interviews. Over half (63 percent) of the MLHIV were calculated to have 'Moderate' score on the 'Consolidated Health Condition', followed by 'Poor' (21 percent) and 'Good' (16 percent) scores. Poor consolidated health condition held significance with greater age, lesser personal and family income, more number of sexual partners and greater frequency of penetration.

The MLHIV respondents started residing in Mumbai since the age of 8 years (median), their sexual fantasies erupted at the median age of 17 (median) and penetrative sexual debut happened at 20 years. However they got married at 26 and were found HIV infected at 33 (median age), after which, they were immediately enrolled on ART at 34 (median age). The spouses were tested after all this, when the MLHIV were 35 years old (median). More than half of the MLHIV claimed to be the 'Initiator' of sexual activity with their spouses, which points towards the patriarchal cultural taboo towards sex.

The spouses of three fourths of the MLHIV were tested HIV positive, with nearly half of them having a CD_4 count of less than 350 (cells/mm^3). Only half of the MLHIV's concordant spouses were initiated on ART, until the time of interview. The incidence of OI and STI amongst in most spouses was observed to be 'less than once', contrary to the multiple frequency of MLHIV's OI and STI incidence.

12.1.c Profile of Spouses of MLHIV (Phase 3)

The purpose of meeting the spouses of MLHIV, was to ascertain further, their responses over disclosure and behaviour change. All spouses met during the Focused Group Discussions were HIV infected and most of them were on ART with an 'average' CD_4 count interval of 200-600 (cells/mm^3). More than half of the spouses had suffered from OI and about one-fourth claimed to have suffered from STI, 'at least once'. Most of the spouses were observed to be 'healthy' during the time of FGD. In case of one third of these concordant couples, their children were also HIV infected.

12.2. FINDINGS ON SEXUAL BEHAVIOUR

This segment collude the findings across the 3 phases on MLHIV's sexual behaviour and seeks to triangulate the understanding of counsellors and spouses along with the MLHIV behaviours.

12.2.1 MLHIV's Queries related to sex

According to the counsellors (irrespective of the counsellor's age), only 43 percent of MLHIV clients *(average mean with standard deviation of 26.8 percent)* had asked them queries related to sex. Especially, one fourth of the counsellors reported that less than 25 percent of the MLHIV clients ask them such queries. It was calculated that MLHIV tend not to ask their queries related to sex to newly appointed counsellors (with less than a year experience), and especially to the female counsellors. More male counsellors were asked questions related to sex irrespective of their years of experience. The major concerns raised by MLHIV include:

a. Concerns in upgrading their knowledge on Sexual Practices
b. Concerns of Safe sex behaviours and Condom use
c. Maintaining relationship with partners outside marriage
d. Concerns related to Procreation

The MLHIV interviews also depicted that most of them preferred to address their sexual concerns with Male counsellors, doctors or MLHIV peer. Gender and age of the counsellor seem to play a cultural barrier in the counsellor - counselee relationship.

The barriers perceived by counsellors in MLHIV not discussing about sex include:

a. Personal Barriers like embarrassment, MLHIV's priority focus on medication, their disinterest in sex, depression and the confidence demonstrated by MLHIV of their knowledge pertaining to sex are the barriers for such discussion.
b. Social Barriers like lower age and opposite gender of counsellors, fear of speaking about private sexual life in public and fear of being stigmatised for the so called 'illicit practices', are not conducive to speak to MLHIV about sex.
c. Structural barriers include high patient load at the testing / treatment centre, lack of privacy, lack of time for individual counselling at the Hospital and inhibition to talk since MLHIV are generally accompanied by spouse or other family members.

12.2.2 MLHIV indulgences in sex outside Marriage

According to MLHIV, 90 percent indulged in sex before marriage with an average (median) of nearly 5 partners. The occupation of the MLHIV in unorganised sector, as well as the HIV positive status of spouse, held strong association with the increasing number of sexual partners outside marriage. Even though this may be a known fact, this study has empirically established the association strongly between these factors. An increase in the number of pre-marital sexual partners of the respondents was found to be directly proportional to their higher educational achievement, good health and that of practicing unprotected sex. After marriage, about 56 percent continued to indulge in extramarital sex with an average (median) of nearly 3 partners. This reduction number of sexual partners outside marriage, is also indicative that marriage can be a variable, which influences 'behaviour change' in MLHIV in terms of partner reduction.

The major reasons for indulgence in pre marital sexual relations included, experimentation, relaxation and enjoyment, peer influence, easy availability or accessibility of sexual partners and influence of alcohol. And the reasons for indulgence in extra-marital sex additionally included, need for variety, dissatisfaction with spouse, restrictions to sex at home, embarrassment in performing varied types of sexual acts with spouse, spousal disinterest in sex, her menstruation period or child bearing phase or menopause, marital conflicts, or in order to maintain HIV negative status of spouse.

More respondents chose brothel based partners for pre-marital sexual indulgences, while more non-brothel based partners were chosen during extra-marital sexual indulgences. Frequenting of visits to the same sexual partners was observed more times in cases non-brothel based partners. There was no significant difference in the use of protected sexual practices in either pre or extramarital sex. A major concern is the fact that many men are not concerned with the risks associated with unsafe sex. Majority of the MLHIV respondents did not use condoms consistently with their pre-marital partners. Many of the respondents interviewed for this study did not use condoms, when having sex with commercial sex workers. Further, a few men perceived that having sex with expensive prostitutes, young girls and girls who live within the neighbourhood or community (non brothel based partner) is safe. Younger MLHIV were found to have more number of sexual partners and indulged in unprotected sex more often than older ones. Even though education is not a positive factor with regard to preventing visits to sexual partners outside marriage, it is seen to be a positive factor for condom use after ART. Such in-depth understanding of MLHIV's problems was not reflected among the interviewed counsellors, who came for training.

12.2.3 Dimensions of Sexual Practices

a. HIV/ STI Assessment of Sexual Partner

Over 91 percent of the consellors 'Never' assessed STI status and 96 percent of them 'Never' assessed the HIV status, of their sexual partners, thus making the respondents vulnerable to re-infection. The major reasons for not doing so were fatalism, ignorance and fear of partner's denial for sex. FGDs with spouses present that STI is a painful incident for both partners and that sex between the married couple is avoided in during symptomatic STI conditions.

Significant association was found between early age of MLHIV's marriage and to the greater incidence of spousal STI. The greater frequency of STI incidence was seen to lower the body weight of the respondent as well as increase the line of ART treatment.

b. Level of Sexual Satisfaction

When the MLHIV were asked to retrospect on the overall level of sexual satisfaction within and outside marriage, most responded that sexual satisfaction was 'Higher' within marriage, compared to that outside marriage, since there exists mutual love, non-influence of alcohol, no fear of physical restrictions of time, space, money, etc, no guilt of 'wrong doing' attached and a sense of possession of spouse, brings greater satisfaction. Further, some respondents have stated that sex outside marriage was mostly due to mere "non availability of sex with married partners". This was contrary to the counsellor's perception that most MLHIV did not have greater level of sexual satisfaction with spouse. According to the counsellors, the MLHIV choose 'Being Faithful' as the prevention strategy, in spite, "because of the education given in ART adherence".

In the FGD with spouses most presented that they have now lost the desire to have sex, while some claimed that they were comparatively less satisfied now in matters of sex, due to the prevailing fear of re-infection.

12.2.4 Sexual behaviours of Men who have sex with Men (MSM)

a. MLHIV who have sex with men

Except for one-fifth of the counsellors, all claimed to know how many of their MLHIV clients practiced homosexual behaviour, irrespective of their gender. More than half of the counsellors estimated that 1-5% of their MLHIV clients would be indulging in MSM behaviour. However, the MLHIV in their interviews admitted that 15 percent of them indulged in MSM behaviours before HIV infection, which reduced to 3 percent after ART onset. This shows that not all MLHIV who practice MSM behaviours report or discuss with the counsellors on the same.

b. Safe sex indulgences of MSM

About 15 percent of the counsellors admitted that they never probed with their MSM clients if they practiced safe sex. Half of the counsellors stated that their MLHIV clients would sadly be practicing unsafe sex with men. Only one third of the counsellors felt assured that their MLHIV clients practiced safe MSM behaviours. The MLHIV interviews revealed that all those who indulged in MSM behaviours even after ART continued to practice unprotected sex. This is a serious concern to be addressed.

c. Bisexuality amongst MLHIV

One third of the counsellors did not know if any of their MLHIV clients were bisexual, while more than half (58 percent) of the counsellors believed that between 1-5 percent of their MLHIV clients could be bisexual. And one-tenth of the counsellors believe that more than 6 percent would be so.

The MLHIV interviews reflect 15 percent of MLHIV to be bisexual, which again surprisingly is beyond the imagination of most counsellors. The spousal knowledge on MLHIV's bisexual behaviour was not explored in the FGD.

d. MLHIV asking Questions asked pertaining to MSM

Nearly half of the counsellors reported that none of their MLHIV clients had ever asked them any query with regards to homosexuality. While others reported that not more than 5 percent of their MLHIV clients, whom they had counselled, had ever asked questions pertaining to homosexuality. The queries of MLHIV with regard to homosexuality have been categorised under the following areas:

- ✰ Seeking knowledge on understanding concepts of MSM
- ✰ Discussing Sexual Problems in practicing homosexuality
- ✰ MLHIV assessing risk behaviours amidst MSM and safe sex related queries
- ✰ Seeking skills in handling relationship crisis arising amongst MSM partners

e. Counsellors Responses to MLHIV queries

Only 70 percent of the counsellor's responses seemed to show confidence in addressing MSM behaviours favourably, with suggesting alternative and safe sexual practices. The responses of remaining counsellors were focussed on abstinence from sex claiming MSM activities to be immoral and their behaviours to be non scientific.

12.2.5 Types of penetrative sexual behaviours practiced by MLHIV

Around one fourth of the counsellors admitted not having explored much on the penetrative sexual practices of their MLHIV clients. More female counsellors did not seem to know about the types of penetrative behaviours practiced by MLHIV.

a. MLHIV indulgence in Vaginal Sex

Around 15 percent of the counsellors had no clue if their MLHIV clients indulged in vaginal sex. Only two third of the counsellors stated that over 80 percent (average median of 90 percent) of their MLHIV clients would be indulging in Vaginal Sex.

However, the MLHIV interviews reveal that almost all respondents (98 percent) performed vaginal sex during every sexual act.

b. MLHIV indulgence in Anal sex

Over one fourth of the counsellors had no clue if their MLHIV clients indulged in anal sex. While one third of the counsellors feel that an average (median) of 3 percent of their MLHIV clients would be indulging in anal sex.

However, the MLHIV interviews reveal that as high as one in ten respondents performed anal sex 'Often' during the sexual act. On the other hand, 42 percent MLHIV had 'never' ever tried anal sex.

c. MLHIV indulgence in Oral sex

Over one fourth of the counsellors had no clue if their MLHIV clients indulged in oral sex. One fifth of the counsellors felt that less than 1 percent of the clients would have indulged in Oral sex. Six out of ten counsellors felt that an average (median) of 2 percent of their MLHIV clients would be indulging in oral sex.

However, the MLHIV interviews admitted that as much one tenth of them performed oral sex 'often' during the sexual act and on the other hand about 53 percent MLHIV had 'never' ever tried oral sex.

As per the MLHIV interviews, most men have performed oral and anal sex with their female counterparts, most of which, were with brothel based partners. However, it is a cause of concern that the counsellors seem to have only a miniscule knowledge of these penetrative indulgences among PLHIV couples and have underestimated the frequency of such practices.

12.2.6 MLHIV's Attitudes towards Male Sexuality

On a 14 point likert scale measuring MLHIV attitudes towards sexuality, it was observed that the respondents were either 'moderately sexist' (74 percent) or 'highly sexist' (25 percent). The sexist attitudes seemed to reduce with longer duration of stay in Mumbai. These sexist attitudes were inflated by higher personal income, better health status or with indulgence in pre/ extra – marital sex. Highly sexist attitudes of MLHIV were observed on the statements mentioned

1. Male sexuality being superior to female sexuality
2. Male sexual urges being stronger than that of females

3. Sex with virgin partner gives greater sexual pleasure for men
4. Age diminishes sexual pleasure in women
5. Use of condoms diminishes sexual pleasure in men
6. Men lose their mental and emotional stability if their sexual needs and fantasies are not satisfied
7. Men should always take initiatives to perform sex

12.3 FINDINGS FROM DISCLOSURE

In the context of HIV infection, familiar concerns about adolescent sexual behaviour are amplified and new ethical dilemmas, pertaining to the disclosure of HIV status to regular extra marital partner and legalization of disclosure have surfaced.

12.3.1 Spousal Disclosure

According to 90 percent of the MLHIV, disclosure was considered as a right of the spouse and 80 percent of the MLHIV opined that there can be a legal binding to this. Such legalisation would help since the spouse is primary caretaker and would be there till the end, it would help prevent the spread of infection, to minimise discord in relationship and would help early diagnosis and treatment of other family members. It should be noted here that this opinion of MLHIV is only related to the disclosure of their HIV status to the primary partner (spouse) and not their sexual partners outside marriage.

As reported by the counsellors, 58 percent (Mean with a standard deviation of 31 percent) {Median = 70 percent} of their MLHIV client's spouses, would have knowledge about the MLHIV's status. About 8 percent of the counsellors 'never' ascertained if their MLHIV clients had disclosed their HIV status to their spouses.

As against the counsellor's perception, 92 percent of the MLHIV respondents claimed that their HIV status was known to their spouses. The discussion below highlights on how the spouses came to know of the MLHIV status and their reactions.

a. Spousal Disclosure Initiated by

92 percent of the MLHIV claimed that their spouses knew of their HIV status. Through the MLHIV interviews, it was calculated that spousal disclosure happened around 2 years after the MLHIV's detection. Further, spousal disclosure was voluntarily initiated by the MLHIV, only in half of the cases. The HCP seem to have revealed the MLHIV status to the spouse directly (without MLHIV consent) in more than one fourth cases, while only in a handful cases, the MLHIV sought the assistance of the HCP towards spousal disclosure. Apart from this, a few spouses had 'by themselves' discovered the status of the MLHIV. It is thus observed that the HCP play a minimal role in spousal disclosure.

Half of the counsellors were of the opinion that the spouse gets to know of their husband's status, in most cases, from 'sources other than their husbands'.

According to the spouses, their MLHIV did not disclose, due to the fear of negative spousal reaction, while some other spouses felt that even their male counterparts did not know of their own HIV status and that the spouses were detected first with HIV infection. The spouses get to know of their HIV status mostly during their illness within the family, or through HCP during illness of MLHIV and only in a few instances through direct disclosure by the MLHIV. The counsellors were thus accurate on their perception about the spouse getting to know of the MLHIV status through other sources.

b. Circumstances of Status Disclosure by MLHIV

According to the counsellors, spousal disclosure by MLHIV would be initiated under the following circumstances (arranged in order of maximum responses):

i. When MLHIV is sick/ admitted and needs spousal care and support

ii. When spouse insists on the need for procreation or during pregnancy

iii. When spouse insists on having sex

The situations, under which voluntary disclosure was initiated by the MLHIV respondent, coincided with the responses of the counsellors. The MLHIV respondents preferred to voluntarily disclose their HIV status, when they were admitted due to illness, or before sexual intercourse, or during pregnancy/child birth or in a few cases when the couple were holidaying.

The spouses also confirmed that the MLHIV initiated disclosure during times of their illness, before marriage or when holidaying. Only a few of the spouses acknowledged the direct/ voluntary disclosure by the MLHIV. Most of the spouses claimed to have discovered their husband's status through HCP, either during their pregnancy or during the illness of their husband. Few of the spouses got to know of their HIV status by reading the MLHIV's blood reports or when these spouses were tested for HIV during their illness or that of their child. These experiences of MLHIV and their spouses are a building block for counsellors to understand when the MLHIV should be advised to disclose their status in consideration of its repercussions.

c. Factors influencing spousal disclosure

The factors influencing disclosure as stated by MLHIV respondents include, sense of responsibility towards spouse, concern for spousal health, need for spousal support in care and treatment, to alleviate distress associated with non-disclosure and to initiate HIV preventive behaviour. All these factors are discerned to be 'Internal' and hence the MLHIV were highly motivated for disclosure.

d. Time taken by MLHIV in disclosing

Nearly half of the MLHIV spent "less than 5 minutes" in disclosing their status to their spouse, while one fourth of them took "about 30 minutes" to do the same. Most of these MLHIV disclosed during their illness and this circumstance was correlated to have had a negative reaction from spouse. Only 8 percent of the MLHIV spent "nearly 2 hours" in disclosure speaking about what the HIV infection, treatment is and how they should be leading their lives hereafter. It is interesting to note that most of the MLHIV who took 'more than an hour' in disclosure have done 'voluntary' disclosure and not with the support/ presence of the HCP. Further most of such MLHIV have experienced a positive impact of disclosure. Thus the counsellor's role in encouraging a detailed spousal disclosure would be more meaningful for the MLHIV's relationship in comparison to a direct disclosure to the spouse.

e. MLHIV's Preparation period for disclosure

Only about a tenth of the MLHIV disclosed their status to their spouses on the same day of their results, while one fourths of the MLHIV took a week and a month respectively towards preparing themselves for disclosure. Over one third of the MLHIV disclosed after a longer duration of time (more than 2 years) and these cases also showed increased frequency of condom use. The amount of time taken for disclosure didn't seem to have a significant correlation with the impact of disclosure, indicating that it is more important to be careful about the "how the disclosure is done" than "when it is done".

f. Words used by MLHIV in disclosure

In understanding how the disclosure was performed by the MLHIV, it was seen that nearly half of the respondents "stated confidently" about their HIV status and "assured the spouse that everything was alright", while only a few took efforts to "explain the infection to their spouses". This style of "explaining the infection" in disclosure, was found successful by the MLHIV, since it reduced their fear and anxiety. A few MLHIV attempted the following satisfactory styles in spousal disclosure: "sounding guilty", "confessing the past", "trying to gain spousal sympathy" or "eliciting mutual support". A few MLHIV 'blamed their spouses' for bringing home the infection.

During the FGD, a couple of spouses expressed the disadvantage of being tested for HIV, before their husbands, thus giving themselves room for being blamed. The spouses were shocked with their husbands and in-laws behaviours, when they were blamed for bringing home the HIV infection, in spite of being so loyal to their husbands.

12.3.2 Feelings associated with spousal disclosure

More than half of the MLHIV felt 'Negative' after their disclosure, which included "feeling ashamed", "guilty", "lonely", "depressed and anxious about health and future". Only one fourth of the MLHIV claimed to have felt 'Positive' (feelings include, "sense of relief", "de-stressed", "content", "pleased" and "peaceful") after their disclosure and the remaining shared 'Mixed' feelings. Positive feelings showed strong associations with longer duration of stay in Mumbai, currently residing with spouse, those who spent more than a week in preparation for disclosure, those who spent greater time spent on disclosure and in those MLHIV where the spouses initiated sexual intercourse. Negative feelings showed associations with older age of MLHIV, presence of STI and indulgence in extramarital relations

12.3.3 Impact of HIV on inter-personal relationship with spouse

According to more than two third of the MLHIV respondents the impact of spousal disclosure has been negative wherein their spouses were shocked to learn about the infection and were anxious about their personal health and the future of their family. Some spouses wept in periodic intervals and did not converse with the respondents for a few days. Episodes of 'periodic anger' and 'blaming the husband for ruining her life' were reported by MLHIV. A tenth of the MLHIV reported of their spousal behaviours like verbal / physical abuse and separation.

In the FGD, no spouse claimed to have reacted 'positively' to disclosure. More spouses seem to have reacted 'negatively', which consisted of behaviours like inducing self harm, demonstrating anger, reduced interpersonal communications, discriminating and blaming the MLHIV. A few spouses reported that after the knowledge of their HIV status, they were either abandoned by their in-laws or faced violence from their male counterparts for bringing home the infection. Some spouses remarked that they reacted 'naively' and gave in to their husbands, since they were in a helpless situation or since they lacked knowledge on HIV or accepting it as a punishment for sins of past life. Later on a few of them started demonstrating greater care and support to the MLHIV, understanding that their option now was to live with it.

12.3.4 Impact of HIV on sexual relationship with spouse

A tenth of the counsellors perceived that there has been no impact of spousal disclosure on their sexual relationship. However, according to the other counsellors, spousal disclosure by MLHIV had the following impact on sexual relationship:

i. Spouses would now ensure condom use by MLHIV

ii. There could be a reduction in frequency of sexual acts

iii. Some spouses discontinue sexual relations and would abstain

iv. Some spouses would allow only foreplay

MLHIV interviews represents 69 percent to have faced 'negative impact' of disclosure on their sexual lives, wherein they had to abstain, restrict their desires to non penetrative or safe sex. After disclosure, spouses showed disinterest in sex, reduced sexual relations or insisted on condom use. In a few cases the respondents were ashamed to initiate sexual advances with spouse after disclosure. The cases of spousal disclosure by HCP showed high associations with a negative impact on the couple's relationship. While the other 31 percent, who shared the 'positive impact' of disclosure on their sexual lives, mentioned how they were happy that sexual intimacy was gradually accepted by spouse, joint decisions were taken towards indulging in safer sexual practices, couple counselling was sought, necessary precautions were being taken to protect their off-springs from HIV. Some respondents mentioned on how the feeling of guilt about past infidelity vanished gradually.

However, one third of the spouses, in FGD, claimed that they have initiated 'sexual abstinence' after the knowledge of their concordant HIV status and a couple of them claimed to have 'comparatively reduced' their sexual indulgences. A few of the spouses pointed out indulgence in 'non-penetrative sexual practices' and a few used protections. A few spouses confessed that they continue to indulge in unprotected sex giving in to their husbands needs or because they had become fatalistic. Some spouses stated that the knowledge of the HIV infection "did not interrupt" their sexual lives and that the couple continue to have sex as they used to have earlier before the knowledge of their HIV status.

Furthermore, the counsellors felt that the spouse indulges in sexual relationships with the MLHIV, in spite of their HIV status disclosure, chiefly due to:

i. Lack of negotiation skills (79 percent)

ii. Spouses feel the need for their sexual desires to be met (38 percent)

iii. Spouse is coerced into sex (36 percent)

iv. Spousal need of procreation (29 percent)

v. In exchange of rewards (cash/ kind) (11.7 percent)

According to MLHIV, the frequency of sexual relations with spouse both before HIV detection and that currently, seem to remain static ie. an average of 4 sexual acts a month. This is indicative that the onset of ART and rejuvenating health would have positively re-ignited the sexual lives of the couple, although there was a dip in sexual relations for some time after HIV detection.

12.3.5 Non Disclosure to Spouses

About 8 percent of the MLHIV had not disclosed their HIV status to their spouses until the time of their interview. The MLHIV's reasons for non disclosure to spouses include wanting to disclose later, fear of upsetting spouse or being disallowed sex, fear of marital discord and accusations of infidelity. The respondents mentioned that they were waiting for a situation like 'childbirth' or 'sickness', so as to disclose their status to spouses. Meanwhile, some MLHIV are making attempts like 'condom use' and 'abstinence' in this interim period of non-disclosure. In preparation for disclosure, some MLHIV iterated the need for 'further counselling support to spouse on health care and support', 'couple counselling for stabilising relationships' and towards 'education of safe practices' and require help in 'mentally preparing oneself for disclosure'.

12.3.6 Disclosure to non spousal sexual partners

About 18 percent the counsellors had no clue if their MLHIV clients had disclosed to their non spousal sexual partners. Nearly half of the counsellors felt that only between 1-20 percent of their MLHIV clients would have disclosed their status to their non-spousal partners. The MLHIV disclosure to non spousal partners was calculated to be 24.3 percent (Mean value with a standard deviation of 27.8) {Median = 20 percent}.

When MLHIV were inquired about non spousal disclosure, 57 percent of them stated that it is the right of their non-spousal sexual partners to know their status in an attempt to protect them from HIV. Also, half of the MLHIV were also in favour of legalisation of non-spousal disclosure, while the others, who did not favour legalisation, feared the negative implications like denial of sex and stigma. Contrary to the counsellor's perception, only a miniscule 6 percent of the MLHIV were found to have actually disclosed their HIV status to their non spousal sexual partners, thus indicating the susceptibility of their sexual partners. It was further observed that these 6 percent have 'Often' shared their status with only those non spousal partners, who were associated with them in a "long term relationship".

The reasons for non disclosure as stated by MLHIV include, performing protected sex, or lack of knowledge of one's own status, or sexual partners responsibility to take care of their health since they are paid in turn, fear of denial in intimacy, or sexual partners not sharing their status although they were into high risk behaviours.

12.4 FINDINGS ON BEHAVIOUR CHANGE

The understanding of behaviour change and the attempts made by MLHIV towards behaviour change were recorded in this segment. Counsellor's interview reveal that their messages on behaviour change to their MLHIV client mostly include Abstinence and Risk reduction focussed messages. It was observed that harm reduction messages (non penetrative sex, safe sex and sex education) and caring for sexual partner's health were not given equal emphasis.

12.4.1 Prevention strategies followed by MLHIV (A-B-C)

Abstinence: Around half of the counsellors perceived that 1-20 percent of their MLHIV clients would be practicing abstinence, as a strategy of behaviour change. This perception was found true as 16 percent of the MLHIV respondents revealed that they have chosen complete abstinence from sex as an HIV prevention strategy after ART.

Being faithful: The counsellors had mixed responses in their beliefs on their MLHIV client's faithfulness, with more number of the counsellors perceiving that more than 40 percent of their MLHIV clients would be faithful to their spouses, after their HIV infection. The MLHIV respondents divulge that 69 percent of them claimed to have reduced their sexual indulgences outside marriage and were now faithful to their spouses.

Consistent condom use: Around half of the counsellors stated that more than 60 percent of the MLHIV consistently used condoms. This was ascertained to be true in the MLHIV interviews, where 64 percent of them claimed consistent use of condoms.

12.4.2 Behaviour Change across the phases of infection

Two thirds of the counsellors were of the view that their MLHIV clients would possibly be having sex 'Occasionally' *(2-3 acts a month)* or 'Rarely' *(2-3 acts in a quarter)*, after the HIV infection. While over one fourth of the counsellors felt that most of their MLHIV clients would be having sex 'Often' *(more than 4 acts a month)*. The counsellors base this data on the evidences from their interactions with MLHIV through their queries during counselling or through interaction with their spouses.

According to MLHIV, the frequencies of sexual desire, non penetrative practices, partners outside marriage, and sexual intercourses outside marriage have decreased considerably after the onset of ART medication as compared to that practiced by the respondent before HIV infection. Behaviours like condom use and status disclosure to sexual partners have increased after the onset of ART, although there is still a large scope for improvement.

12.4.4 Safe Sex Practices

Most of the counsellors (89 percent) iterated that their clients were having unsafe sex even after being detected HIV positive. Amongst them 14 percent counsellors opined that their clients 'Rarely' practiced safe sex, in spite of regular counselling and MLHIV being aware of the risks. Only 19 percent of the counsellors felt that their MLHIV clients indulged in safe sex 'Very Often'. It was perceived that a major chunk of MLHIV, who practice safe sex, do not do so on 'every' occasion, thus increasing the threat in the spread of the infection.

Most of the MLHIV (95 percent) equated safe sex with condom use. Only a few knew that it also includes avoiding multiple partners (15 percent) and indulging in non penetrative (9 percent) sex. The major hurdles faced in implementing safe sex include alcohol influence, lack of knowledge on safe sex and skin infections. Only a few spouses agreed to indulgence in non-penetrative sex as a measure of safe sex.

Although interpersonal intimacy is a normal milestone in adolescent development, lapses in precautions during intercourse could result in the transmission of HIV to partners and offspring. Engaging in intimate touch or non penetrative sex, without intercourse appeared to be an uncommon form of sexual expression amongst MLHIV.

12.4.5 Condom Use Behaviours

a. Condom use by MLHIV after HIV infection

Use of condoms, after the HIV infection, is the most focused strategy of safe sex practice in counselling trainings, yet the counsellors had mixed opinions on the actual use of condoms by MLHIV. Only one fourth of the counsellors thought that 'most' of their MLHIV clients used condoms.

In the interviews with MLHIV, incidence of condom use rose 12 times to 62 percent after onset of ART. Unsafe intercourse was associated with discomfort using condoms, reluctance to disclose HIV status, and anger or anxiety when thinking about HIV. Condoms are a distressing reminder of HIV infection for affected individuals. Introducing condoms in a sexual relation can raise difficult questions from partners, necessitating disclosure of HIV status. Ultimately, emotional adjustment to HIV infection and willingness to inform sexual partners may be important determinants of condom use.

Only few of the spouses reported that they used condoms during their sexual relations post the knowledge of their HIV status.

b. Reaction of sexual partner to condom use

About two thirds of the MLHIV claim that most of their sexual partners (within and outside marriage) complimented their condom use, while in case of 17 percent MLHIV respondents; the sexual partners objected the use of condoms. In the FGD, most spouses shared that they would promote condom use as it was considered safe and would protect them from an increase in viral load.

c. Difficulties faced in condom use

According to MLHIV the difficulties faced in condom use include

a. Individual level issues in non-condom use include lack of trust in condoms, non-disclosure of status to sexual partner, ignorance, forgetfulness, lack of proper knowledge on use of condoms and discomfort in using condoms.

b. Issues faced with sexual partners include, suspicion by partner, partners objection in using condoms claiming that they don't have any infection, causes irritation on partners skin, monogamous/ faithful partner, fatalism in partners about infection.

c. Social and structural issues include religious issues, embarrassment to purchase or pick up condoms and peer pressure on not to use. Concerns were also on cost and quality of condoms, slippages, reduced pleasure, non availability.

12.4.6 Substance use Behaviours

When the MLHIV were asked about their substance use behaviours before sexual activity, all of them claimed only the intake of alcohol as a practice. It was found that the frequency in use of alcohol 'After onset of ART' was six times lower than that 'Before ART'. Variables like higher age, higher education, higher income and good health status were also closely associated with the reduction of alcohol use.

According to these MLHIV respondents, alcohol intake helped prolonged sexual performance, gave courage to take risks, reduced inhibitions to have sex outside marriage and to perform non-traditional acts. Alcohol, in most cases was consumed before sexual activity with 'commercial' sexual partners (76 percent) or with 'non commercial' partners (37 percent). Only one-fourth of them used alcohol, before sexual indulgence, with their spouses. The FGD with spouses indicate that the husbands do insist on sex under the influence of alcohol but most spouses reported that they would not permit sexual relations in such circumstances either.

12.4.7 Impact of ART on sexual behaviour

After the onset of ART, the MLHIV have consciously 'reduced multiple sexual indulgences' (67 percent), have 'curbed their sexual excitements' (63 percent) or have 'initiated protected practices' (41 percent). Around one fourth of the respondents stated that after being initiated on ART, they feel dislike for sex, decrease in sexual satisfaction, early ejaculation, inability to maintain penile erection and feeling of impotence. Quite a few studies quoted in the literature review chapter have also pointed out these.

The onset of ART comparatively reduced the MLHIV's sexual desires, number of sexual partners outside marriage, frequency of non-penetrative acts, frequency of sexual indulgences and MSM behaviours, in comparison to the behaviours before the HIV detection. On the other hand the onset of ART positively enhanced the use of condoms and frequency of disclosure

12.4.8 Behaviour Changes post ART

Although one third of the counsellors never asked their MLHIV about their sexual behaviours post HIV detection, the others perceived that the frequency of penetrative sex by MLHIV, were 'rare' or 'occasional'.

The MLHIV stated that after ART the following behaviours have changed namely Alcohol Intake, high risk sexual activities, initiating abstinence, condom use, spending time with family, peer and community involvement, focus on non-penetrative sex and on spiritual involvements. Complete sexual abstinence after onset of ART was reported by 16 percent of MLHIV.

The spouses claim to have lost their sexual satisfaction post HIV detection. The use of condom was practiced consistently only by a few spouses although all knew of the relevance of condom use as a preventive strategy.

12.4.9 Factors influencing behaviour change

According to the Counsellors, the major factors influencing behaviour change in MLHIV would be as categorised below:

a. Internal factors like feeling of guilt and in repentance of illicit behaviour, fear of acquiring other OI and STI, fear of increase in viral load or re-infection, fear of complications in ART, focus on improving health.

b. Sexual Partner focussed factors include prevention of HIV to partner, demonstrate love and commitment to partner and re-building trust in spouse

c. Social factors include concern for future of children and family

d. Structural factors include religious involvement, greater understanding developed on HIV, influence of counselling support provided by them.

In the MLHIV interviews, the respondents acknowledged the counselling education at the ART, NGO, ICTC and that in support group meeting as major factors, which influenced them to change their behaviours. Additionally factors like reading IEC materials, attending religious services, self determination to stay healthy for family and children, fear of re-infection with HIV, STI or OI and guilt feelings about the past, have also been instrumental in bring about behaviour change. MLHIV rated male counsellors, doctors and male peers as persons, whom they feel can be approached for discussions on sex and sexuality related issues

The entire hypotheses set for the study were all proven true. These were

Objective: To study the socio economic profile, health and sexual practices of the HIV infected respondents and their spouses

1. Earlier the age in sexual initiation greater the chances to have multiple sexual partners

2. Men indulge into unsafe sexual relations without the knowledge of the HIV status

3. The first exposure for the respondent's knowledge about HIV begins with their HIV test

4. MLHIV rarely ascertain the STI or HIV status of their sexual partners before sexual intercourse
5. Factors like age, income and partners outside marriage have an impact on the health of the respondent

Objective: To trace the process and consequences of disclosure

6. Longer the time taken in spousal disclosure, lesser the negative impact on one's own feelings as well as better relationship with the spouse
7. HIV status Disclosure to spouse was more prevalent after ART onset
8. HIV status Disclosure to other sexual partners was minimal

Objective: To study the affect of the 'HIV positive status' and 'ART' on sexual behaviour

9. Frequency of sexual indulgences decreased comparatively after the onset of ART.
10. Condom use with sexual partners increased after ART
11. The onset of ART has influenced the extent of consumption of alcohol use by reducing it
12. Factors related to personal profile such as education, income and health status has a significant association with the reduction in alcohol consumption.

All the above proven hypotheses points towards one factor: The significant role of the counsellor in providing crucial care and support to MLHIV. Further, the facilitative role played by the counsellor in transforming behaviours of the MLHIV, is evident from the study findings.

The above mentioned findings have lead the researcher to formulate practical "Counsellor - Counselee Road Map" as mentioned in the next segment for its primary stakeholder the 'counsellor', who play a very significant role in the life of MLHIV towards initiation of any transformation in their lives.

12.5 COUNSELLOR COUNSELLE ROAD MAP

Understanding the Socio Economic Background of the MLHIV

Nearly half of the MLHIV respondents have not completed their secondary education, implying the need for counsellors to focus lesser on reading materials/ pamphlets as tools and emphasise more on the use of illustrations and audio visuals towards educating them on HIV and behaviour change. The verbal communication with such persons will also have to be in a simplified fashion.

Half of the sample also were not employed in 'secured' occupational settings and were leading a hand-to-mouth existence based on their daily wages or were dependent on their spouses/ children to supplement their family income. This dependency of MLHIV on his family members would have certainly diminished their self esteem, for they have to be at the compassion of their family members for finance as well as in aspects of decision making. In such circumstances the counsellor has to proactively involve the family members in the disclosure, care and treatment process, since the MLHIV will not be in a position to elicit such support. Education on low cost nutritional recipes and remedial health care holds great importance in such cases. Avenues for alternate and supplementary economic options need to be explored along with counselling.

Half of sample was observed to be breadwinners for their family with a mean monthly income of Rs.5000. In such situations, any recurring illness or an increase in care, support or treatment costs will only add-up to the financial crunch within the family. The situation is worsened if the MLHIV stands to lose his employment due to his illness. Thus the family members have to be prepared well in advance to hunt for job opportunities, to supplement the main source of income, in order to be able to balance their future economic demands and sharing financial responsibilities in the family.

Assessment of MLHIV Health Status

Nearly half of the MLHIV have suffered from recurring OI and STI, indicating poor health conditions, which adversely affects the body weight, observed healthiness, CD_4 count as well as the regime of ART. During such infections, the MLHIV also seem to abstain from any sexual indulgences. This is thus the stage when the family may suspect the infection and hence the MLHIV clients need to be well prepared for disclosure in such circumstances. Also, the ratio of frequent OI and STI amongst the couples seems similar and it seems that the contagious infections are transmitted due to physical proximity and unhygienic practices. Thus the symptoms of an OI in a PLHIV should alert the counsellor on educating them on the measures of preventing its spread to their spouses, irrespective of concordant/ discordant status.

A fourth of the MLHIV had not tested their spouses for HIV, as yet, and another one fourth had not re-tested their HIV negative spouses in the last six months. These are both presumed to be discordant conditions, which in reality may not be the case and the counsellors need to encourage HIV and CD_4 testing of MLHIV's spouses on regular intervals towards better care in early detection.

Of those HIV tested spouses, there are HIV Concordant couples, who are both on ART. These couples would also need special attention of the counsellor in positive prevention, treatment adherence, positive living and especially to help these couples build up a strong support system for their children. The training institutes need to add the following areas to the curriculum of Counselling Concordant couples on ART and focus on addressing issues of discordant couples.

The counsellor also needs to address the concerns of PLHIV couples, who choose not have children, to cope with the stigma they face in this regard. The MLHIV who had children, were concerned about the future vulnerability of their children after their death, which also needs to be looked into. This is also an area where curriculum needs to be built on how to prepare such couples.

With the rising number of separation/ divorces and remarriages amongst PLHIV, counselling on marital concord is the need of the hour. Such a counselling needs to address barriers like lack of trust, communication gaps, resentment, oppressive patriarchal practices, fatalistic approach towards life in the event of HIV, interference and discrimination by the in-laws, responsible management of finance and household chores. It is important for the counsellors to develop healthy ways of building fidelity in relationship, managing anger/ unresolved arguments and anxiety, responding to criticism and complaints within the relationship and discussing unmet needs of either partner. In family counselling, the involvement of parents and in-laws as peacemakers should change the blame scenario and associated stigma that the spouse has to cope with. Pre marital counselling endeavours need to be thought about by AIDS Control Organisations for youth living with HIV and also for those wanting to re-marry.

Figure 43: Chronological events in the life of MLHIV

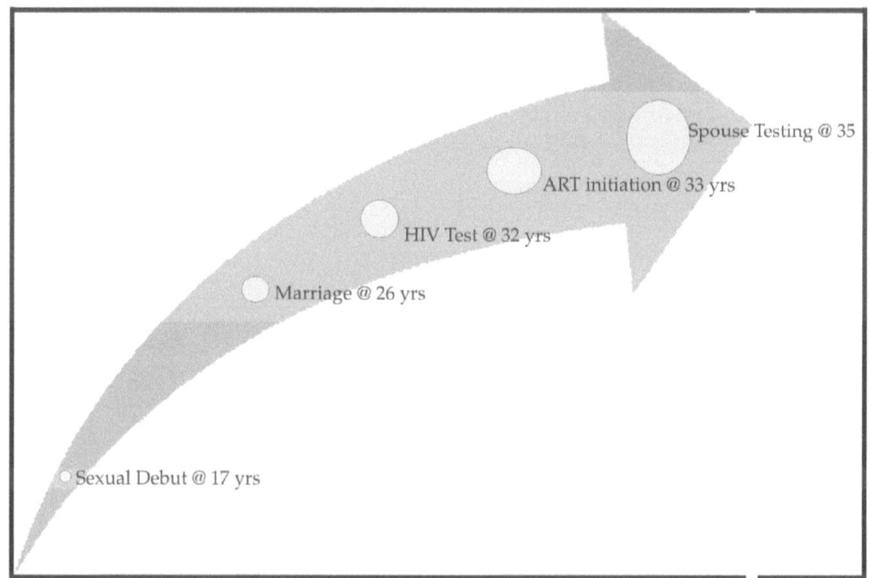

As seen in the chronological depiction above, 10 year long gap was observed between the age of sexual debut and the HIV test. This finding points the need for vigilance in identifying high risk behaviours amongst all adolescent clients and preventing them in its early stages. The HIV testing also needs to be encouraged before marriage. Moreover, the duration between the 'HIV test' and 'ART initiation' was observed to be less than a year, indicating that most persons have tested themselves only when it was high time to start ART. It is also important for the AIDS Control Organisations to lay a check on this trend and to reverse it.

Additionally, the age of ART onset in the sample was 33 years, which is a very early age for onset of treatment based on the average life-span for the treatment's 'survival mortality'. The significance of early HIV detection and proper care to postpone treatment is the need of the hour. NACO has initiated several programs targeting the teen-age population. The efficacy of these programs and their impact has to be consistently assessed and redesigned periodically. The collaboration with sectors like education, entertainment, media and employment is very crucial here.

It is of greater concern to observe Spouse testing happening 4 years later to the detection of one's own infection. This delay offers no room for damage control and hence partner notification and partner testing are to be considered tenants in every Post test – Positive result counselling session.

Sexual Behaviours of MLHIV

The illustration below is a snapshot of the findings from MLHIV's sexual behaviours.

Figure 44 Sex outside marriage

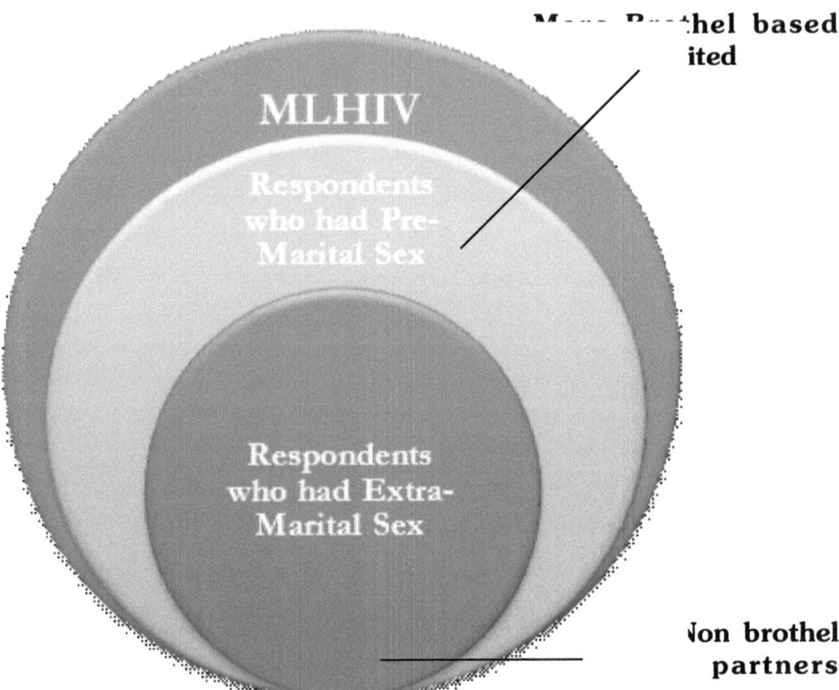

The MLHIV's infidelity in within marriage due to mismatch in sexual preferences and expectations within the couple are areas which need resolution, in order to reduce risk behaviours outside marriage. An environment needs to be created amongst the couple to discuss commitment, compatibility and emotional connectivity with the couple.

It was seen that condoms have equally not been used in both Pre and Extra marital relations, either due to ignorance or due to the perception that the partner looked safe or due to fatalism. The counsellors in the interview have perceived a greater use of condoms and reduced sexual indulgences, which is contrary to the practices of MLHIV.

The barriers explained by the MLHIV due to which condoms were not used were mostly noted to be myths and misconceptions amongst the MLHIV. More often, difficulties in condom use seem to be 'perceived' by MLHIV than that 'encountered' when practiced. It is important to clarify with the MLHIV that sexual relations with 'non-brothel based partners' is also a high risk behaviour. In this context, counsellors re-iteration and emphasis on "consistent condom education and skills in using", is strongly recommended, by means of in-depth discussions. In an attempt to mitigate re-infection and super-infection, the spouses also have also to be educated not just on 'negotiating condom use' but also on complimenting the use of condoms by their MLHIV. This will help in consistency of condom practice.

Besides condoms, the other tools of safe sex need to be introduced to the PLHIV. A fatalistic approach on safe sexual practices is cited often in spousal relationship; especially among older couples. MLHIV, who had higher education and those with higher income seem to practice unprotected sex indicating fatalistic approach towards the infection. This is a state of mind that has to be changed into a reason to lead healthier lives. Channelizing sexual energy into meaningful and creative activities is also a possibility to address the 'fatalistic' attitude.

The prevalence of anal sex seems to be higher than that perceived by the counsellors. The counsellors should know that MLHIV performed anal and oral sex more with female partners (than with other men), especially brothel based, as this was perceived to be a safe sex method deriving greater pleasure. The training institutes need to play an active role in piercing the stereotype of linking anal and oral sex to homosexual couples. There is a need for MLHIV to be better informed about the risks in anal sex and for their misconceptions on anal sex to be clarified.

The penetrative sexual debut of the sample started at a very early age of 14 years. Amongst them, the MLHIV, who have married at a very young age (even before the legal age of marriage), were also observed to have experimented with Pre-marital sex. This study thus overrules the myth that the males in adolescent (early) marriages do not have pre-marital indulgences. It is therefore important for every counsellor to do a thorough risk assessment even with adolescent males. Sexuality counselling be provided for PLHIV interested in Re-marriage or marriage after the knowledge of self's HIV status.

As compared to sexual relations outside marriage, the level of sexual satisfaction was observed to be 'high' within marriage, for reasons of mutual love, non-influence of alcohol, no fear of physical restrictions like time, space, money, or no guilt of 'wrong doing' attached and also the sense of possessing of spouse. These reasons can be used as good citations to encourage sex within marriage and encouraging behaviours on fidelity with spouses. It is thus vital to educate clients that sexual satisfaction is a psychological phenomenon. The MLHIV will further need education on various types of safe sexual practices, which can derive pleasure. Also, the spouses need to be encouraged to play a proactive role in initiating sexual advances, foreplay and afterplay, in order to compliment the MLHIV's expectations from a sexual act and thus leading to greater satisfaction within marriage.

The counsellor's interviews show discomfort of many counsellors to proactively interact with the PLHIV on their sexual behaviours and concerns. On the other hand, MLHIV interviews state that they prefer to consult the only the Counsellors (especially males), Doctors and Peer Educators to discuss their queries pertaining to sex and hence any initiative taken by the MLHIV to discuss about their sexual queries are to be capitalised as potential opportunities to discuss their sexual lives and behaviours.

The capacity of the counsellor to handle such myriad shades and nuances of sexual relations as well as related problems, need to be looked into. There could be a team approach of the counselling and testing centres in addressing these issues. The centre can also become a hub of activities and workshops for MLHIV, wherein, experts from relevant fields can be invited for animation and input.

Types of Sexual Partners

About one sixth of the respondents had indulged in sex with other men before the HIV infection and only one admitted to having sex with a transgender, but none wanted to be identified as a homosexual. All of them mentioned that they were predominantly a "heterosexual" and "sex with men was for fun, experimentation or under pressure". Such bisexual behavioural traits are difficult to identify and may not be discussed upfront by the MLHIV (as seen in the counsellors interviews too) and will need sensitive probing. The training institute thus needs to be aware that classification of men into 'homo' and 'hetero' are not explicit and that behaviours have overlapping shades.

The onset of ART seems to have reduced the homosexual behaviours of one third of MLHIV respondents. This may be because of inadequate knowledge of safe homosexual behaviours, fear of treatment reactions or may also be because of the prevention education instilled by the intervening agencies. However the sustenance of this decision and relapse is a concern, which needs to be addressed with harm reduction education. Furthermore, counsellors should take caution, as interviews show that one-third of the counsellors tend not to respond in favour of homosexual behaviour.

The mean intervals on sexual behaviours as reported by MLHIV, across their three stages of HIV infection are as categorised figure 43.

Although there have been some improvements in behaviours after the onset of ART, there needs to be greater focus on education in the following areas (as highlighted)

- ☆ Non penetrative practices
- ☆ Consistent condom use
- ☆ Disclosure to sexual partners and positive prevention
- ☆ Protected sexual intercourses with spouse
- ☆ Avoid the use of alcohol before sex

It was observed that the onset of ART has immediate impact on the MLHIVs risky indulgences, however with gradual increase in time and health, the MLHIV start active indulgences in sex. Such a relapse in risk behaviours of older ART clients

Figure 45 Phases of HIV Infection

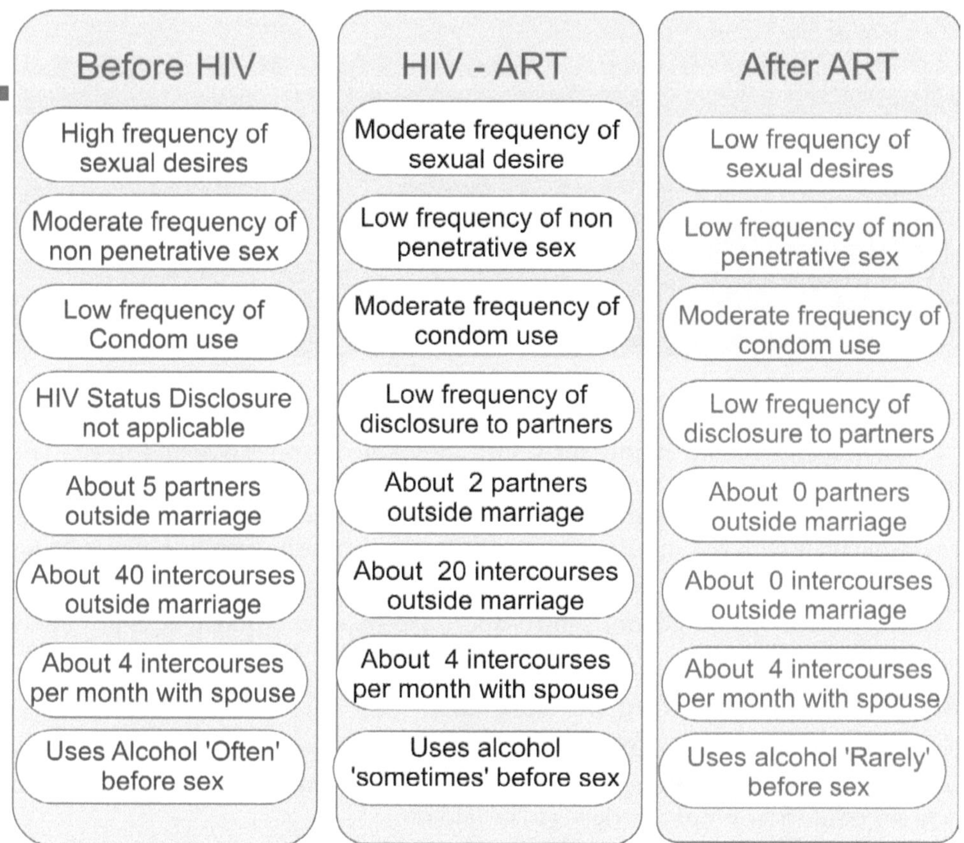

in good health has to be assessed by the counsellors. As an impact on ART, some MLHIV have also complained of dislike for sex, decrease in sexual satisfaction, early ejaculation, erection problems and feeling of impotence. There is need to probe further if this is due to the ART medications or a psychological impact of HIV status. It is also important to identify factors such as higher education, income and health have a greater influence on extent of alcohol consumption before sexual activity.

Counsellors need to educate MLHIV on how addiction to alcohol and its intake before the sexual activity hinders their relationship with spouses, leading to conflicts.

The counsellor thus needs to understand and respond to the clients according to their stages of infection since the sexual needs are different from those on ART. After ART onset the attitude of MLHIV towards penetrative sexual practices changes to needs of companionship and that of mutual care and support.

Sexist Attitudes

The attitudes of most MLHIV were found to be sexist on the areas mentioned graphically.

Figure 46 Sexist Attitudes prevailing amongst MLHIV

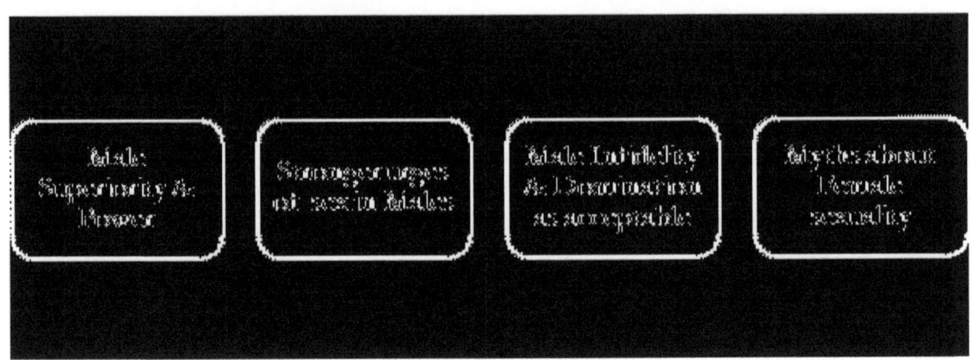

The MLHIV having highly sexist attitudes were the ones who indulged in sex outside marriage, had more number of sexual partners and did not use condoms. This is a pointer towards special attention required for such men, who seem sexist, in assessing their high risk indulgences and mitigating these by bringing about change in their chauvinistic perspectives.

Workshops on gender sensitisation, violence on women, equality issues, and other such themes related to sexist attitudes would be of value in this context.

MLHIV's understanding on Safe Sex

The understanding of MLHIV as well as counsellors on "Safe Sex" practice was limited to: condom use, reduction in sexual partners or risky penetrative practices. In safe sex education, emphasis needs to be laid on

- ✓ Non penetrative practices,
- ✓ Establishing communication and warmth within relationship
- ✓ Assessments of STI and HIV infections amongst the partner
- ✓ Abstaining alcohol intake before sexual indulgence

A shift from anal to oral sex services in commercial sex may be considered as one possible risk reduction strategy for male and transgender sex workers who cannot negotiate condom use in anal sex.

The spouses seem to face an even worse stigma of childlessness than the stigma of condom use. This education of safe pregnancy techniques is also to be considered when discussing about safe sex practices.

Factors influencing Behaviour Change

The MLHIV validate the interplay of following actors as key agents of behaviour change in their lives:

Figure 47 Factors influencing Behaviour Change

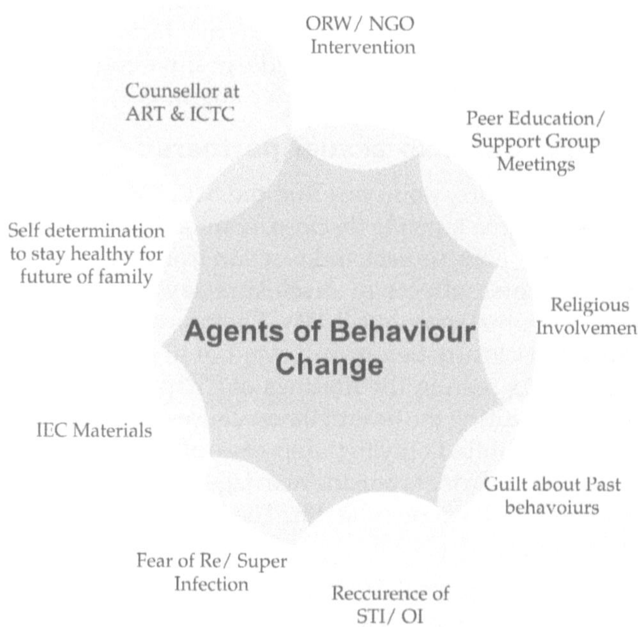

The above illustration points out that Internal factors like motivation, guilt, self determination, self reconciliation and altruism, play a vital role in behaviour change. Also the maintenance of healthy spousal relationship is a key agent in behaviour change. When the objective of behaviour change is focused on spouse, children and for family, better results were observed in its sustenance. The rights of the sexual partner should not be overlooked when educating behaviour change using the "Stages of Change Model".

The role of spirituality and exercise as a way of life, have been proven effective in behaviour change education in the West and can be imitated. Behaviour change messages carry more impact when delivered by counsellors (especially ART) and peers. MLHIV do not change their risky behaviours on the basis of an intellectual awareness rather, the determinant of sustained change lies in being a member of a community organisation (ART Peer Group, Positive People's Network, PLHIV Support Group), which actively promotes and supports such changes.

Behaviour change messages must give people realistic and sustainable choices from amongst which individuals and couples can choose according to their preferred sexual practices and the life circumstances. Behaviour change theories show that proper and timely communication from various stakeholders, is an integral part of the behaviour change process, than that compared to unilateral effort to change.

Thus interplay needs to be established between intrinsic factors (like trust, motivation, overcoming fear, reconciliation, love and commitment to partner) and external factors like health of sexual partner, future of children and family, structural factors including religious involvement, education on HIV. In other words, behaviour change is the outcome of combination of both internal and external factors working in harmony with one another. This interplay will help rekindle positive energy within individuals to strengthen and sustain any behaviour change attempts.

Disclosure of HIV status to sexual partners

Findings from disclosure, point out that the MLHIV's understanding on the rationale for disclosure, time taken to disclose, manner in which disclosure is done are key aspects that decide the impact and reaction from spouses. The counsellor's role in mitigating adverse effects of disclosure lay in tactfully handling the aforementioned life circumstances of MLHIV. The counsellors should aim towards encouraging spousal disclosure before any event of ill health in order to reap the benefits of disclosure. As seen in the findings of Chapter 9, any delay in spousal disclosure, or disclosure during the time of illness causes negative impact. Disclosure education should not be limited only to the spouses of MLHIV, for it puts to risk not just the lives of their sexual partners outside marriage, in the event of unsafe practices, but also poses risk to MLHIV's own health. The Johari Window approach can be used as a tool of disclosure.

The MLHIV's fears in spousal disclosure that needs to be addressed include: perceived accusations of infidelity, fear of being disallowed sex or marital discord. The MLHIV on ART who had not yet disclosed to their spouses had no plan on when and how to disclose. This is an area where the ICTC counsellors should play a significant role in preparing every MLHIV for spousal disclosure, even before their ART onset, so that ART adherence can also be enabled. Most of these MLHIV have sought support in couple counselling to enhance marital relationships post disclosure.

Circumstances of disclosure

In most occasions, disclosure has happened in medically critical circumstances like during illness of the MLHIV or during pregnancy of their spouse. In these circumstances the MLHIV are left with no option but to disclose and such circumstances are not conducive to a healthy reaction of the spouse. The MLHIV should be encouraged not to wait till such critical circumstances for disclosure and should be prepared on how to create an enabling environment conducive to a healthy disclosure.

Initiating Disclosure

As seen below, most respondents have voluntarily initiated disclosure and only a few seek the support of the HCP. Both the MLHIV and Spousal FGD highlight that quite a few of the spouses get to know of their husbands status through the HCP during illness or pregnancy, during their own HIV test, or discovered on suspicion.

Figure 48 Disclosure Initiatives of MLHIV

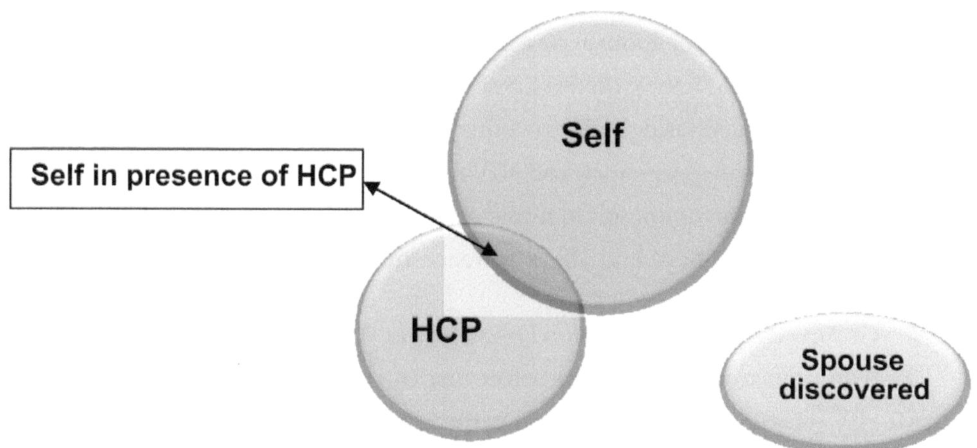

The direct disclosure by HCP or spousal discovery of HIV status seems to have had a harmful impact on the marital relationship. When disclosure is made to the spouse, it will be helpful, if the spouse is well informed on how to handle the MLHIV and their relationship in the context of HIV status. In view of this, proactive initiative of the counsellor is encouraged in helping clients taking initiatives towards timely disclosure before the spouse discovers or before the HCP needs to disclose.

The feelings after disclosure show that a large number of the MLHIV suffered from negative feelings like feeling ashamed to face spouse, guilt of illicit behaviours, feeling lonely, depressed, anxious and hopelessness. These feelings may indicate non acceptance of spouse or even the fear of spousal reaction. The correlations show that MLHIV who felt negative after disclosure had indulged in extramarital sex. Hence in such cases, the counsellors will have to primarily address the MLHIV's guilt conscience, in order to normalise his feelings.

It is obvious that spousal disclosure may have immediate negative reactions to the extent of physical violence and abandonment. The common negative impact of spousal disclosure on sexual relations include, sexual abstinence, reduced sexual contacts and demonstration by spouse on decreased interest in sex or feeling ashamed to have sex. However, it has to be understood that such discriminatory spousal behaviours determine lack of knowledge on safe sexual behaviours and stigma associated with HIV. In such situations, towards building marital concord, the counsellor role is to educate the spouse on both protected penetrative practices as well as non penetrative practices. There is a need for building up a healthy communication on sex between the couple, taking joint decisions towards safe sexual indulgences and child bearing, forgiving the past behaviours and helping the MLHIV overcome his guilt.

The factors influencing spousal disclosure as stated by the respondents that can be helpful for the counsellor to motivate other MLHIV include

- ☆ MLHIV's responsibility and concern towards the primary partners health and to prepare her for her deteriorating health
- ☆ MLHIV's need for spousal care and support to cope with treatment
- ☆ Benefits in alleviating distress, associated with non-disclosure
- ☆ Benefits of facilitating HIV preventive behaviours and risk reduction
- ☆ Benefits of safe pregnancy and HIV negative child
- ☆ Show benefits for oneself in terms of internal peace and concord
- ☆ Consider the ORW and Peers to reach out to the spouses for experience sharing.
- ☆ Group education sessions on Disclosure at ART Centre
- ☆ Significance of self disclosure before disclosure by others or partner discovery

MLHIV who have spent more time in the 'disclosure event', were seen to have more positive impact of disclosure and this finding points out that the content of disclosure has to be laden with the pros and cons of HIV status and planning for life hereafter. The MLHIV should be encouraged to have a substantial discussion with spouses for disclosure and should be empowered to deal with anticipated spousal reactions. If the counsellor cannot find time, they have to identify and build other support systems. The MLHIV needs to be trained also on the words/ styles that can be used for the disclosure event.

Thus the key ingredients in effective spousal disclosure as identified in this study are as depicted below:

Figure 49 Factors influencing effective Spousal disclosure

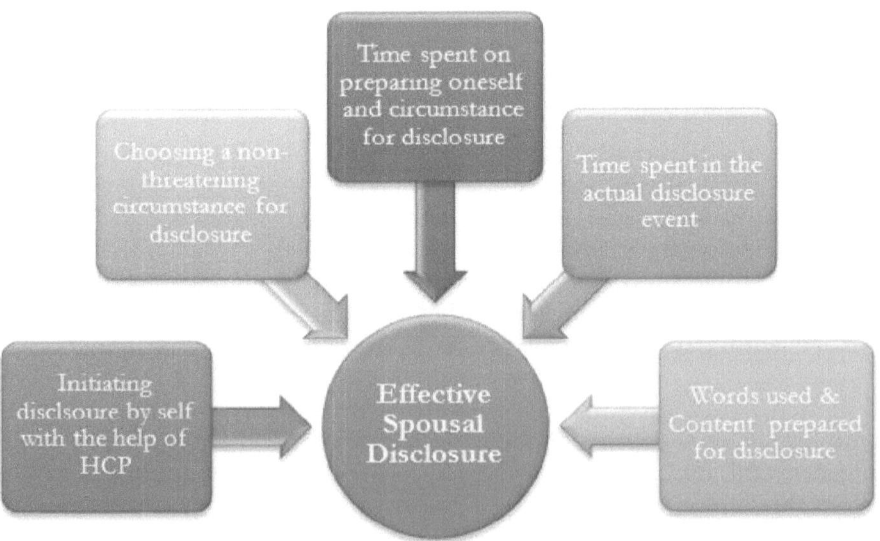

As much as it is important to disclose about one's HIV status to the spouse, disclosure to other sexual partners also holds high significance. The MLHIV needs conscientisation on the right to good health of their non spousal sexual partners too. In conditions where disclosure is not possible for the MLHIV, unprotected sexual relations should be highly advocated in the interest of preventing the spread of HIV in the society. The intensive strategies used for spousal disclosure may not be required in cases of other sexual partners due to the short-lived nature of their physical contacts. But it should be understood that in such cases the counsellor may not have a direct role of interaction with the non-spousal partner and the MLHIV's capacity has to be built in handling the disclosure event. The study also points out the ease in which, some MLHIV disclosed their status to regular non spousal partners and the same can be encouraged.

Thus the above recommendations and suggestions offered to the counsellors, is with the hope of building an effective mutual relationship with the PLHIV, in order to respond to their sexual health needs. An open discussion on this issue will lead to further discoveries, untouched by this study and essential in addressing the sexual concerns of the PLHIV. This road map is also a building block parent bodies and other stakeholders intervening in the field of HIV to construct an ongoing education curriculum for counsellors. Additional recommendations to stakeholders are highlighted below.

12.6. Recommendations from Counsellors to Training Institutions:

The need for more training on crucial knowledge in assessing sexual behaviours of MLHIV is loud and clear from the counsellors, based on their suggestions on required training inputs as mentioned in Chapter 7, is reiterated and summarised in brief here:

1. Skill based workshops on how to question clients on their sexual practices and on how to educate MLHIV on positively channelizing sexual desires.
2. Session on Reproductive health covering content like sexual health and hygiene, understanding human anatomy and its functions, Impact of sexual behaviour on physiology, Sexual behaviour during menstruation and on Contraception
3. Session on Sexuality covering types of sexual orientations and sexualities, Types of having sex, Good practices regarding sex and Risky behaviours.
4. Knowledge and Skills in conducting a sex education for PLHIV during ART group meetings, handling sexuality related queries of adolescence and children, communicating about sex with PLHIV who are not as educated,
5. Orientation to the practices of sexual minorities, education on how to identify a transgender or a homosexual, addressing issues and concerns of sexual minorities and bringing about behaviour changes in bisexuals.
6. In depth education on safe sex strategies, inclusive of its stages, types, safe sex between concordant and discordant couples, condom negotiation skills, convincing partner into safe sex, Use of foreplay for orgasm, Ways to masturbate.

7. Techniques of behaviour change, disclosure and promoting monogamy
8. The counsellors have shown keen interest to know of updates in the field of medical and social researches conducted on PLHIV, MSM and TG.
9. Sharing of Success stories and good practices practiced by counsellors in eliciting information on Sexuality and in bringing about behaviour change of their clients.
10. Need to demonstrate the content and manner of spousal disclosure, in order to make men comfortable for early disclosure.

The key to the success of behaviour change in gay communities is attributed to peer-education programs. These peer educators carried messages that were being communicated effectively in the highly personalised context of small group meetings. It created more impact when conveyed horizontally, by peers, than when they are conveyed vertically, by sources of authority to "the masses", and that individuals who are given the power to make decisions about their own lives in the context of a supportive community are far more likely to adopt and maintain appropriate behaviours. Such peer educators need to be trained by the counsellors and linked to MLHIV practising high risk behaviours. Only such conscious efforts for ongoing education can encourage in raising the consciousness of MLHIV's and behaviour change actions.

Accordingly if the following considerations are initiated, there will be a significant dip in incidence of new infections and sexual health of the PLHIV will also be simultaneously ensured. This study would thus like to propose some areas for future researchers to explore on the issue, in order to contribute a crucial role in expanding the theoretical framework of this issue.

12.7. Recommendations for future researchers

1. Explore the conflict areas related to sexual dynamics within concordant and discordant couples and identify the skills related to marriage counselling for such couples. An in-depth interview with MLHIV and their spouses triangulating a few NGO / Hospital based counsellors as key informants. A comparative analysis of sexual dynamics can be measured amongst the couples who know each other's status and those who do not know. It can be ascertained if factors like couple's age, years of marriage, income, ART initiation, health conditions and sexual practices influence such dynamics.
2. An Interview with spouses of MLHIV on the same areas covered by this study (ie. practices, partners, pleasure/ pain aspects, power relationships) to understand comprehensively their sexual behaviours and gender related concerns of women. It can further bring to light the reproductive health concerns and nature and frequency of infections amongst the spouses. The study results become meaningful with an inclusive criterion of spouses who are not widows and MLHIV's good health conditions.
3. Assess the gender based training needs of counsellors and identify the gaps in relation to their effective counselling skills. This study can be performed by the training institutes so as to develop communication skills of all

counsellors, irrespective of gender, in imparting information on reproductive and sexual health

4. Study and explore the negotiation skills of spouses while engaging in safe sexual practices. It will be interesting to observe of differences in negotiation skills between rural and urban spouses, employed and home based spouses and also based on educational achievement of women. How the intervening agencies have helped empower their negotiations skills can also be deliberated.
5. Assessment of the counsellor-initiated disclosure process in the field and its impact on the marital relations of spouses. It needs to be understood on how often the counsellor has to disclose the status and under what circumstances the PLHIV are willing to initiate disclosure. The counsellor's preparation and process for disclosure can be explored to identify how it can be strengthened further. It also needs to be ascertained whether disclosure has an association with ART onset. Thus the training institute would come to know if the skills in disclosure need to be imparted with greater focus on ART counsellors.
6. A longitudinal study to assess the consistency in the behaviour change of the MLHIV. This will help understand if behaviour change is only a short lived practice, with the early years of ART or if these have been consistently sustained. The factors influencing and retarding sustenance of behaviour change efforts will certainly be tools of education for the intervening agencies.
7. A study on myths and misconceptions amongst PLHIV on sexual matters and their ideas on patriarchy. This study can include the assessment of non sexist attitudes of MLHIV, as a part of their behaviour change.

Conclusion

The control of the disease HIV and AIDS is very much dependent on the effectiveness of the counsellors, who are in direct contact with the PLHIV, and can enable their decision making. The findings of this study depict that the PLHIV have high regard for the messages and inputs provided by the counsellors towards behaviour change and most of them are taking initiatives to implement them. It is important to understand here that unless the information is re-enforced in the counselling set up at different time intervals, fatalism may develop amongst MLHIV leading to relapse. The MLHIV peer support is also seen as an influential channel for sustenance in behaviour change, which needs to be capitalised.

Care and Support for PLHIV is the need of the hour in India, considering the dip in incidence rates of new infections. In this context, this study offers great significance in designing the paradigm for the sexual health and rights of PLHIV, which needs to be given adequate mileage in the national program and the sensitive issue of sexuality be addressed with utmost care. Only such a considerate initiative from the counsellors as well as the training institutions will help reach the ultimate goal of HIV counselling in building better lives and a healthy future for PLHIV.

ANNEXURE 1

BIBLIOGRAPHY

Author & Year	Details
AARP, 2004	Close relationships among older Americans : an analysis of the portrayal of close relationships in AARP magazine between 1966 and 2003 Dept. of Sociology, University of North Carolina at Chapel Hill, 2004
Acharya, 1992	Peace culture amidst power conflicts.[S.I.] : Fellowship Of, 1992
Adam Carr,1991	The emergence of the paedophile in the late twentieth century Taylor & Francis, Australian Historical Studies, 36, no. 126 (2005): 272-295
Aggleton, 1996	AIDS Education and Prevention An Interdisciplinary Journal National Institutes of Health Volume 23, 2011ISSN: 0899-9546
AIDS Care, 2004	Meta-analytic Examination of Online Sex-Seeking and Sexual Risk Behavior Among Men Who Have Sex With Men, September 2006 - Volume 33 - Issue 9 - pp 576-584, doi: 10.1097/01.olq.0000204710.35332.c5
Aldrich et al., 2000	Who's who in gay and lesbian history, Volume 2, Routledge, 2000, ISBN 0415159822, 9780415159821
Alfred, 1981	Sex differences in reports of illness and disability: A preliminary test of fixed role obligation hypothesis Journal of health and Social Behaviour 1981, Vol 22 (June)
Alphonse et. al., 2010	A Quest for a Way to Enhance the Process of CounselingUnpublished: College of Social Work, Nirmala Niketan, Mumbai
Altman, 2000	Sexuality and Globalization Journal of NSRC Sexuality Research & Social Policy, January 2004 Vol. 1, No. 1 National Sexuality Resource Center, San Francisco State University http://nsrc.sfsu.edu, last accessed on Jan 2010
Altman & Taylor, 1973	Communication in interpersonal relationships: Social Penetration Theory. In M. E. Roloff and G. R. Miller (Eds.), Interpersonal processes: New directions in communication research, 257-277. Newbury Park, CA: Sage
Antagana, 2000	Sexual behaviour of PLHIV in Yaounde, Cameroon, Africa Journal Magrebin, A. Réa. - VOL IX - P. 22, Yaoundé B.P : 5408, République de Cameroun
Armistead et. al., 1999	African-American women and self-disclosure of HIV infection: Rates, predictors, and relationship to depressive symptomatology. AIDS and Behaviour, 1999; 3:195-204.
Assiter, 1988	Feminist perspectives in philosophy Indiana University Press, 1988, ISBN: 0253204615, 9780253204615
Babcock, 1998	Applying the Trans-theoretical Model to Female and Male Perpetrators of Intimate Partner Violence: Gender Differences in Stages and Processes of Change Violence and Victims Volume 20, Number 2, 2005 , pp. 235-250(16), Springer Publishing Company
Bailey & Hart, 2006	Sexual risk behaviour of men who have sex with men: emerging patterns and new challengesCurrent Opinion in Infectious Diseases: February 2010 - Volume 23 - Issue 1 - p 39–44 doi: 10.1097/QCO.0b013e328334feb1, HIV infection and AIDS: Edited by Martin Fisher
Bandura, 1997	Social Cognitive Theory: An Agentic Perspective Annu. Rev. Psychol. 2001.52:1-26, Department of Psychology, Stanford University, Stanford. California 94305-2131

Becker, 1974	"The Health Belief Model and Personal Health Behavior." Health Education Monographs 2:324–473. COPYRIGHT 2002 The Gale Group Inc.
Bem, 1965	An Experimental Analysis of Beliefs and Attitudes. Unpublished Doctoral Dissertation, University of Michigan.
Berer, 2003	Sex sexuality, sexual healthReproductive Health Matters, Vol. 6, No. 12, Nov., 1998, Sexuality Published by: Reproductive Health Matters, Issue Stable URL: http://www.jstor.org/stable/i291539, last accessed on July 1009
Blumstein & Schwartz 1983	The Role of Sexual Behavior in the Identification Process of Gay and Bisexual Males The Journal of Sex Research, Vol. 37, No. 2 (May, 2000), pp. 123-132
Borcher, 1999	Parents' Perception Towards Disclosure Of Their HIV Positive Unpublished University Of Science And Technology, Michigan.
Bordo,1994 ideas	Essentialism and Punishment in the Icelandic Women's Movement: all (no matter how liberating in some contexts or for some purposes) are condemned to be haunted by a voice from the margins, either already speaking or presently muted but awaiting the conditions for speech, that awakens us to what has been excluded, effaced, 'damaged'. European Journal of Women's Studies May 1995 2: 171-183,
Bouhnik, 2002	Highly active antiretroviral treatment does not increase sexual risk behaviour among French HIV infected injecting drug users J Epidemiol Community Health 2002;56:349–353, Dr Y Obadia, ORS-PACA, 23 rue Stanislas Torrents, 13006 Marseille, France
Bourdieu, 1998	Passeron. 1977. Reproduction in Education, Society and Culture. London: Sage. Cambridge University Press
Bowes & Dickinson 1991	Violence Against Women and HIV/AIDS: Setting the Research Agenda Meeting Report Gender and Women's Health World Health Organisation Conference 23-25 October 2000, Geneva, Switzerland
Brett Kahr, 1999	The History of Sexuality: From Ancient Polymorphous Perversity to ModernGenital Love J Psychohist 26,4:764-78
Bruyn et al.,1995	Facing the Challenges of HIV/AIDS/STDs: A Gender-based Response. Royal Tropical Institute, SAfAIDS, and the WHO Global Programme on AIDS.
Bunell et al., 2004	Changes in sexual behavior and risk of HIV transmission after antiretroviral therapy and prevention interventions in rural Uganda ISSN 0269-937 2006 Lippincott Williams & WilkinsUganda Virus Research Institute, P.O. Box 49, Entebbe, Uganda.
Bunting, 2001	Sustaining The Relationship: Women's Caregiving In The Context Of HIV Disease Health Care Women Int. 2001 Jan-Feb;22(1-2):131-48. Department of Community Nursing, Medical College of Georgia, Augusta 30912-4250, USA.
Cade et al., 2002	Unsafe Sex among HIV Positive Individuals: Cross-sectional and Prospective Predictors J Community Health. 2010;35(2):115-123. © 2010 Springer Science+Business Media
Caldwell, 2000	Resistances to behavioiural change to reduce HIV/AIDS infection in predominantly heterosexual epidemics in third world countries Canberra: Australian National University, National Centre for epidemiology and Population Health
Caraël, 1997	Baseline for the evaluation of an AIDS programme using prevention indicators: a case study in Ethiopia. National AIDS Control Programme, Ministry of Health, Addis Ababa, Ethiopia. Bull World Health Organ. 1996;74(5):509–516
Carl, 1986	A telling dilemma HIV disclosure between male (homo)sexual partners Published by Sigma Research © November 2004, ISBN: 1 872956 78 5

Carovano, 1992	More than mothers and whores: Redefining the AIDS prevention needs of women. International Journal of Health Services 21(1): 131-142.
Carrier, 1989	Sexual behavior and the spread of AIDS in Mexico. Medical Anthropology Quarterly, 10, 129-142.
Catania, et al., 2001	How many HIV infections cross the bisexual bridge? An estimate from the United States. AIDS, 11, 1031-37, The Haworth Press
Chesney and Smith, 1999	Critical delays in HIV testing and care. The potential role of stigma. American Behavioral Scientist, 42, 1162-1174.
Ciccarone et al., 2003	Sex Without Disclosure of Positive HIV Serostatus in a US Probability Sample of Persons Receiving Medical Care for HIV Infection, Research And Practice, June 2003, Vol 93, No. 6 American Journal of Public Health
Cleveland et al, 1985	Women and Men in organisation: Sex and Gender issues at work Lawrence Elbarum associates ltd., Industrial Avenue, Mahwah, NJ, 07430
Coates, 1998	"You Must Do the Test to Know Your Status": Attitudes to HIV Voluntary Counseling and Testing for Adolescents Among South African Youth and Parents doi: 10.1177/1090198106286442 Health Educ Behav February 2008 vol. 35 no. 1 87-104
Coleman, 1992	Is your patient suffering from compulsive sexual behavior? Psychiatric Annals, 22(6) 320-325.
Connell, 1995	Masculinities Cambridge: Polity.
Cornwall, 1994	"What is participatory research?" Social Science and Medicine 41(12): 1667 - 1676
Crandall & Coleman 1992	AIDS-related stigmatization and the disruption of social relationships. Journal of Social and Personal Relationships 9, 163-177.
Crawford, Travers 1999	Reading AIDS: A content analysis of homosexuality in young adult fiction. "Reducing Inequities through Participatory Research and Community Empowerment." Health Education & Behavior 24(3): 344 - 356.
Culpert, 1968	The Interpersonal Process of Self-Disclosure: It Takes Two to See OneNew York: Renaissance Editors.
Cunnhinga, 1981	When children molest children: Group treatment strategies for young sexual abusers. Orwell VT: Safer Society press
Dandona et al., 2005	High risk of HIV in non-brothel based female sex workers in India. BMC Public Health. 87 (5).
Das, 2000	Male Sexual behavior in Orrissa, New evidence and issues, Pune, India
David et al., 2002	Gender Dimensions of HIV Status Disclosure to Sexual Partners: Rates, Barriers and Outcomes: A Review Paper Department of Gender and Women's Health (GWH) Family and Community Health (FCH) World Health Organization
deMause, 1974	The history of childhood New York Psyhcohistory press
Derlega et al., 1993	Self-Disclosure Newbury Park, CA: Sage
Desai, 2000	'Queer Theory and Alternative Sexualities' Paper presented at Seminar Series on Homosexuality in African Literary Studies, University of Cambridge, Cambridge.
Deutsch., 1973	The Resolution of Conflict: Constructive and Destructive Processes. New Haven, CT: Yale University Press
Devillly., 2005	Estimating means and percentages in a complex sampling survey: application to a French national survey on sexual behaviour (ACSF). Stat Med 1997; 16:397–423.

DiClemente., 1995 HIV prevention for adolescents: Utility of the Health Belief Model. AIDS Education and Prevention, 3 (1), 50-59.

Dover., 1988 Classical Greek Attitudes to Sexual Behavior, Greek Homosexuality and Initiation, in Dover, K. J. (Ed.) The Greeks and their Legacy: Collected Papers. Volume II: Prose Literature, History, Society, Transmission, Influence. Oxford [etc.]: Blackwell, p115-34

Duck and Pittman, 1994 Social and personal relationships. In M. L. Knapp & G. R. Miller (Eds.) Handbook of interpersonal communication (pp. 676–695). Thousand Oaks, CA: Sage.

Eisele et al., 2008 "High levels of risk behavior among people living with HIV Initiating and waiting to start antiretroviral therapy in Cape Town South Africa." AIDS Behavior 12(4): 570-7.

Ekstrand, et al., 1999 Mode effects in surveys of gay men: A within-individual comparison of responses by mail and by telephone. Journal of Sex Research, 36, 67-75.

Elford, 2000 Combination therapies for HIV and sexual risk behavior among gay men. Journal of Acquired Immune Deficiency Syndromes, 23, 266_71.

Elias et al., 1995 Transforming AIDS prevention to meet women's needs: A focus on developing countries Social Science and Medicine, 40(7), 93 1-943.

Elkhal, 2010 Pannexin-1 hemichannel-mediated ATP release together with P2X1 and P2X4 receptors regulate T-cell activation at the immune synapse. Blood. 2010 Nov 4;116(18):3475-84. Epub 2010 Jul 21. PubMed PMID: 20660288;

PubMed Central PMCID: PMC2981474.

Elwood et al., 2003 Reasons for HIV disclosure/nondisclosure in close relationships: Testing a model of HIV–disclosure decision making. Journal of Social and Clinical Psychology, 23(6), 747-67.

Fakir, 2004 'The people shall govern.' Idasa Roundtable Discussion. Cape Town:

Festinger, 1957 A theory of cognitive dissonance. Stanford, CA: Stanford University Press.

Fisher & Adams, 2003 Experience with and Internet-based, theoretically grounded educational resource for the promotion of sexual and reproductive health. Sexual and Relationship Therapy, 18, 293-308.

Foreman, 1998 AIDS and Men, Taking Risks or Taking Responsibility? London: Panos/Zed Books.

FPAI, 2005 Reproductive and Sexual Health and Rights 4th Asia Pacific Conference on Exploring New Frontiers...APCRSH 2007, Hyderabad • India http://www.epos.in/public/docs/4apcrsh2007_abstract_1.pdf, July 2009

Gagnon and Parker, 1995 Concieving Sexuality New York: Routledge

Girardi, 2004 Retaining Core Staff: The impact of human resource practices on organizational commitment. Journal of Comparative International Management, 8(2), 23-42.

Glaser, 1988 Raising PCP's Awareness to Patient Culture: PEAs as Cultural Agents SE Louisiana U

Gorbach et al., 2004 Don't ask, don't tell: Patterns of HIV disclosure among HIV positive men who have sex with men with recent STI practicing high risk behaviour in Los Angles and Seattle.Sex Transmitted Infections, 80(6), 512–517

Gouldner,1960 The norm of reciprocity: A preliminary statement. American Sociological Review, 25, 161-178.

Greeff, 2008	Disclosure of HIV status: Experiences and perceptions of people living with HIV/AIDS and nurses involved in their care in Africa.Qualitative Health Research,18: 311–324.
Greeley, 1991	Faithful attraction: Discovering intimacy, love, and fidelity in American marriage. New York: Doherty.
Green, 1995	Sex, love and seropositivity: balancing the risks. In: P. AGGLETON, P. DAVIES & G. HART teds), AIDS: safety, sexuality and risk (pp. 144-158). London: Taylor & Francis.
Gregson, 2006	HIV decline associated with behavior change in eastern Zimbabwe. Science 2006; 311:664–666.
Gunter R., et. al., 2008	Privacy in E-commerce: Stated behaviour versus actual behaviour. Communications of the ACM, 48, 101–106.
Halkitis & Wilton, 2006	Barebacking identity among HIV-positive gay and bisexual men: Demographic, psychological, and behavioral correlates. AIDS, 19(S1), 27–36.
Harrison et al., 1992	Self-reported childhood and adolescent sexual abuse among adult homosexual and bisexual men. Child Abuse & Neglect, 16, 855–864.
Hays et al., 1992	Disclosing HIV seropositivity to significant others AIDS 7, 425-531
Heise, 1995	Conceiving sexuality: Approaches to sex research in a postmodern world. 'Violence, sexuality, and women's lives' New York & London: Routledge.
Heise and Elias, 1995	"Transforming AIDS prevention to meet women's needs: a focus on developing countries." Social Science and Medicine 40(7): 933-943.
Holt et al., 1998	The role of disclosure in coping with HIV infection. AIDS Care, 10(1): 49-60.
Hunt, 1974	Sexual Behavior in the 1970s Chicago: Playboy Press
Ichikawa & Natpratan, 2006	Substance use and sexual behaviours of Japanese men who have sex with men: a nationwide internet survey conducted in Japan.BMC Public Health. [serie en Internet] 2006 [citado 2 Jul 2008];6:[aprox. 41 p.]. http://www.pubmedcentral.nih.gov/ articlerender.fcgi?tool=pubmed&pubmedid =17002800
Jackson, 2002	Aids Africa: Continent in Crisis SA faids, Harare.
Jourard, 1975	Self-disclosure: An experimental analysis of the transparent self. New York: Wiley.
Kalichman & Nachimson, partners.	Self-efficacy and disclosure of HIV positive serostatus to sex 1999 Health Psychology, 18, 281-287
Kalichman et al., 2003	Sensation seeking, alcohol use and sexual risk behaviours among men receiving services at a clinic for sexually transmitted infections. Journal of the Study of Alcohol, 64: 564-569.
Katz, 1997	Mom I've got something to tell you – disclosing HIV infectionJournal of Advanced Nursing, 25(1): 139-143.
Katz; Ullrich et al., 2003	Concealment of homosexual identity, social support and CD4 cell count among HIV-seropositive gay men. Journal of Psychosomatic Research, 54, 205–212.
Kelly, 1995	AIDS prevention and treatment: Psychology's role in the health crisis Clinical Psychology Review, 8, 255-284.
Kerr, 1991	African Popular Theatre from Pre-Colonial Times to the Present Day James Currey, London
Keuls, 1985	The Reign of the Phallus: sexual politics in ancient Athens 1985 Cambridge Mass

Kinsey et. al., 1948 Sexual Behavior in the Human Male Philadelphia: Saunders.

Klein, 1999 Resistance of personal risk perceptions to debiasing interventions, Health Psychology, 14(2): 132–40

Kline, 1994 HIV-Infected women and sexual risk reduction: The relevance of existing models of behavior change.AIDS Education and Prevention, 6(5), 390-402.

Klitzman, 2004 Moral Secrets: truth and lies in the age of AIDS Baltimore, Johns Hopkins University Press.

Kopytoff, 1990 Women's roles and existential identities' in Beyond the Second Sex: new directions in the Anthropology of gender. Philadelphia: University of Pennsylvania Press

Kurdek, 1991 Differences between heterosexual nonparent couples and gay, lesbian, and heterosexual parent couples. Journal of Family Issues, 22, 727-754

Laryea & Gien, 1993 The Impact of HIV-Positive Diagnosis on the Individual, Part 1: Stigma, Rejection and Loneliness. Clinical Nursing Research. 2 (3), 245-266.

Latkin, 1999 Drug network characteristics as a predictor of cessation of opiate use among adult injection drug users: A prospective study. American Journal of Drug and Alcohol Abuse, 25, 463_/473.

Laumann et al., 1994 The social organization of sexuality: Sexual practices in the United States. Chicago, IL: University of Chicago Press.

Leickness,1999 HIV/AIDS and society Human Sciences Research Council, Cambridge Mass

LeMoncheck, 1997 Loose Women, Lecherous Men. New York and Oxford: Oxford University Press.

Lepper, Greene, & Nisbett, 1973 Rethinking the value of choice: A cultural perspective on intrinsic motivation. Journal of Personality and Social Psychology, 76, 349-366

Lurie et al., 2003 Who infects whom? HIV-1 concordance and discordance among migrant and non-migrant couples in South Africa. AIDS, 17 (15), 2245-2252.

Maman, 2000 The intersections of HIV and violence: directions for future research and interventions. Social Science and Medicine, 2000; 50:459-78

Mane et al.,1994 "Effective communication between partners: AIDS and risk reduction for women." AIDS. Vol. 8 (supp. 1), S325-S331

Manjar, 2007 Sexual Health of Women in UP (unpublished) Centre for Advanced Study, AMU, Aligarh (U.P.)

Manniche., 1987 Low back pain: what is the long-term course? A review of studies of general patient populations. Eur Spine J 2003;12:149-65

Margolese., 2002 Engaging in psychotherapy with the orthodox Jew: A critical review. American Journal of Psychotherapy, 37

Marks & Crepaz., 2001 HIV-positive men's sexual practices in the context of self-disclosure of HIV status. Journal of Acquired Immune Deficiency Syndrome, 27(1): 79-85

Martin et al., 2007 Healthcare-Based Interventions for Sexual Violence Victims: A Review of the Literature. Submitted to Trauma, Violence & Abuse: A Review Journal, April 17, 2006

Masenja., 1993 'Sacrificing female bodies at the alter of male privilege: Journal of theology and religion in Africa 27(1), 98"122.

Mason et al.,1995 Culturally sanctioned secrets? Latino men's nondisclosure of HIV infection to family, friends, and lovers Health Psychology, 14, 6–12

Matovu, 2007 "Voluntary HIV counselling and testing acceptance, sexual risk behaviour and HIV incidence in Rakai, Uganda". AIDS 19: 503-511.

McLeroy, 1988 — An ecological perspective on health promotion programs. Health Ed Quarterly 1988, 15(4): 351-377

MDACS, 2008 — Mumbai District AIDS Control Organization http://www.mdacs.org/submenu.php?cid=21&pcatid=21, last accessed on July 2010 Meystre-

Agustoni, 2006 — Evaluation of the AIDS Prevention Strategy in Switzerland Mandated by the Federal Office of Public Health: Sixth Synthesis Report 1996-1998. Lausanne: Institut universitaire de médecine sociale et preventive

Michael, 2004 — How does disclosure affect HIV prevention Center for AIDS Prevention Studies (CAPS) and the AIDS Research Institute, University of California, San Francisco

Miles. 1994 — Textual harassment: desire and the female body. In the good body: Asceticism in contemporary culture (pp. 49–63). New Haven, CT: Yale University Press

Moore, 1991 — Beyond shame: Reclaiming the abandoned history of radical gay sexuality. Boston: Beacon Press.

Morrell, 2001 — The times of change: Men and masculinity in South Africa. In R. Morrell (Ed.), Changing men in southern Africa (pp. 3–37). London: Zed Books

MSACS, 2007 — Annual Report 2006-2007 http://www.eha-health.org/resources/doc_view/4-annual-report-2007.html, Last visited on December 2009

Nachegam 2003 — HIV/AIDS and antiretroviral treatment knowledge, attitudes, beliefs, and practices in HIV-infected adults in Soweto, South Africa. J Acquir Immune Defic Syndr. 2005;38:196–201

NACO, 2007 — Operational Guidelines for Integrated Counseling and Testing Centres National AIDS Control Organization, Government of India, July 2007

NACO, 2010 — Operational Guidelines For Community Care Centres And Comprehensive Care and Support Centres National, National AIDS Control Organisation Ministry of Health and Family Welfare Government of India New Delhi

Naidoo, 2007 — Disclosure of HIV status: Experiences and perceptions of people living with HIV/AIDS and nurses involved in their care in Africa. Qualitative Health Research,18: 311–324.

Nair, 2004 — Developing Strategies That Tackle the Root Causes of Stigma: Building Action on Sound Analysis Abstract 119. in PEPFAR Annual Meeting. 2006. Durban, South Africa

NFHS, 2005 — National Family Health Survey (NFHS 3),2005–2006, National Fact Sheet. India: . International Institute for Population Sciences and ORC Macro; 2005 2006. http://www.nfhsindia.org/nfhs3.html (Accessed 1 October, 2009)

Nicole Crepaz et al ., 2004 — The Effectiveness of Individual-, Group-, and Community-Level HIV Behavioral Risk-Reduction Interventions for Adult Men Who Have Sex with Men A Systematic Review, Task Force on Community Preventive Services

Nussbaum, 1999 — Communication and aging. Lawrence Eribaum Associates

Nyblade, 2000 — Population-Based HIV testing and counselling in rural Uganda: participation and risk characteristics. Journal of Aquired Immune Deficiency Syndromes, 2001; 28:463-470.

O'Brien et al., 2003 — Prevalence and correlates of HIV serostatus disclosure. Sex Transm Dis. 2003;30:731–735.

O'Leary., 2001 — Effects on Sexual Risk Behavior and STD Rate of Brief HIV/STD Prevention Interventions for African American Women in Primary Care Settings Am J Public Health. 2007;97:1034–1040. doi:10.2105/AJPH.2003.020271

Ogilvie., 2004 — Fertility intentions of women of reproductive age living with HIV in British Columbia, Canada. AIDS 2007; 21:S83–S88

Ortner and Whitehead., 1989 Stigma and Social Exclusion Healthcare London Routledge

Oishi et al., 2005 The nonobvious social psychology of happiness Psychological Inquiry, 16, 162-167.

Panda, 2002 Interface between drug use and sex work in Manipur. Natl Med J India. 2001 Jul-Aug;14(4):209-11.

Parker, 1995 Conceiving sexuality: Approaches to Sex Research in a Postmodern WorldNew York: Routledge

Parsons et al., 2005 Barebacking among Internet-based male sex workers Journal of Gay and Lesbian Psychotherapy, 9(3/4), 89–110.

Paxton, 2002 The Paradox Of Public HIV Disclosure Australian Research Centre in Sex, Health and Society, La Trobe University, Australia AIDS Care 14(4): 559-67 (2002)

Pearce & Sharp, 1973 Self-disclosing communication. Journal of Communication, 23, 409-425.

Pennebaker et al., 1988 Disclosure of traumas and immune function: health implications for psychotherapy. Journal of Consulting and Clinical Psychology 56, 239–245.

Petosa, 1991 Using health belief model to predict safer sex intentions among adolescents Health education quarterly 18(4) 462-476

Petrak, et al., 2001 Factors associated with self-disclosure of HIV serostatus to significant others British Journal of Health Psychology, 6, 69–79.

Pitt, 1992 "Company policy and AIDS in Zimbabwe," Journal of Social Development in Africa 6:53-70.

Podesia, 1998 Star/1 TE. Liver transplantation in cystic fibrosis Lancet 1989:1: 107.

Pomeroy, Martin, & Gebhard, 1953 Sexual Behavior in the Human Female Philadelphia: Saunders

Porche, 2004 The State of Science: Violence and HIV Infection in Women. Journal of the Association of Nurses in AIDS Care, 2003. 14(6): p. 56-68.

Priyamvada, 2007 Explanations of Domestic Violence in India and the United States: A Comparative Analysis Unpublished Doctoral Dissertation, University of Michigan.

Prochaska, 1992 Measurement of condom and other contraceptive behavior change among women at high risk of HIV infection and transmission. Paper presented at the IX International Conference on AIDS (Abstr PO-D38-4416), Berlin, Germany.

Pukar, 2004 Male sexuality and HIV, Naz Foundation International, January 2004, Issue 44, Palingswick House, 241 King Street, London W6 9LP, UK.

Rao, 1991 Child sexual abuse of Asians compared with other populations. Journal of the American Academy of Child and Adolescent Psychiatry, 31, 880–886

Roazen, 1969 Heresy: Sandor Rado and the psychoanalytic movement. Northvale: Jason Robinson Inc

Robles, 1998 Sexual identity formation and AIDS prevention. AIDS and Behavior 10:531-539.

Rosemary, 2006 Sexual Desire and Arousal Disorder in Women. New England Journal of Medicine, 354 (14), 1498-1506.

Rossiaud, 1984 Medieval Prostitution New York: Blackwell

Rutz et al., 1997 Long-term effects of an educational program for general practitioners given by the Swedish Committee for the Prevention and Treatment of Depression Acta Psychiatrica Scandinavica, 85, 83–88.

Ryan., 1984 Lesbian and gay youth: Care and counseling. New York: Columbia University Press.

Sadovsky., 1991 Androgen therapy for effects of aging in older men. American Family Physician, 72, 170–171.

Saffren., 1999 Depression, hopelessness, suicidality, and related factors in sexual minority and heterosexual adolescents. Journal of Consulting and Clinical Psychology, 67(6), 859-866.

Seidler., 1991 Reason, desire, and male sexuality', in P Caplan (ed) The Cultural Construction of Sexuality London: Routledge

Serovich & Greene, 1993 Perceptions of family boundaries: The case of disclosure of HIV testing information. Family Relations, 42, 193-197.

Sgombich et al., 2004 Sexual behaviours and condom use among people living with HIV/AIDS in Chile. Ab. ThOrD1451. XIV International AIDS Conference, Barcelona, July 2002

Shajahan and Cavanagh, 1998 Admission for depression among men in Scotland, 1980-95: retrospective study', British Medical Journal

Shehan et al., 2005 Vital Statistics Ireland: Findings from the All-Ireland Gay Men's Sex Survey, 2000. Dublin: Gay Health Network.

Srivasatava, 1994 Factors that influence the believing of Child sexual abuse disclosures Department of Psychology and the Graduate School of the University of Oregon

Stall, 2000 Intertwining Epidemics: A review of research on substance use among men who have sex with men and its connection to the AIDS epidemic. AIDS and Behavior, 4, 2, 181–192.

Steiner, 1994 Measuring feminine gender identity in homosexual males. Arch. Sex. Behav. 3:249-60

Stevens, 1998 Attachment orientations, social support, and conflict resolution in close relationships. Theory and Close Relationships (pp. 166–188). New York, NY: Guilford Press.

Stillion, 1995 Suicide Across the Life Span: Premature Exits. Hemisphere, New York.

Stirratt, 2006 I have something to tell you: HIV serostatus disclosure practices of HIV-positive gay and bisexual men with sex partners. American Psychological Association; Washington, DC: 2006. pp. 101–120.

Stone, 1987 The course of borderline personality disorder. American Psychiatric Press Review of Psychiatry inc. Washington DC; 8, 103-122.

Strauss, 2002 Basics of Qualitative Research. Newbury Park, CA: Sage Publications

Strecher et al., 1997 Do tailored behavior change messages enhance the effectiveness of health risk appraisal? Results from a randomized trial. Health Education Research, 11(1), 97–105.

Sweat, 1995 Reducing HIV incidence in developing countries with structural and environmental interventions. AIDS 1995, 9 (suppl. A):S251-S257.

Tannahill, 1980 Sex in history. New York: Stein & Day

Tawil, 1995 Enabling approaches for HIV/AIDS prevention: can we modify the environment and minimize the risk? AIDS 1995, 9:1299-1306.

Taylor, 1973 Point of view and perception so causality, Journal of Personality and Social Psychology, 32, 439-445

Thibaut & Kelley, 1959 Communications and persuasion: Psychological studies in opinion change, New Haven, CT: Yale University Press

Thomas S., 2007 — Sexual Behaviour Of HIV Infected Men On ART, J.J. Hospital Unpublished: Certificate Course I n Advanced Research Methodology, College Of Social Work, Nirmala Niketan, Mumbai University

Thomas et al., 2007 — Identifying Opinion Leaders to Promote Behavior Change University of Southern California, Alhambra, Published online before print June 29, 2007, doi: 10.1177/1090198106297855 Health Educ Behav December 2007 vol. 34 no. 6 881-896

Ullrich et al., 2003 — Concealment of homosexual identity, social support and CD4 cell count among HIV-seropositive gay men. Journal of Psychosomatic Research, 54, 205–212.

UNAIDS, 2004 — Joint United Nations Program on AIDS [UNAIDS] 2002: Nigeria: Epidemiological Fact Sheets, 2002 Update. http://www.unaids.org/html/pub/Publications/Factsheets01/Nigeria_EN_pdf.pdf

UNAIDS, 2001 — The impact of Voluntary counseling and testing: A global review of the benefits and challenges .http://www.unaids.org

UNAIDS, 2003 — HIV prevalence and associated risks in young men who have sex with men. Journal of American Medical Association, 284, 198-204

UNAIDS, 1999 — Gender and HIV/AIDS: Taking Stock of Research and Programs. Geneva.

Valleroy et al., 2000 — HIV prevalence and associated risks in young men who have sex with men. Young Men's Survey Study Group. Journal of American Medical Association, 284, 198-204

Van de Velde et al., 2004 — AIDS-related health behavior: coping, protection motivation and previous behavior. Journal of Behavioral Medicine, 14, 429-51.

Wainberg,1998 — Public health implications of antiretroviral therapy and HIV drug resistance. JAMA. 1998 Jun 24;279(24):1977–1983.

Weiss, Gupta, 1998 — Bridging the Gap: Addressing Gender and Sexuality in HIV Prevention. Washington, DC: International Center for Research on Women.

WHO, 1999 — Groups at Risk: WHO Report on the Epidemic, 1996.Geneva, Switzerland: World Health Organization

Wight, 2006 — Parental influences on young people's sexual behaviour: A longitudinal analysis Medical Research Council, Social and Public Health Sciences Unit, 4 Lilybank Gardens, Glasgow G12 8RZ, UK

Wilkinson, 1997 — Tuberculosis and HIV: current status in Africa AIDS 11 (suppl B):S115-S123.

Xia, 2006 — Social Influence and Individual Risk Factors of HIV Unsafe Sex among Female Entertainment Workers in China Xiushi Yang, Old Dominion University; AIDS Educ Prev. 2010 February; 22(1): 69–86. doi: 10.1521/aeap.2010.22.1.69

Zea, 2007 — Predictors of Disclosure of HIV-Positive serostatus among Latino Gay Men. Journal of Cultural Diversity and Ethnic Minority Psychology, Vol. 13, 304-312.

Znoj, 2010 — Sexual risk behaviour in emerging adults: Gender– specific effects of hedonism, psychosocial distress, and sociocognitive variables in a 5-year longitudinal study. AIDS Educ.Prev. 22, (2)148-159.

ANNEXURE 2

Questionnaire for Counsellors

Profile

1. Sex : Male / Female
2. Age : __________
3. Religion : __________
4. Education : __________
5. Centre : VCTC / PPTCT / DIC / ART / CCC / NGO
6. Training Status : Trained / Untrained
7. Period of experience as a Counselor: __________

Sexual Behaviour

1. Out of **every 10** Male clients counseled, how many have queries related to sexual performance or sexuality related issues? ____________

Can you enlist some of their sexuality related queries/ concerns?

2. What do you think are some of the barriers faced by Male PLHA in asking you questions pertaining to Sexual practices?

3. How often do most HIV infected men continue to have sex with their wives/ other sexual partners? **Very Often / Often / Occasionally / Rarely / Never**

Can you support the above answer with some evidence?

How much percentage of the above is safe sex? ____________

4. How many of the male HIV infected cases indulge in sex with men? _______

Do they often indulge in safe behaviour? Yes / No

How many cases have so far asked you questions related to homosexuality?

____

What are some of the questions raised in relation to homosexuality?

What was your response to these questions?

5. How many of your clients who appear to be Heterosexual also be Homosexual? ______

Can you give evidence of their bisexuality?

6. How many of your HIV infected males could involve in these kinds of sexual practices:

a. Vaginal Sex : _________ %

b. Oral Sex : _________ %

c. Anal Sex : _________ %

Behaviour Change

7. An HIV infected male, expresses his intent on having sex with his spouse/ sexual partner and asks you how to go about it. What would be you response?

8. An HIV infected male **on ART**, expresses his intent on having sex with his spouse / sexual partner and asks you how to go about it. What would be you response?

9. How many of the male PLHA clients you have counseled so far, follow the below behavior change strategies:

a. Abstinence : _______ %

Why do these clients choose this strategy?

b. Being Faithful : _______ %

Why do these clients choose this strategy?

c. Consistent condom use : _______ %

Why do these clients choose this strategy?

10. "Safe sex" is the only method in prevention of HIV through the sexual route. What are the components of Safe Sex Counseling according to you?

Disclosure

11. According to you, how many the male clients have disclosed their HIV status

a. to their wives before sexual intercourse? __________ %

b. to other sexual partners __________ %

When do men generally disclose their HIV status?

a. When partner's insist on having sex

b. When partner expresses the need for procreation

c. When the male is sick/ admitted and needs spousal care & support

d. Men rarely disclose and the spouse gets to know from other sources

e.

What is the average length of time that men require to disclose results to sexual partners?

12. What do you think is the impact of disclosure to spouse on sexual relations?

a. The spouse discontinues to have sexual intercourses anymore

b. The spouse allows only foreplay

c. There is a reduction in the frequency of sexual act

d. The spouse continues to have sexual intercourses after a while (as earlier)

e.

13. If the sexual partner knows of the clients HIV status and yet continues to have sex, the common reasons could be:

a. Coercion into sex by the male

b. Being paid in cash or kind for sex

c. The partner feels that his/her sexual desires need to be met

d. For Procreation

e. Lack of partner's negotiation skills (to say NO)

f.

What has been the impact of counseling on disclosure and sexual behaviour change?

a. Social involvement of HIV positive men after ART

b. Public Disclosure of status enhances social involvement

c. Incidence of self disclosure with a sexual partner

Training

14. If offered a training on Safe Sex Counseling, what are some of the areas of "sexuality- related" counseling that you would like us to focus on?

ANNEXURE 3

Interview Schedule for MLHIV

<Scholarship support by National AIDS Control Organization (NACO)>

Sexual Behaviour, Disclosure and Behaviour Change amidst HIV infected men

PhD Thesis, University of Mumbai

Mr. Sony Thomas

September 2009

Introduction

I, Mr. Sony Thomas am a research student at the College of Social Work, an academic institution that trains students in the field of social work. The College also trains Counselors across the country to help change lives of PLHIV. Through this Interview amidst **Male** PLHIV in Mumbai, I am interested to discover more about the sexual behavior, disclosure related practices and the components of behavior change. I'm interviewing 100 male persons from the ART Centres in Mumbai. Your honest responses and insights will help intervening organizations, to effectively build tools to educate HIV infected persons on issues related to handling one's own sexuality. I anticipate your whole hearted cooperation in this study.

Questionnaire no # : Date of interview

:

RESPONDENT's CONSENT FORM

Please remember:

1. Participation is entirely **Voluntary** and you reserve the right to terminate/ resign at any time during the interview or choose not to respond to parts of the interview, without any justification. This gesture shall be respected.
2. Some questions may probe into your personal life situations and I shall handle those with utmost sensitivity. You can be sure that your answers, together with the answers of others, will be used only in tables in the analysis of information from all respondents. You need not disclose your name/ contact information for this interview.
3. Your **Answers** will be treated as private and confidential and none of your individual answers will be available to anyone at any time. Hence your truthful and frank response, is highly regarded and respected in the welfare of other male PLHIV.
4. You responses are not being graded on this interview, neither will any of your responses effect your relationship with the ART centre.
5. This interview may an hour of your time. Please take your time and answer carefully.

Inclusion criteria

The respondent should

i. Have been on ART for at least 6 months

ii. Be of age between 24 - 50 years

iii. Be a resident of Mumbai

Respondents Undertaking

I am convinced with the cause of this research and am willing to associate in this process and share my knowledge and experiences for the purpose under no pressure.

Signature of respondent: ________________ Date: ___________

Signature of interviewer: ______________________ Date: ___________

Personal profile

1 **Current Age** : ____________

2 **Since what age have you been residing in Mumbai** : __________

3 **Educational achievement**

1 Less than primary education

2 Primary Education completed

3 Secondary Education completed

4 Higher Secondary completed

5 Graduate and above

4 **Occupation**

1 Currently unoccupied

2 Daily Wage labourer

3 Home Based work

4 Service

5 Business

6 Any other _______________

5 **Personal Income**

1 _______________

2 No Income

6 **Any other earning members in the family**?

Who *Income*

_________________________ _________________________

_________________________ _________________________

7 **Marital status**

1\. Unmarried Goto 14

2\. Married

8 At what age did you first get married? : __________

9 Have you remarried? : Yes / No

1\. Yes

2\. No Goto 11

10 Age of re-marriage

: ____________

11 Are you currently living together with your spouse

1. Yes — Goto 13
2. No

12 If No, What is the reason of not living with your spouse

1.	Spouse in village	Age of separation	: __________
2.	Spouse expired	Age of loss of spouse	: __________
3.	Spouse divorced	Age of Divorce	: __________

13 How many children do you have : __________

Respondent's Health Status

14 **CD4 count (last 6 months)**

1 ____________
2 Not Tested

15 **ART Status**

1 on First line
2 on Second line
3 Discontinued ART

16 **Reported Body weight :** __________

17 **Observed Healthiness**

1 Feels Healthy
2 Feels Weak

18 **How often did you suffer from STIs?**

1 Very Often
2 Often
3 Sometimes
4 Rarely
5 Never

19 **How often do you suffer from Opportunistic Infections?**

1 Very Often

2 Often

3 Sometimes

4 Rarely

5 Never

20 **What were these Opportunistic Infections that you suffered from?**

____

____

Spousal Health Status

21 **When was your spouse last tested for HIV**

1. ________________ (month, year)

2. Not yet tested

22 **What is your spouse's HIV status**

1 Negative Goto 28

2 Positive

23 If Positive, what was her CD4 count (checked last 6 months)

1. ________________

2. Not yet tested

24 ART Status

1 On ART

2 Not on ART

25 If on ART

1 on First line

2 on Second line

3 Discontinued ART

26 How often do she suffer from Opportunistic Infections

1 Very Often

2 Often

3 Sometimes

4 Rarely

5 Never

27 What were these Opportunistic Infections?

____

____

28 How often did she suffer from STIs?

1 Very Often

2 Often

3 Sometimes

4 Rarely

5 Never

SECTION 2 : Respondents SEXUAL BEHAVIOUR

Age Chronology

29 Age of Onset of ART medication : __________

30 Age of HIV+ test result : __________

31 Age of Knowledge on HIV/AIDS : __________

32 Age of 1st sexual intercourse : __________

33 Age of 1st sexual feelings onset : __________

Pre Marital Sex

34 Have you indulged in sexual practices before marriage?

1 Yes

2 No Goto 42

35 If so, How many sexual partners did you have before marriage? :

____

36 What were your sexual preferences at that time? ö

37 How often did you practice penetrative sex before marriage?

1. Very Often
2. Often
3. Sometimes
4. Rarely

38 What provoked you for Pre-marital sex?	Often	Sometimes	Rarely
Experimentation with sex/ Curiosity			
Peer Influence			
Need for relaxation/ enjoyment			
Just happened under Alcohol/ Drug Influence			
Media/ Porn film influence			
It just happened in an intense relationship			
Easy access/ availability of sex			
Any other			

39 Who were your sexual partners before marriage?	Often	Sometimes	Rarely
Brothel based partner			
Non brothel based partner			

40 How frequently according to you, have you indulged in protected sex, before marriage?

1 Every time

2 Most times

3 Sometimes

4 Rarely

5 Never

41 What are the reasons for not protecting yourself every time?

____

____

Extra marital sex

42 Have you indulged in sexual relations outside marriage?

1 Yes

2 No

43 What were your preferences while selecting sexual partners outside marriage? And why did you choose them? ö

44 How many sexual partners did you have after marriage?: ___________

45 How often did you practice penetrative sex in extramarital relations?

1. Very Often
2. Often
3. Sometimes
4. Rarely

46	What provoked you to extra marital sex?	Often	Sometimes	Rarely
1	Experimentation / Curiosity			
2	Peer Influence			
3	Need to relax/ enjoy			
4	Just happened under Alcohol/ Drug Influence			
5	Media/ Porn film influence			
6	Restrictions to sex at home due to presence of parents/ children			
7	Dissatisfaction with spouse			
8	Wanted a change/ variety			
9	Embarrassment to perform varied types of sexual act			
11	Spousal Disinterest in sex			
12	Menstruation periods of spouse			
13	Child-bearing phase of spouse			
14	Menopause of spouse			
15	HIV-ve status of spouse			
16	Marital Conflict			
17	Any Other			

47	Your extramarital sexual partners were:	Often	Sometimes	Rarely
	Brothel based partner			
	Non brothel based partner			

48 Can you share more about your non-brothel based partners?

____

49 How frequently did you have protected sex in extramarital sex?

1. Every time — Goto 51
2. Most times
3. Sometimes
4. Rarely
5. Never

50 What are the reasons for not protecting yourself every time

____

For all your sexual partners outside marriage

51 What efforts have you taken to check for STI status?

____

52 How often did you check for partner's STI before sexual relations

1. Every time — Goto 54
2. Most times
3. Sometimes
4. Rarely
5. Never

53 What are the reasons for not ascertaining partners STI status every time?

____

____

54 How often did you check for partner's HIV status before sexual relations

1. Every time — Goto 56
2. Most times
3. Sometimes
4. Rarely
5. Never

55 What are the reasons for not ascertaining partners HIV status every time?

____

____

56 Level of satisfaction	Highly	Moderately satisfactory	Notsatisfactory satisfactory
Rate the level of satisfaction you felt in having sex **outside** marriage (pre/extra)			
Rate the level of satisfaction you felt in having sex **within** marriage			

57 If your level of 'satisfaction of sex' outside marriage is higher than that of within marriage, what could be the reason?

____

____

58 Who usually initiates sexual intercourse within marriage?

1 Always Me

2 Sometimes Me and sometimes Wife

3 Never Me

4 Not applicable

59	Types and frequency of sexual behaviors	Often	Sometimes	Rarely	Never
i	Vaginal Sex				
ii	Oral Sex				
iii	Anal Sex				
iv	Non penetrative sex and Self Simulation				
v	Sexual desires/ Fantasies				

Scores: 1. Never 2. Rarely 3. Sometimes 4. Often 5. Very Often

60	Incidences	Before HIV detection	After HIV – before ART	After ART onset
i	Incidence of experiencing Sexual desires/ Fantasies			
ii	Incidence of performing Masturbation or Non penetrative sex			
iii	Incidence of Use of condoms during every act			
iv	Incidence of HIV status disclosure to sexual partner	Not applicable		

Fill actual Numbers

61	Frequency Approximation	Before HIV detection	After HIV – before ART	After ART onset
i	Total number of sexual partners			
ii	Total number of sexual intercourses			
iii	Total number of sexual intercourses with Male/ TG partners			

Respondent's perceptions on Male Sexuality

1. Strongly agree 2. Agree, 3. Disagree, 4. Strongly Disagree

No.	Statement	Opinion Score
62	Male sexuality is always superior to female sexuality	
63	Male sexual urges are stronger than the sexual urges in females	
64	Male sexual expressions are not to be considered immoral	
65	Male sexual behavior has a greater degree of societal sanction	
66	Male sexual behavior need not be controlled as such, like female sexual behavior	
67	Men to men sexual expressions are acceptable as pleasure activities	
68	Having multiple sexual partners, for a man is socially important	
69	Sex with a virgin partner gives greater pleasure and satisfaction	
70	Age doesn't diminish sexual desires in men, unlike women	
71	Use of Condom diminishes the sexual pleasure in men	
72	Men lose their mental and emotional stability if their sexual needs and fantasies are not satisfied	
73	Elder male peers influence the awareness on sexual activity	
74	Men should always take initiatives to perform sex	

DISCLOSURE

75 Do you think that your wife/ sexual partner has a right to know about your HIV status? 1. Yes 2. No

76 Should Disclosure to spouse be made compulsory by law? Give reasons

1. Yes, ____________________
2. No, ____________________

Spousal Disclosure

77 Did you disclose your HIV status to your **Spouse**

1. Yes Goto 82
2. No

If not Disclosed

78 Why did you choose not to disclose

1. Was preparing myself to disclose later
2. Fear of upsetting spouse
3. Fear of accusations of infidelity
4. Fear of loss of support/ rejection/ marital discord
5. Fear of being disallowed sex
6. Any other

79 What efforts do you make to prevent HIV transmission if you do not disclose?

80 What help would you require to enter into the process of disclosure?

81 When do you plan to disclose?

1. Before sexual intercourse
2. During pregnancy / child birth
3. During sickness
4. When you both were holidaying
5. Any other Goto 89

If Disclosed

82 How do you feel after having disclosed your HIV status to your spouse?

83 What are some reasons which made you disclose your status to spouse? *Multiple choice*

1. Sense of responsibility/ concern for partner's health
2. To prepare spouse for failing health /severe illness
3. Need for social support to cope with treatment
4. To alleviate the distress associated with non-disclosure
5. Under doctors/ counselors insistence
6. To facilitate HIV-preventive behavior
7. Any other

84 Who initiated the disclosure?

1. Self initiated — Goto 85
2. Health care Provider initiated (anonymous third party)
3. Me in presence of Health care Provider
4. Spouse discovered my HIV status

85 If self initiated, When did you disclose of the HIV status

1. Before sexual intercourse
2. During pregnancy / child birth
3. During sickness / AIDS
4. When you both were holidaying
5. Any other

Can you explain how did u disclose your status to your spouse?

86 Time required : ____

87 Words used : ____

____

88 Response of partner : ______________________

89 What was the negative impact of Disclosure on your sexual relations with spouse?

90 What according to you were the Positive impact/ benefits of disclosure to spouse?

91 What would be the further assistance you would require in the process of disclosure?

92 **Disclosure to other sexual partners**

Do you consider that it is the right of your sexual partner to know of your HIV status? Give reasons

1. Yes, ______________________
2. No, ______________________

93 Should status disclosure to sexual partners outside marriage be made compulsory by law? Give reasons

1. Yes, ______________________
2. No, ______________________

94 How often did you disclose your HIV status before sex with your other sexual partner/s

1. Every time Goto 96
2. Most times
3. Sometimes
4. Rarely
5. Never

95 If not Every time, why did you choose not to disclose your HIV status

1. Performed protected sex
2. Afraid that the partner won't permit sex
3. Partner was also infected
4. Since I pay for sex, its their responsibility to take care
5. Partners could anyways be HIV infected due to their high risk behaviors
6. Any other

96 Have you disclosed to sexual partners with whom you have been associated for a long period of time?

1. Yes
2. No

97 Can you explain When and How did u disclose your status to your partners other than wife

____

____

98 What are your suggestions to encourage disclosure to other sexual partners among positive people?

____

____

BEHAVIOUR CHANGE

99 Explain what is safe/ protected sex according to you?

100What are some of the hurdles you face in practicing safe sex?

101What kind of support do you need to sustain your decision to practice safe sex?

102Did the initiation of ART impact your sexual performance?

1. Yes
2. No Goto 104

103 If yes, what was the impact of ART

Multiple response

1. Observing complete Abstinence
2. Reduced multiple sexual indulgences
3. Had to curb sexual excitements
4. Dislike for sex
5. Decrease in sexual satisfaction
6. Feeling of impotence/ sexual dysfunction
7. Unable to maintain erection
8. Early ejaculation
9. Protected sexual practices
10. Any other

104How does your sexual partner react to condom use

1. Compliments condom use
2. Suspects the need for condoms
3. Objects the use of condoms

105What are some of the difficulties you face in the use of condoms?

____

____

106Have you been consuming any substances to enable the sexual act **before you started ART**

1. Very Often
2. Often
3. Sometimes
4. Rarely
5. Never

107Have you been consuming any substances to enable the sexual act **after you started ART**

1. Very Often
2. Often
3. Sometimes
4. Rarely
5. Never

Give your opinions on the following

108 Alcohol consumption during sexual activity is helpful in *Multiple choice*

1. Providing courage to take risks
2. Increased and prolonged sexual performance
3. Reduces inhibitions on having sex outside marriage
4. Reduces inhibitions in performing non-traditional sexual acts
5. Any other

109 Alcohol/ drugs is often consumed before having sex with *Multiple choice*

1. Spouse
2. Commercial sexual partner
3. Non Commercial sexual partner
4. Male partners

110 What are some of your behaviour patterns that have changed post ART? **Give reasons** *Multiple choice*

1. Complete Abstinence from sex ____________________
2. Abstinence of extramarital sex____________________
3. Reduced High risk activities____________________
4. Reduced Alcohol/ Drug intake____________________
5. Consistent condom use____________________
6. Greater focus on Non penetrative sex ________________
7. Have become more Spiritual____________________
8. Spends greater time with family____________________
9. Greater Social/ community involvement____________________
10. Active participation in peer networks ____________________
11. Any other

111 Whom do you attribute your behaviour change to? **Give reasons**

Multiple choice

1. Counseling at Testing Centre
2. Counseling at ART Centre
3. NGO Outreach/ Community interventions programs
4. Peer Education/ support group meetings
5. Reading IEC materials
6. Religious involvement

7. Self need to stay healthy for family and children
8. Incidence of STI or Opportunistic infections
9. Fear of HIV re-infection
10. Guilt about illicit past
11. Any other

112 With whom would you feel most comfortable discussing you sexual problems *Rank priority*

Male Counselors

Female Counselors

Doctor

Male PLHIV / Peer

Other non HIV infected Male Colleagues

Any other

113 How would you rate yourself with regard to change in sexual behavior and safe sex practiced in your life?

1. Excellent
2. Very Good
3. Good
4. Not so good
5. Very bad

ANNEXURE 4
FGD Guide for spouses of MLHIV
PhD Thesis, University of Mumbai
CONSENT FORM (Participants copy)

Introduction

I, Mr. Sony Thomas am a research student at the College of Social Work, an academic institution that trains students in the field of social work and also trains Counselors across the country to help change lives of PLHIV. I am interviewing Male PLHIV in Mumbai, and am interested to discover about their sexual behavior, disclosure related practices and the components of behavior change.

I am also looking at the spousal perception of male sexual behavior change and on the dimensions of disclosure, for which I shall be arranging a discussion with HIV infected and affected women between 24 – 50 years and residing in Mumbai

Please remember:

1. Participation is entirely **voluntary** and you reserve the right to resign at any time during the interview or choose not to respond to parts of the interview. This gesture shall be respected.
2. Some questions may probe into your personal life situations and I shall handle those with utmost sensitivity. You can be sure that your answers, together with the answers of others, will be used only in the analysis of MLHIV behaviors. You need not disclose your name/ contact information for this interview. If you are interested to know about the findings/ outcome of the study, I shall share with CHIRAG project a copy of the same, which will be made available for your reading.
3. Your responses are not being graded on this interview, neither will any of your responses effect your relationship with the spouses or service providers.
4. Your truthful and frank response, is highly regarded and respected in the welfare of my area of research interest for sexual well being of MLHIV. This discussion may take an hour of your time.
5. There shall be no financial remuneration provided for participating in this study.

Respondents Undertaking

I am convinced with the cause of this research and am willing to associate in this process and share my knowledge and experiences for the purpose under no pressure. I anticipate your whole hearted cooperation in this study. I am assured of the confidentiality of the names shared during this discussion will not be used in the study and I am well aware that there shall be no compensation for being a part of the study.

Signature of respondent: ____________________ Date: ___________

FGD areas

1. How did your male counterparts disclose their HIV status to you
2. How long after the HIV test was disclosure initiated
3. What according to you are some of the perceived reasons for disclosure by MLHIV
4. Can you explain how has their disclosure affected your sexual intimacy and activities in early days and in a later stage
   a. Frequency of penetrative sex
   b. Increased tension – period of discord – how did concord happen
5. Hindrances / efforts made in safe sex practices with spouse and its experiences
6. How do you perceive pleasure in non penetrative sexual activities

1st FGD with HIV infected Women

Date	: 20th March 2010
Time	: 3 to 4:30pm
Venue	: CHIRAG office, Bhandup
No of participants	: 10 women
Researcher	: Mr. Sony Thomas
Assisted by	: Ms. Meghna Jethva, Research Officer of GFATM Saksham, in the presence of Ms. Jyoti, Centre Cordinator of CHIRAG

2nd FGD with HIV infected Women

Date	: 10th April 2010
Time	: 2 to 3:00pm
Venue	: CHIRAG office, Sion-Dharavi
No of participants	: 11 women
Researcher	: Mr. Sony Thomas
Assisted by	: Ms. Meghna Jethva, Research Officer of GFATM Saksham, in the presence of Ms. Vandana Parmar, Centre Cordinator of CHIRAG

ANNEXURE 5

NACOs Approval for fellowship

No. T. 11020/20/2008-NACO (R&D)
Government Of India
Ministry of Health and Family Welfare
Department of AIDS Control Organization

9th Floor, Chandralok Building,
36 Janpath, New Delhi 110001
19th March 2009

To.
Principal,
College of Social Work, Nirmala Niketan,
University of Mumbai, 38, New Delhi Marine Lines,
Mumbai-400 020

Subject: 'Award of NACO Research Fellowship on HIV/AIDS' for the year 2008-09'

Sir,

This is to inform you that Mr. Sony Thomas, Research Scholar from College of Social Work, Mumbai has been selected for NACO-Research Fellowship Scheme for his study entitled:

Sexual Behaviour, disclosure and Behaviour Change amidst HIV Infected Men

An amount of Rs. 1,50,000/- (Rupees One Lakh Fifty Thousand Only) has been sanctioned and is being released through the Head of Institution.

As per scheme the concerned Scholar should proceed with the study under supervision of his guide, and submit progress report to NACO. On submission of a copy of the completed dissertation, a 'Fellowship Certificate' will be awarded to him,

(Dr. S. Venkatesh)
Deputy Director General (Research)

Copy for Information to:-

Mr. Sony Thomas
College of Social Work, Nirmala Niketan,
University of Mumbai

SYNOPSIS

Title of Thesis	: **Sexual Behaviour, Disclosure and Behaviour Change amidst HIV infected men**
Name of Candidate	: **Mr. Sony Thomas**
Degree	: **Doctor of Philosophy in faculty of ARTS**
Subject	: **Social Work**
Registration Number & date	: **No. Th./ 8777 of 2008, dated 27th June 2008**
Research Guide	: **Dr. Mary Alphonse,**
	Principal
	College of Social Work, Nirmala Niketan
Signatures	:

I append herewith that this work is based on the discovery of new facts done independently

____

Mr. Sony Thomas

I certify that the statements made in this thesis are correct

____

Dr. Mary Alphonse

SYNOPSIS

Introduction

HIV insinuates itself silently and enters into the blood stream of newer and young individuals each day. Ever since the last three decades, instead of the trend of infection reversing itself, there has been an exponential acceleration in the number of deaths each year. A major route of transmission of the HIV infection has been identified as sexual intercourse contributing over 90 percent of the epidemic transmission in the country (UNAIDS, 2004). Sexual behaviours of high risk groups have frequently been blamed for rapid spread of the disease. In this context this study throws light on the relevance of understanding sexual behaviours of Men living with HIV (MLHIV), in the context of reversing the epidemic under Millennium Goals. Male sexual behaviour has received considerable attention in the past decade because of the crucial role that men play in the HIV epidemic. Current global statistics show that there are more men who are afflicted with the disease. For this reason, sexual behaviour change is a major focus of HIV prevention efforts and understanding changes in behaviour is important for both predicting the future path of the epidemic and for developing policy.

Disclosure of one's HIV status helps the sexual partners to negotiate safer sexual practices and to indulge into lower risky behaviours. HIV status disclosure is believed to be cornerstone firstly in prevention of the infection from PLHIV to the uninfected population and secondly to help prevent PLHIV from acquisition of 'super-infection'. Behaviour change post the knowledge of one's HIV status is the only vaccine to curb the spread of HIV from infected populations into the general community and also behaviour change strategies are quintessential for the PLHIV to regain health and live longer.

The counsellors play a very significant role in mitigating the spread of the epidemic and handling the consequence of the infection on the PLHIV. The findings of this study will enhance their perspectives on halting the epidemic and the welfare of PLHIV. The study aims to throw light on the process of initiating and sustaining behaviour change in the context of sexual indulgences and disclosure to sexual partners.

Study Rationale

The presence of HIV takes toll on the individual's nutrition, hygiene, exercise, recreation, rest, medical care, housing, employment, sexuality and spiritual aspects. Intervening organizations have been addressing varied socio-economic issues of PLHIV. However, sexuality issues of PLHIV are yet to receive a human face. PLHIV are at a risk of being denied their right to control their fertility, occasionally by coercive efforts, with the intention of preventing transmission to sex partners and to the new born. In an attempt to curb the infection, PLHIV are generally educated to abstain from illicit sexual behaviours or homosexual acts, or avoid pregnancy or advised against marriage for those contemplating it and lastly are forced to repress their sexual thoughts or to practice safer sex, with the use of condoms (Nyblade, 2000). Counselling on sexuality for PLHIV is often centred on complete abstinence or the use of protection. Such prohibitive recommendation reinforces a sense of decreased self-esteem, leading to negative repercussions on all aspects of sexual life (Matovu, 2004). A few literatures reviewed, show that some PLHIV perceive pain in practicing sexual abstinence and feel responsible to use condoms out of choice (Crepaz, 2004). Sexuality is a natural urge, which needs to be channelized either through fantasies, foreplay or through actual sexual intercourse. A loving, passionate, emotionally and physically satisfying sex life is not something that can be denied to PLHIV. The purpose of sexual union is both procreation and pleasure. Condom use is strongly critiqued by PLHIV networks and MSM groups as an unviable long term strategy. Safer sex practices seem to be shorn off by PLHIV under the pretext of their priorities of procreation, intimacy needs in new wed-locks, and inaccessibility of condoms (Bulletin, 2000). The efforts to prevent HIV have to be connected with a vision of a better world rather than just the goal of universal condom use. A world has to be envisioned, where every PLHIV, lives with respect and satisfactory sexual life. As people live longer with HIV, the focus should be on improving quality of life. (Kelly, 1998)

Researches show that MLHIV start their sexual careers early in adolescence and generally before the age of marriage (Dandona, 2005). Reproductive health issues and Family planning techniques are little known at this stage of life. High risk sexual indulgences and multiple sexual partners are experimented in this stage for curiosity and experimentation. All these factors put them at a risk to unwanted pregnancies and STI/HIV. Furthermore, the infidelity in sexual behaviour makes them vectors in the spread of HIV epidemic. Hence the prevention of the epidemic focuses on bringing about a behaviour change amongst men.

Some literatures in India, point out that the frequency of sexual relations initiated by men on ART has reduced drastically and so has the practice of multiple partners. Conditions like recurring symptomatic illness, sexual and erectile dysfunctions have further barred PLHIVs interest in sexual indulgence (Dandona, 2005). However, little is known about the modification of sexual behaviour in response to new therapies among PLHIV. On the contrary, concerns have also been raised that these treatment improvements may increase the opportunities for continued or relapse to risk behaviours among male PLHIV, and that they may create a new threat for public health through transmission of HIV viral strains that have already acquired genetic resistance characteristics against actual treatments. (Elford, 2000)

The substantive rationale for choosing men on ART as sample for this study is to assess their sexual histories in a biographical fashion, which will serve as a point of reference to study behaviour changes over a period of time at these three main time periods, namely, sexual behaviour 'Before the HIV infection', 'After the HIV test but before the onset of ART' and that 'After the onset of ART'. Comparative analysis, aimed to be 'within cases', will provide better indicator of conceptualising the individual's behaviour change over a period of time than that 'across cases'.

Self Disclosure is not just a vital component for timely health seeking behaviours like testing and treatment but also a ground for enabling the practice of safer sex, in an attempt to prevention of the epidemic.

Counselling in the field of HIV has proven to be the most effective tool in building up the survival rates of PLHIV. The case history explorations done by the counsellor in assessment of the risk behaviours of the clientele and the remedial behaviour change measures suggested have certainly contributed towards the quality of life of PLHIV as well as in the reduction in the incidence of new infections, at large. Ongoing capacity building of counsellors based on advances made in research and evidences of successful behaviour change models are the need of the hour to ensure better services to PLHIV.

STUDY OBJECTIVES

The study has been divided into 3 phases based on its 3 different units of analyses as the sample, namely counsellors, MLHIV and the spouses of interviewed MLHIV. This research has been framed on the following objectives, to explore with the sample:

PHASE 1: Hospital Based Counsellors

1. To study the counsellors understanding about their MLHIV clients in areas pertaining to sexual behaviour, disclosure and behaviour change

PHASE 2: MLHIV on ART

Sexual Behaviour

2. To study the socio economic profile, health and sexual practices of the HIV infected respondents and their spouses
3. To understand the respondents perception of male sexuality

Disclosure

4. To trace the process and consequences of disclosure
5. Ascertain factors influencing disclosure and the barriers in disclosure

Behaviour Change

6. To study the affect of the 'HIV +ve status' and 'ART' on sexual behaviour
7. Ascertain the factors influencing sexual behaviour change

PHASE 3: Spouses of MLHIV

8. To study the spousal perception on their husband's to disclosure and behaviour change initiatives.

The study findings shall open doors to understand the influencing factors of disclosure and the process of behaviour change. As an outcome of this research, a Road Map shall be prepared for the Counsellor on sexuality related counselling areas for MLHIV, which will be recommended to National AIDS Control Organisation (NACO) in training its counsellors and shall be disseminated to other intervening agencies in the field of HIV.

METHODODOLOGY

As a precursor to this study, the researcher had carried out a qualitative study on 'Sexual behaviour, Disclosure and Behaviour Change of men on ART', in Mumbai, with an urge to understand the concepts and variables emerging in sexual behaviour and its patterns amidst MLHIV on ART. This pre-cursor research used a *'Biographical Method'* to capture the 'mosaic' nature of sexual histories of the male PLHIV, through a *'Non Random Purposive Sampling Method.'* Herein, 8 MLHIV were interviewed in depth and by triangulation through a FGD with the ORWs in the field of HIV, various variables were coined. The findings of this pioneering initiative helped conceptualise the design of the present study.

Based on the objectives of this study and the areas for probing, the researcher divided the collection of primary data of this study into three phases as under. Each phase has been arranged in a linear fashion and the information gathered and variables identified in each phase helped snowball the paradigm of exploration for the next phase.

Phases	sample	Method	Vision
Phase 1	Hospital based Counsellors	Quantitative	Understand counsellor's perception of MLHIV behaviours and their training needs in counselling MLHIV
Phase 2	MLHIV on ART	Quantitative	To study dimensions and extent of sexual behaviours among MLHIV
Phase 3	Spouses of MLHIV	Qualitative	Affirm the spousal experiences and responses to MLHIV behaviours

In each of these cases Non random purposive Sampling technique was used with sample sizes as under

Phases	Study Population	Study Universe	Sample Size	Tool Used
Phase 1	Hospital based Counsellors in Maharashtra	75 ART Counsellors 749 ICTC counsellors in Maharashtra (MSACS, 2007)	85 counsellors of Maharashtra (67 ART, 18 ICTC)	Questionnaire
Phase 2	MLHIV on ART in Mumbai	4152 MLHIV registered on ART in Mumbai (MSACS, 2007)	152 MLHIV on ART in Mumbai	Interview Schedule
Phase 3	Spouses of MLHIV residing in Mumbai	42 spouses of MLHIV who are associated with organisation CHIRAG	21 spouses of MLHIV in Mumbai	FGD Interview Guide

Scope and limitations of the study

This study proposal was submitted to NACO research division for Ethical clearance and the study was also awarded the NACO Research fellowship for the year 2008-09. This recognition is certainly helpful to advocate the study findings for macro policy interventions.

The other scope and limitations of this study are:

Phase 1: The counsellors participating were from ICTC and ART Centres giving a holistic understanding of the counsellor's perspective. Most of the counsellors interviewed were from the ART background and hence they would have had a greater understanding of their male clients due to their greater exposure to follow-up counselling. The interview with counsellors helped conceive the framework for devising variables in assessing the interview with MLHIV. The views expressed by counsellors in 2009, may perhaps have changed over a period of time. The counsellors undertaking induction training may not have interacted with all their clients and their statements may reflect their generalisation for their clients.

Phase 2: The researcher's prior association and rapport with the interviewed MLHIV, through the CHIRAG project, influenced their frank responses. Most of the MLHIV at the end of the interview stated that they had never ever talked about their sexual behaviours so explicitly to anyone before. There is also a fair possibility that the researcher may have missed a certain aspects of their experiences if they had wilfully kept some information undisclosed or even understated their actual sexual behaviours in fear of being identified as overtly sexual. The study findings refer to the MLHIV practices and behaviour change attempts until May 2010.

Phase 3 : MLHIV respondent's spouses were purposefully chosen and the results have to be viewed in the context of their experiences on disclosure and behaviour changes as witnessed amongst their husband. The FGD was limited to the domain of their sexual interaction with their husbands.

None of the findings of this study can be generalized as they are not from a representative sample. However, the study holds a strong significance in the absence of information available in this area. It is a pointer for further need of exploration and experimentation.

MAJOR FINDINGS

A. Respondents Profile

In better understanding the findings of the study an overview of the respondent's profiles across the 3 phases have been summarized herein.

Profile of Counsellors from ICTC/ART

The 85 counsellors were interviewed while they came for their training in counselling at CSWNN Institute. The sample may not representative of the population. However, their responses indicated lot of their issues related to sexuality counselling. These issues are triangulated with the findings from other groups of respondents in the study.

Around one third of the interviewed counsellors were females. Of these, 15 percent of the respondents were fresh graduates and were new in the field of counselling with less than 25 years of age. Over half of the counsellors were in the age bracket 26 – 30 years, with a mean age of 29 years. More men seem to be employed in this profession than women and at more or less the same age. Around three fourths of the counsellors were post graduates in Social Work discipline.

Profile of MLHIV on ART

Through purposive sampling method these 152 MLHIV respondents were selected. Most men interviewed in this study fell in the age bracket of 30 to 50 years, with a mean age of 38 years. They have been residing in Mumbai since 20 to 40 years, with an average 29 years of stay. Only one third of the MLHIV had completed secondary education while nearly half of them were educated less than the primary level. More than half of the MLHIV were either into service or business, while others were daily wage labourers or did home based work and about 7 percent of the MLHIV were unemployed during the time of the interview. The MLHIV's educational achievement was directly proportional to their occupation.

Apart from one tenth respondents, who did not have a personal income, the mean income of the others was found to be around Rs.5000/- . In most cases (89 percent), the respondent's total family income was less than Rs.10,000/-. It was calculated that the respondent's personal income was supplemented by additional family income in only 29 percent cases, while all other respondents were the only source of income in their family.

The mean age of marriage amongst the MLHIV was calculated to be 26 years, even as 15.8 percent have married before the legal age of marriage ie.21 years. Moreover, 8 percent of the respondents had re-married, since their first spouse had either died of AIDS or had separated. Over three fourths of the respondent resided with their spouses in Mumbai, while the spouses of others were either in the village, expired or divorced. One fourth of the respondents had either one, two and three children respectively, while 14 percent of the respondents did not have a child yet.

About half of the MLHIV had a CD4 count of less than 350 (cells/mm^3) at the time of the interview and they also looked healthy with their body weight ranging from 50-70 kg. Most (86 percent) were on first line ART and more than half of the MLHIV complained from the incidence of STI and OI, at least 2 or more times. Over half (63 percent) of the MLHIV were calculated to have 'Moderate' Consolidated Health, followed by 'Poor' (21 percent) and 'Good' (16 percent).

The MLHIV respondents started residing in Mumbai at the median age of 8 years, their sexual fantasies erupted at the median age of 17 and sexual debut happened at 20 years. However they got married at 26 and were found HIV infected at 33 (median age), wherein they were immediately enrolled on ART at 34 (median age). The spouses were tested after all this, when the MLHIV were 35 years old (median). More than half of the MLHIV claimed that they initiated sexual relations within marriage.

The spouses of three fourths of the MLHIV were tested positive with nearly half of them having a CD4 count of less than 350 (cells/mm^3). However, less than half of the spouses tested positive were initiated on ART. The incidence of OI and STI amongst more than half of the spouses was observed to be less than once, contrary to the frequency of MLHIV's OI/STI incidence.

Profile of Spouses of MLHIV

All spouses met during the Focused Group Discussions were HIV infected and most of them were on ART with a CD_4 count more than 200 (cells/mm^3). More than half of the spouses had suffered from OI and about one-fourth claimed to have suffered from STI at least once. Most of the spouses were observed to be healthy during the time of FGD.

B. FINDINGS ON SEXUAL BEHAVIOUR

MLHIV's Queries related to sex

According to the counsellors (irrespective of the counsellor's age), only 44 percent of MLHIV clients *(average mean with standard deviation of 26.8 percent)* had asked them queries related to sex. Especially, one fourth of the counsellors reported that less than 25 percent of the MLHIV clients ask them such queries. It was calculated that MLHIV tend not to ask their queries related to sex to newly appointed counsellors (with less than a year experience), and especially to female counsellors. Most male counsellors were asked questions related to sex irrespective of their years of experience. The major concerns raised by MLHIV include:

a. Concerns related to upgrading their knowledge on Sexual Practices

b. Concerns related to Safe sex behaviours and Condom use

c. Concerns related to maintaining relationship with partners outside marriage

d. Concerns related to Procreation

The MLHIV interviews also depict that most of them prefer to address their sexual concerns with Male counsellors, Doctors or MLHIV peer.

The barriers perceived by counsellors in MLHIV not discussing about sex include:

a. Personal Barriers like embarrassment, priority focus on medication, disinterest in sex, depression and greater confidence in oneself about knowledge pertaining to sex.

b. Social Barriers like lower age and opposite gender of counsellors, fears of speaking about private sexual life in public and fear of being stigmatised for illicit practices.

c. Structural barriers include high patient load at the testing/ treatment centre, no space for privacy, lack of time for individual counselling at the Hospital and inhibition to talk since MLHIV are generally accompanied by spouse or other family members

MLHIV indulgences in Sex outside Marriage

According to MLHIV, 89 percent indulged in sex before marriage with an average (median) of nearly 5 partners. The occupation of the MLHIV in unorganised sector, as well as the HIV positive status of spouse, held strong association with the increasing number of sexual partners outside marriage. Even though this may be a known fact, this study has empirically established the association strongly between these factors. An increase in the number of pre-marital sexual partners of the respondents was found to be directly proportional to their higher educational achievement, good health and that of practicing unprotected sex. After marriage, only 56 percent indulged in extramarital sex with an average (median) of nearly 3 partners. This reduction number of sexual partners outside marriage is also indicative that marriage is a variable which influences 'behaviour change' in MLHIV.

The major reasons for indulgence in pre marital sexual relations included, experimentation, relaxation and enjoyment, peer influence, easy availability or accessibility of sexual partners and influence of alcohol. And the reasons for indulgence in extra-marital sex additionally included, need for variety, dissatisfaction with spouse, restrictions to sex at home, embarrassment in performing varied types of sexual acts with spouse, spousal disinterest in sex, menstruation period or child bearing phase or menopause of spouse, marital conflicts, or in order to maintain HIV negative status of spouse

More respondents chose brothel based partners for pre-marital sexual indulgences, while non-brothel based partners were chosen during extra-marital sexual indulgences. Frequenting of visits to the same sexual partners was more observed in cases non-brothel based partners. There was no significant difference in the use of protected sexual practices in either pre or extramarital sex. A major concern is the fact that many men are not concerned with the risks associated with unsafe sex. Many of the respondents interviewed for this study did not use condoms, when having sex with commercial sex workers. Further, a few men remarked that having sex with expensive prostitutes, young girls and girls who live within the neighbourhood or community (non brothel based partner) is safe. Younger MLHIV were found to have more number of sexual partners and indulged in unprotected sex more often than older ones. Even though education is not a positive factor with regard to preventing visits to sexual partners outside marriage, it is seen to be a positive factor for condom use after ART. Such in-depth understanding of MLHIV's problems was not reflected among the interviewed counsellors, who came for training.

Dimensions of Sexual Practices

a. HIV/ STI Assessment of Sexual Partner

Over 91 percent of the respondents 'Never' assessed STI status and 96 percent of them 'Never' assessed the HIV status, of their sexual partners, thus making the respondents vulnerable to re-infection. The major reasons for not doing so were fatalism, ignorance and fear of partner's denial for sex. FGD with spouses present that STI is a painful incident for both partners and that sex between the married couple is avoided in such conditions.

b. Level of Sexual Satisfaction

In retrospection on the level of sexual satisfaction, most respondents reported that sexual satisfaction was 'Higher' within marriage, compared to that outside marriage, since there exists mutual love, non-influence of alcohol, no fear of physical restrictions of time, space, money, etc, no guilt of 'wrong doing' attached and a sense of possession of spouse, brings greater satisfaction. Further, some respondents have stated that sex outside marriage was mostly due to mere "non availability of sex with married partners".

FGD with spouses present that most of the spouses have lost their desire to have sex and others claimed that they are comparatively less satisfied sexually currently, due to the prevailing fear of re-infection. Most counsellors did not think that the MLHIV had greater sexual satisfaction with spouse but stated that it was certainly a factor influencing the MLHIV's decision on choosing the prevention strategy of "Being Faithful".

Understanding behaviours of Men who have sex with Men (MSM)

a. MLHIV who have sex with men

Except for one-fifth of the counsellors, all others, irrespective of their gender, claimed to know how many of their MLHIV clients practiced homosexual behaviour. More than half of the counsellors claimed that 1-5% of their MLHIV were indulging in MSM behaviour. However, the MLHIV in their interviews admitted that 15 percent of them indulged in MSM behaviours before HIV infection, which reduced to 3 percent after ART onset. This shows that not all MLHIV who practice MSM behaviours report or discuss with the counsellors on the same.

b. Safe sex indulgences of MSM

About 15 percent of the counsellors admitted that they never probed with their MSM clients if they practiced safe sex. However, half of the counsellors stated that their MLHIV clients would sadly be practicing unsafe sex with men. Less than one third of the counsellors felt assured that their MLHIV clients practiced safe MSM behaviours. The MLHIV interviews revealed that all those who indulged in MSM behaviours even after ART continued to practice unprotected sex. This is a serious concern that needs to be addressed.

c. Bisexuality amongst MLHIV

More than half (58 percent) of the counsellors believed that between 1-5 percent of their MLHIV clients could be bisexual, while one-tenth of the counsellors believe that more than 6 percent would be so. The MLHIV interviews reflect 15 percent of MLHIV to be bisexual, which again surprisingly is beyond the imagination of most counsellors. The spousal knowledge on MLHIV's bisexual behaviour was not explored in the FGD.

d. MLHIV asking Questions asked pertaining to MSM

Nearly half of the counsellors reported that none of their MLHIV clients had ever asked them any query with regards to homosexuality. While 41 percent of them reported that '1 to 5 percent of their MLHIV clients', whom they had counselled, had ever asked questions pertaining to homosexuality. The queries of MLHIV with regard to homosexuality have been categorised under the following areas:

a. Seeking knowledge on understanding concepts of MSM
b. Discussing Sexual Problems
c. MLHIV assessing risk behaviours amidst MSM and safe sex related queries
d. Seeking skills in handling situations arising amongst MSM partners

e. Counsellors Responses to MLHIV queries

Only 70 percent of the counsellor's responses seemed to show confidence in addressing MSM behaviours, with suggesting alternative and safe sexual practices. The responses of remaining counsellors were focussed on abstinence from sex claiming MSM activities to be immoral and their behaviours to be non scientific.

Types of penetrative sexual behaviours by practiced by MLHIV

Around one fourth of the counsellors admitted not having explored much on the penetrative sexual practices of their MLHIV clients. More female counsellors did not seem to know about the types of penetrative behaviours practiced by MLHIV.

a. MLHIV indulgence in Vaginal Sex:

Around 15 percent of the counsellors had no clue if their MLHIV clients indulged in vaginal sex. Only two third of the counsellors stated that over 80 percent of their MLHIV would be indulging in Vaginal Sex (average median of 90 percent MLHIV). However, the MLHIV interviews reveal that almost all respondents (98 percent) performed vaginal sex during every sexual act.

b. MLHIV indulgence in Anal sex

Over one fourth of the counsellors had no clue if their MLHIV clients indulged in anal sex. While one third of the counsellors feel that only up to 20 percent of their MLHIV would be indulging in anal sex (Average median of 3 percent MLHIV). However, the MLHIV interviews reveal that as much as one in ten respondents performed anal sex 'Often' during the sexual act. On the other hand 42 percent MLHIV had never ever tried anal sex.

c. MLHIV indulgence in Oral sex

Over one fourth of the counsellors had no clue if their MLHIV clients indulged in oral sex. Six out of ten counsellors felt that between 1-20 percent of their MLHIV would be indulging in oral Sex (Average median of 2 percent MLHIV). However, the MLHIV interviews reveal that only one tenth of them performed oral sex 'often' during the sexual act and on the other hand about 53 percent MLHIV had never ever tried oral sex.

MLHIV Attitudes towards Male Sexuality

On a 14 point likert scale measuring MLHIV attitudes towards sexuality, it was observed that the respondents were either 'moderately sexist' (74 percent) or 'highly sexist' (25 percent). The sexist attitudes seemed to increase with respondent's income, health and their indulgences in pre/extramarital sex and also with their short duration of residence in Mumbai. Highly sexist attitudes were observed on the statements mentioned below

1. Male sexuality being superior to female sexuality
2. Male sexual urges being stronger than that in females
3. Sex with virgin partner gives greater sexual pleasure for men
4. Age diminishes sexual pleasure in women
5. Use of condoms diminishes sexual pleasure in men
6. Men lose their mental and emotional stability if their sexual needs and fantasies are not satisfied
7. Men should always take initiatives to perform sex

C. FINDINGS ON HIV STATUS DISCLOSURE

In the context of HIV infection, familiar concerns about adolescent sexual behaviour are amplified and new ethical dilemmas, such as those pertaining to the disclosure of HIV status to regular extra marital partner and legalization of disclosure surface.

Spousal Disclosure

According to 90 percent of the MLHIV, disclosure was considered as a right of the spouse and 80 percent of the MLHIV opined that there can be a legal binding to this. Such legalisation would help since the spouse is primary caretaker and would be there till the end, it would help prevent the spread of infection, to minimise discord in relationship and would help early diagnosis and treatment of other family members. It should be noted here that this opinion of MLHIV is only related to the disclosure of their HIV status to the primary partner and not their sexual partners outside marriage.

About 8 percent of the counsellors 'never' ascertained if their MLHIV clients had disclosed their HIV status to their spouses. More than half of the counsellors believe that at least 'more than 60 percent' of their MLHIV clients would have disclosed their HIV status to their spouses. As reported by the counsellors, 58 percent of their MLHIV clients (Mean with a standard deviation of 31 percent) {Median = 70 percent}, seems to have disclosed their HIV status with their spouses. Contrary to the counsellor's perception, 92 percent of the MLHIV respondents actually claimed to have disclosed their status to their spouses

a. Spousal Disclosure Initiated by

Half of the counsellors were of the opinion that the spouse gets to know of their husband's status, in most cases, from 'sources other than their husbands'.

The MLHIV interviews also project that disclosure was voluntarily initiated by the MLHIV himself, only in half the cases. The HCP revealed the status to the spouse directly in more than one fourth cases, while only in a handful cases did the MLHIV seek the assistance of the HCP for disclosure. In a few cases, the spouses discovered the status of the MLHIV.

According to few spouses, their MLHIV did not disclose their HIV status due to the fear of spousal reaction, while some other spouses felt that even their male counterparts did not know of their own HIV status and that the spouses were detected first with HIV infection.

b. Circumstances of Status Disclosure by MLHIV

According to the counsellors, spousal disclosure by MLHIV occurs under the following circumstances in order of maximum responses:

i. When MLHIV is sick/ admitted and needs spousal care and support

ii. When spouse insists on the need for procreation or during pregnancy

iii. When spouse insists on having sex

The situations, under which voluntary disclosure was initiated by the MLHIV respondent, coincided with the responses of the counsellors. Additionally, the MLHIV respondents preferred to disclose their HIV status, before sexual intercourse or in a few cases when the couple were holidaying.

The spouses also confirmed that the MLHIV initiated disclosure during times of their illness, before marriage or when holidaying. Only one third of the spouses claimed that their MLHIV husbands disclosed their HIV status to them directly. Most of the spouses discovered their HIV status through HCP during pregnancy or during the illness of their husbands. Few of the spouses got to know of their HIV status by reading the MLHIV blood reports or when these spouses were tested during their illness or that of their child.

c. Factors influencing spousal disclosure

The factors influencing disclosure as stated by MLHIV respondents include, sense of responsibility to spouse, concern for spousal health, need for spousal support in care and treatment, to alleviate distress associated with non-disclosure and to initiate HIV preventive behaviour. All these factors are seen to be 'Internal' and hence they were highly motivated.

d. Time taken by MLHIV in disclosing

Nearly half of the MLHIV spent "less than 5 minutes" in disclosing their status to their spouse, while one fourth of them took "about 30 minutes" to do the same. Most of these MLHIV disclosed during their illness and was observed to have had a negative reaction from spouse. Eight percent of the MLHIV spent "nearly 2 hours" in disclosure speaking about what the HIV infection, treatment is and how they should be leading their lives hereafter. It is interesting to note that most of the MLHIV who took 'more than a hour' in disclosure have done 'voluntary' disclosure and not with the support (in the presence) of the HCP. Further most of such MLHIV have experienced a positive impact of disclosure.

e. MLHIV's Preparation Period for disclosure

Only about a tenth of the MLHIV disclosed their status to their spouses on the same day of their results, while one fourths of the MLHIV took a week and a month respectively towards preparing themselves for disclosure. Over one third of the MLHIV disclosed only after a longer duration of time. The period of time taken for disclosure didn't seem to have a significant correlation with the impact of disclosure, indicating that it is more important to be careful about the "manner" in which disclosure is done than "when" it is done.

f. Words used by MLHIV in disclosure

Nearly half of the respondents "declared confidently their HIV status" and "assured the spouse that everything was alright", while only a few took efforts to "explain the infection to their spouses". This style of "explaining the infection" in disclosure was found successful by the MLHIV and can be promoted. A few MLHIV tried to "sound guilty" and "confessed their past" to their spouses, or "tried to gain spousal sympathy" and elicited "mutual support". A few MLHIV 'blamed their spouses' for bringing home the infection.

During the FGD, a couple of spouses expressed the disadvantage of being tested for HIV, before their husbands, thus giving themselves room for being blamed. The spouses were shocked with their husbands and in-laws behaviours, when they were blamed for bringing home the HIV infection, in spite of being so loyal to their husbands.

Feelings associated after spousal disclosure:

More than half of the MLHIV felt 'Negative' after their disclosure, which included "feeling ashamed", "guilty", "lonely", "depressed and anxious about health and future". Only one fourth of the MLHIV claimed to have felt 'Positive' (feelings include, "sense of relief", "de-stressed", "content", "pleased" and "peaceful") after their disclosure and the remaining few remarked that they had 'Mixed' feelings.

Impact of HIV on spousal relationship

According to more than two third of the MLHIV respondents the impact of spousal disclosure has been negative wherein their spouses were shocked to learn about the infection and were anxious about their personal health and the future of their family. Some spouses wept for long and did not converse with the respondents for a few days. Episodes of 'periodic anger' and 'blaming the husband for ruining her life' were reported by MLHIV.

In the FGD, no spouse claimed to have reacted 'positively' to disclosure. More spouses claim to have reacted 'negatively', which consisted of behaviours like threatening to induce self harm, demonstrating anger, discrimination and accusing the husband. Some spouses remarked that they reacted 'naively' and gave in to their husbands, since they were in a helpless situation or since they lacked knowledge on HIV.

A few spouses reported that after the knowledge of their HIV status, they were either abandoned by their in-laws or faced violence from their male counterparts for bringing home the infection. More spouses, who knew of their husband's HIV status, reduced interpersonal communications and reacted negatively to the MLHIV, while only a few reacted naively and demonstrated greater care and support to the MLHIV.

Impact of HIV on sexual relationship with spouse

According to one tenth counsellors, it was perceived that there would have been 'No' impact of spousal disclosure on their sexual relationship. However, according to the other counsellors, spousal disclosure by MLHIV had the following impact on sexual relationship:

i. Spouse ensures condom use by MLHIV

ii. Reduction in frequency of sexual act

iii. Spouse discontinues sexual relations

iv. Spouse allows only foreplay

According to MLHIV, the frequency of sexual relations with spouse both before HIV and that after ART, seem to remain static ie. an average of 4 sexual acts a month.

MLHIV interviews represents 69 percent to have faced 'negative impact' of disclosure on their sexual lives, wherein they had to abstain, restrict their desires to non penetrative or safe sex. After disclosure, spouses showed disinterest in sex, reduced sexual relations or insisted on condom use. In a few cases the respondents were ashamed to initiate sexual advances with spouse after disclosure. While the other 31 percent, who shared the 'positive impact' of disclosure on their sexual lives, mentioned how they were happy that sexual intimacy was gradually accepted by spouse, joint decisions were taken towards indulging in safer sexual practices, couple counselling was sought, necessary precautions were being taken to protect the off-springs from HIV. Some respondents mentioned on how the feeling of guilt about past infidelity vanished gradually.

However, one third of the spouses, in FGD, claimed that they have initiated 'sexual abstinence' after the knowledge of their concordant HIV status and a couple of them claimed to have 'comparatively reduced' their sexual indulgences. A few of the spouses pointed out indulgence in 'non-penetrative sexual practices' and a few used protections. A few spouses confessed that they continue to indulge in unprotected sex giving in to their husbands needs or because they had become fatalistic. Some spouses stated that the knowledge of the HIV infection "did not interrupt" their sexual lives and that the couple continue to have sex as they used to have earlier before the knowledge of HIV.

Furthermore, the counsellors felt that the spouse indulges in sexual relationships with the MLHIV, in spite of their HIV status disclosure, chiefly due to the following reasons:

i. Lack of negotiation skills (78.8 percent)

ii. Spouses feel the need for their sexual desires to be met (37.6 percent)

iii. Spouse is coerced into sex (36.4 percent)

iv. Spousal need of procreation (29.4 percent)

v. In exchange of rewards (cash/ kind) (11.7 percent)

Non Disclosure to Spouses

About 8 percent of the MLHIV had not disclosed their HIV status to their spouses until the time of their interview. The MLHIV's reasons for non disclosure to spouses include wanting to disclose later, fear of upsetting spouse or being disallowed sex, fear of marital discord and accusation of infidelity. The respondents mentioned that they are waiting for a situation like 'childbirth' or 'sickness', so as to disclose their status to spouses. Meanwhile, some MLHIV are making attempts like 'condom use' and 'abstinence' in this interim period of non-disclosure. Some MLHIV iterated the need for 'further counselling support to spouse on health care and support', 'couple counselling for stabilising relationships' and towards 'education of safe practices' and help in 'mentally preparing oneself for disclosure'.

Disclosure to other sexual partners

About 18 percent the counsellors did not know if their MLHIV clients had disclosed to their non spousal sexual partners. Nearly half of the counsellors felt that only between 1-20 percent of their MLHIV clients would have disclosed their status to their non-spousal partners. The MLHIV disclosure to non spousal partners was calculated to be 24.3 percent (mean value with a standard deviation of 27.8 percent) {Average median = 20 percent}.

When MLHIV were inquired about non spousal disclosure, 57 percent of them stated that it is the right of their non-spousal sexual partners to know their status in an attempt to protect them from HIV. Also, half of the MLHIV were also in favour of legalisation of non-spousal disclosure, while the others, who did not favour legalisation, feared the negative implications like denial of sex and stigma. Contrary to the counsellor's perception, only a miniscule 6 percent of the MLHIV were found to have actually disclosed their HIV status to their non spousal sexual partners, thus indicating the susceptibility of their sexual partners. It was further observed that these 6 percent have 'Often' shared their status with only those non spousal partners, who were associated with them in a "long term relationship".

The reasons for non disclosure as stated by MLHIV include, performing protected sex, or lack of knowledge of one's own status, or sexual partners responsibility to take care of their health since they are paid in turn, fear of denial in intimacy, or sexual partners not sharing their status although they were into high risk behaviours.

FINDINGS ON BEHAVIOUR CHANGE

The understanding of behaviour change and the attempts made by MLHIV towards behaviour change were recorded in this segment. Counsellor's interview reveal that their messages on behaviour change to their MLHIV client mostly include Abstinence and Risk reduction focussed messages. It was observed that harm reduction messages (non penetrative sex, safe sex and sex education) and caring for sexual partner's health were not given equal emphasis.

Prevention strategies followed by MLHIV (A-B-C)

Abstinence:

Around half of the counsellors (51 percent) perceived that 1-20 percent of their MLHIV clients would be practicing abstinence, as a strategy of behaviour change. This perception was found true as 16 percent of the MLHIV respondents revealed that they have chosen complete abstinence from sex as an HIV prevention strategy after ART.

Being faithful:

The counsellors had mixed responses in their beliefs on their MLHIV client's faithfulness, with more number of the counsellors perceiving that more than 40 percent of their MLHIV clients would be faithful to their spouses, after their HIV infection. The MLHIV respondents reveal that 69 percent of them claimed to have reduced their sexual indulgences outside marriage and were now faithful to their spouses.

Consistent condom use:

Around half of the counsellors stated that more than 60 percent of the MLHIV consistently used condoms. This was ascertained to be true in the MLHIV interviews, where 64 percent of them claimed consistent use of condoms.

Behaviour Change across the phases of infection

Two thirds of the counsellors were of the view that their MLHIV clients would possibly be having sex 'Occasionally' *(2-3 acts a month)* or 'Rarely' *(2-3 acts in a quarter),* after the HIV infection. While over one fourth of the counsellors felt that most of their MLHIV clients would be having sex 'Often' *(more than 4 acts a month)*. The counsellors base this data on the evidences from their interactions with MLHIV through their queries during counselling or through interaction with their spouses.

According to MLHIV, the frequencies of sexual desire, non penetrative practices, partners outside marriage, and sexual intercourses outside marriage have decreased considerably after the onset of ART medication as compared to that practiced by the respondent before HIV infection.

Behaviours like condom use and status disclosure to sexual partners have increased after the onset of ART, although there is still a large scope for improvement.

Safe Sex Practices

Most of the counsellors (89 percent) iterated that their clients were having unsafe sex even after being detected HIV positive. Amongst them 14 percent counsellors opined that their clients 'Rarely' practiced safe sex, in spite of regular counselling and MLHIV being aware of the risks. Only 19 percent of the counsellors felt that their MLHIV clients indulged in safe sex 'Very Often'. It was perceived that a major chunk of MLHIV, who practice safe sex, do not do so on 'every' occasion, thus increasing the threat in the spread of the infection.

Most of the MLHIV (95 percent) equated safe sex with condom use. Only a few knew that it also includes avoiding multiple partners (15 percent) and indulging in non penetrative (9 percent) sex. The major hurdles faced in implementing safe sex include alcohol influence, lack of knowledge on safe sex and skin infections. Only a few spouses agreed to indulgence in non-penetrative sex as a measure of safe sex.

Although interpersonal intimacy is a normal milestone in adolescent development, lapses in precautions during intercourse could result in the transmission of HIV to partners and offspring. Engaging in intimate touch or non penetrative sex, without intercourse appeared to be an uncommon form of sexual expression amongst MLHIV.

Condom Use

a. Condom use by MLHIV after HIV infection

Use of condoms, after the HIV infection, is the most focused strategy of safe sex practice in counselling trainings, yet the counsellors had mixed opinions on the actual use of condoms by MLHIV. Only one fourth of the counsellors felt that 'most' of their MLHIV clients used condoms.

In the interviews with MLHIV, incidence of condom use rose 12 times to 62 percent after onset of ART. Unsafe intercourse was associated with discomfort using condoms, reluctance to disclose HIV status, and anger or anxiety when thinking about HIV. Condoms are a distressing reminder of HIV infection for affected individuals. Introducing condoms in a sexual relation can raise difficult questions from partners, necessitating disclosure of HIV status. Ultimately, emotional adjustment to HIV infection and willingness to inform sexual partners may be important determinants of condom use.

Only few of the spouses reported that they used condoms during their sexual relations post the knowledge of their HIV status.

b. Reaction of sexual partner to condom use

About two thirds of the MLHIV claim that most of their sexual partners (within and outside marriage) complimented their condom use, while in case of 17 percent MLHIV respondents; the sexual partners objected the use of condoms. In the FGD, most spouses shared that they would promote condom use as it was considered safe and would protect them from an increase in viral load.

c. Difficulties faced in condom use

According to MLHIV the difficulties faced in condom use include

a. Individual level issues in non-condom use include lack of trust in condoms, non-disclosure of status to sexual partner, ignorance, forgetfulness, lack of proper knowledge on use of condoms and discomfort in using condoms.

b. Issues faced with sexual partners include, suspicion by partner, partners objection in using condoms claiming that they don't have any infection, causes irritation on partners skin, monogamous/ faithful partner, fatalism in partners about infection.

c. Social and structural issues include religious issues, embarrassment to purchase or pick up condoms and peer pressure on not to use. Concerns were also on cost and quality of condoms, slippages, reduced pleasure, non availability whenever required.

Use of Substances before sexual activity

When the MLHIV were asked about their substance use behaviours before sexual activity, all of them claimed only the intake of alcohol as a practice. It was found that the frequency in use of alcohol 'After onset of ART' was six times lower than that 'Before ART'. Variables like higher age, higher education, higher income and good health status were also closely associated with the reduction of alcohol use.

According to these MLHIV respondents, alcohol intake helped prolonged sexual performance, gave courage to take risks, reduced inhibitions to have sex outside marriage and to perform non-traditional acts. Alcohol, in most cases was consumed before sexual activity with 'commercial' sexual partners (76 percent) or with 'non commercial' partners (37 percent). Only one-fourth of them used alcohol, before sexual indulgence, with their spouse.

The FGD with spouses indicate that the husbands do insist on sex under the influence of alcohol but most spouses reported that they do not permit sexual relations in such circumstances.

Impact of ART on sexual behaviour

After the onset of ART, the MLHIV have consciously 'reduced multiple sexual indulgences' (67 percent), have 'curbed their sexual excitements' (63 percent) or have 'initiated protected practices' (41 percent). Around one fourth of the respondents stated that after being initiated on ART, they feel dislike for sex, decrease in sexual satisfaction, early ejaculation, inability to maintain penile erection and feeling of impotence. Quite a few studies quoted in the literature review chapter have also pointed out these.

Behaviour Changes post ART

The MLHIV stated that after ART the following behaviours have changed namely Alcohol Intake, high risk sexual activities, initiating abstinence, condom use, spending time with family, peer and community involvement, focus on non-penetrative sex and on spiritual involvements. Complete sexual abstinence was reported by 16 percent of the respondents.

Factors influencing behaviour change

According to the Counsellors, the major factors influencing behaviour change in MLHIV would be as categorised below:

a. Internal factors like feeling of guilt and in repentance of illicit behaviour, fear of acquiring other OI and STI, fear of increase in viral load or re-infection, fear of complications in ART, focus on improving health.

b. Sexual Partner focussed factors include prevention of HIV transmission to partner, demonstrate love and commitment to partner and re-building trust in spouse

c. Social factors include concern for future of children and family

d. Structural factors include religious involvement, greater understanding developed on HIV, influence of counselling support provided by them.

In the MLHIV interviews, the respondents acknowledged the counselling education at the ART, NGO, ICTC and that in support group meeting as major factors, which influenced them to change their behaviours. Additionally factors like reading IEC materials, attending religious services, self determination to stay healthy for family and children, fear of re-infection with HIV, STI or OI and guilt feelings about the past, have also been instrumental in bring about behaviour change.

The following hypothesis set for the study were all proven true

1. Earlier the sexual initiation greater is the multiple sexual partners
2. Men have multiple sexual partners before the knowledge of their HIV status
3. The HIV test would be the first exposure to their education on HIV
4. Men would have rarely ascertained the STI or HIV status of their sexual partners before sexual intercourse
5. Longer the duration of living with HIV, greater the comfort level of HIV status disclosure to spouse
6. HIV status Disclosure to spouse will be more prevalent after ART onset
7. HIV status Disclosure to other sexual partners will be minimal
8. Frequency of sexual indulgences would have comparatively decreased after the onset of ART.
9. Condom use with sexual partners would have increased after ART

Conclusion

Care and Support for PLHIV is the need of the hour in India, considering the dip in incidence rates of new infections. In this context, this study offers great significance in designing the paradigm for the sexual health and rights of PLHIV, which needs to be given adequate mileage in the national program and the sensitive issue of sexuality be addressed with utmost care. The control of the disease HIV and AIDS is very much dependent on the effectiveness of the counsellors, who are in direct contact with the PLHIV, and can enable their decision making. The findings of this study depict that the PLHIV have high regard for the messages and inputs provided by the counsellors towards behaviour change and most of them are taking initiatives to implement them. It is important to understand here that unless the information is re-enforced in the counselling set up at different time intervals, fatalism may develop amongst MLHIV leading to relapse. The onus of these study findings are attributed to the counsellors, whose skills in counselling on sexuality and disclosure will have to be nurtured. This study ends with a Road Map for the counsellors training curriculum, on how to address the needs and concerns of various groups on sexuality. Only such a considerate initiative from the counsellors as well as the training institutions will help reach the ultimate goal of HIV counselling in building better lives and a healthy future for PLHIV.